T0263244

Psychiatric Aspects of Critical Care Medicine: Update

Editor

JOSÉ R. MALDONADO

CRITICAL CARE CLINICS

www.criticalcare.theclinics.com

Consulting Editor
JOHN A. KELLUM

July 2017 • Volume 33 • Number 3

ELSEVIER

1600 John F. Kennedy Boulevard • Suite 1800 • Philadelphia, Pennsylvania, 19103-2899

http://www.theclinics.com

CRITICAL CARE CLINICS Volume 33, Number 3
July 2017 ISSN 0749-0704, ISBN-13: 978-0-323-53126-9

Editor: Katie Pfaff
Developmental Editor: Casey Potter

Critical Care Clinics (ISSN: 0749-0704) is published quarterly by Elsevier Inc., 360 Park Avenue South, New York, NY 10010-1710. Months of issue are January, April, July, and October. Business and Editorial Offices: 1600 John F. Kennedy Blvd., Suite 1800, Philadelphia, PA 19103-2899. Customer Service Office: 6277 Sea Harbor Drive, Orlando, FL 32887-4800. Periodicals postage paid at New York, NY and additional mailing offices. Subscription prices are $221.00 per year for US individuals, $584.00 per year for US institution, $100.00 per year for US students and residents, $263.00 per year for Canadian individuals, $732.00 per year for Canadian institutions, $309.00 per year for international individuals, $732.00 per year for international institutions and $150.00 per year for Canadian and foreign students/residents. To receive student/resident rate, orders must be accompanied by name of affiliated institution, date of term, and the signature of program/residency coordinator on institution letterhead. Orders will be billed at individual rate until proof of status is received. Foreign air speed delivery is included in all *Clinics* subscription prices. All prices are subject to change without notice. POSTMASTER: Send address changes to *Critical Care Clinics*, Elsevier Periodicals Customer Service, 11830 Westline Industrial Drive, St. Louis, MO 63146. **Customer Service: 1-800-654-2452 (US). From outside of the US, call 1-314-447-8871. Fax: 1-314-447-8029. E-mail: journalscustomerservice-usa@ elsevier.com (for print support) or journalsonlinesupport-usa@elsevier.com (for online support).**

Reprints. For copies of 100 or more of articles in this publication, please contact the Commercial Reprints Department, Elsevier Inc., 360 Park Avenue South, New York, NY 10010-1710. Tel.: 212-633-3874; Fax: 212-633-3820; E-mail: reprints@elsevier.com.

Critical Care Clinics is also published in Spanish by Editorial Inter-Medica, Junin 917, 1ᵉʳ A, 1113, Buenos Aires, Argentina.

Critical Care Clinics is covered in *MEDLINE/PubMed (Index Medicus), EMBASE/Excerpta Medica, Current Concepts/ Clinical Medicine, ISI/BIOMED,* and *Chemical Abstracts.*

Contributors

CONSULTING EDITOR

JOHN A. KELLUM, MD, MCCM
Professor of Critical Care Medicine, Medicine, Bioengineering and Clinical &
Translational Science, Director, Center for Critical Care Nephrology; Vice Chair for
Research, Department of Critical Care Medicine, University of Pittsburgh School of
Medicine, Pittsburgh, Pennsylvania

EDITOR

JOSÉ R. MALDONADO, MD, FAPM, FACFE
Professor of Psychiatry and, by courtesy, of Internal Medicine, Surgery, and Emergency
Medicine; Medical Director, Psychosomatic Medicine Service; Medical Director,
Emergency Psychiatry Service, Stanford University School of Medicine, Stanford,
California

AUTHORS

ANDREA AMENT, MD
Fellow, Psychosomatic Medicine, Department of Psychiatry, Stanford University School of
Medicine, Stanford, California

OSCAR JOSEPH BIENVENU, MD, PhD
Associate Professor, Department of Psychiatry and Behavioral Sciences, Johns Hopkins
University School of Medicine, Baltimore, Maryland

JOSEPH H. DONROE, MD, MPH
Assistant Professor of Medicine, Department of Internal Medicine, Yale University School
of Medicine, New Haven, Connecticut

STEPHEN J. FERRANDO, MD
Department of Psychiatry, Westchester Medical Center, New York Medical College,
Valhalla, New York

ZACHARY FREYBERG, MD, PhD
Departments of Psychiatry and Cell Biology, University of Pittsburgh, Pittsburgh,
Pennsylvania

RENEE M. GARCIA, MD
Clinical Instructor, Division of Psychosomatic Medicine, Department of Psychiatry and
Behavioral Sciences, Stanford Hospital and Clinics, Stanford, California

TED-AVI GERSTENBLITH, MD
Instructor, Department of Psychiatry and Behavioral Sciences, Johns Hopkins University
School of Medicine, Baltimore, Maryland

EARL DE GUZMAN, MD
Fellow, Psychosomatic Medicine, Department of Psychiatry, Stanford University School of Medicine, Stanford, California

STEPHANIE M. HARMAN, MD
Clinical Associate Professor, Department of Medicine, Stanford University School of Medicine, Stanford, California

KIRK A. HARRIS, MD
Assistant Professor, Department of Psychiatry, Rush University, Chicago, Illinois

SHEILA C. LAHIJANI, MD
Assistant Professor, Department of Psychiatry and Behavioral Sciences, Stanford University School of Medicine, Palo Alto, California

HOCHANG B. LEE, MD
Associate Professor, Department of Psychiatry, Yale School of Medicine, New Haven, Connecticut

JOSÉ R. MALDONADO, MD, FAPM, FACFE
Professor of Psychiatry and, by courtesy, of Internal Medicine, Surgery, and Emergency Medicine; Medical Director, Psychosomatic Medicine Service; Medical Director, Emergency Psychiatry Service, Stanford University School of Medicine, Stanford, California

SAHIL MUNJAL, MD
Department of Psychiatry, Westchester Medical Center, New York Medical College, Valhalla, New York

MARK A. OLDHAM, MD
Assistant Professor, Department of Psychiatry, Yale School of Medicine, New Haven, Connecticut

RYAN PETERSON, MD
Psychosomatic Medicine Fellow, Department of Psychiatry, Yale School of Medicine, New Haven, Connecticut

WALTER PIDDOUBNY, MD
Psychosomatic Medicine Fellow, Department of Psychiatry, Yale School of Medicine, New Haven, Connecticut

J.J. RASIMAS, MD, PhD, FAPM
Director of Consultation, Liaison Psychiatry, Hennepin County Medical Center, Associate Professor of Psychiatry and Emergency Medicine, Penn State College of Medicine, Hershey, PA; University of Minnesota, Minneapolis, Minnesota

PETER A. SHAPIRO, MD
Professor, Department of Psychiatry, Columbia University Medical Center, College of Physicians and Surgeons, Columbia University; Director, Consultation-Liaison Psychiatry Service, New York-Presbyterian/Columbia University Medical Center, New York, New York

YELIZAVETA SHER, MD
Clinical Assistant Professor, Department of Psychiatry and Behavioral Sciences, Stanford University Medical Center, Stanford, California

COURTNEY M. SINCLAIR, BA
Veterinary and Biomedical Sciences, University of Minnesota, Saint Paul, Minnesota

JEANETTE M. TETRAULT, MD
Associate Professor of Medicine, Department of Internal Medicine, Yale University School of Medicine, New Haven, Connecticut

PAULA ZIMBREAN, MD
Associate Professor, Departments of Psychiatry and Surgery (Transplant), Yale New Haven Hospital, New Haven, Connecticut

Contents

> Traumatic brain injury (TBI) is an alteration in brain function, or other evidence of brain pathology, caused by an external force. TBI is a major cause of disability and mortality worldwide. Posttraumatic amnesia, or the interval from injury until the patient is oriented and able to form and later recall new memories, is an important index of TBI severity and functional outcome. This article will discuss the updates in the epidemiology, definition and classification, pathophysiology, diagnosis, and management of common acute neuropsychiatric sequelae of traumatic brain injury that the critical care specialist may encounter.

> Older adults account for half of intensive care unit (ICU) admissions and ICU days, and approximately 2 in 5 older adults in the ICU have preexisting cognitive impairment (PCI). PCI identification is important for risk stratification and may influence ICU utilization and decision-making surrogacy. PCI is overlooked in more than half of patients without screening; however, screening instruments can identify PCI in less than 5 minutes. Management of PCI in the ICU involves addressing associated neuropsychiatric symptoms. Nonpharmacological interventions should be considered the mainstay of treatment; psychotropics may be considered, although available data on their efficacy is limited.

> Delirium is the most common psychiatric syndrome found in the general hospital setting, with an incidence as high as 87% in the acute care setting. Delirium is a neurobehavioral syndrome caused by the transient disruption of normal neuronal activity secondary to systemic disturbances. The development of delirium is associated with increased morbidity, mortality, cost of care, hospital-acquired complications, placement in specialized intermediate and long-term care facilities, slower rate of recovery, poor functional and cognitive recovery, decreased quality of life, and prolonged hospital stays. This article discusses the epidemiology, known etiological factors, presentation and characteristics, prevention, management, and impact of delirium.

CRITICAL CARE CLINICS

Preface

Psychiatric Aspects of Critical Care Medicine: Update

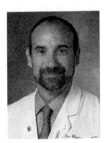

José R. Maldonado, MD, FAPM, FACFE
Editor

Critical care units are fast-paced, stressful environments. They are places where patients are taken to be put back together, but often it is also where they suffer and die. It is likewise a challenging place for medical personnel, carrying a high degree of professional burnout and medical personnel posttraumatic stress disorder (PTSD). This issue represents an ambitious effort to bring together the information that critical care personnel (eg, intensivists, anesthesiologists, surgeons nurses, and medical psychiatrists) need to understand the complex and diverse neuropsychiatric and ethical problems they and their patients face together, every day in the intensive care unit (ICU).

Drs DeGuzman and Ament (Stanford) discuss the epidemiology and neurobiology of traumatic brain injury (TBI), with a special focus on the neurobehavioral sequelae of head trauma, including details regarding TBI's phases of recovery, the evaluation of the resultant neurocognitive sequelae, and a discussion of a rational approach to the management of the behavioral and psychiatric symptoms following trauma.

As the US population ages, clinicians have to deal with an aging brain. Drs Oldham, Piddoubny, Peterson and Lee (Johns Hopkins) provide us with an excellent review of the presentation and detection of preexisting cognitive impairment in the critical care setting and provide the foundation for the management of the behavioral and psychiatric symptoms of cognitive impairment in the clinical setting.

Delirium or acute brain failure is the single most common neurobehavioral disorder experienced by medically ill patients, and no place has a higher incidence than the critical care unit. The occurrence of delirium affects patient's morbidity and mortality, affects the safety of patients and providers alike, and has profound implications regarding long-term outcome. Dr Maldonado (Stanford) conducts a comprehensive review of the epidemiology, etiologic factors, characteristics, and methods of diagnosis and summarizes the evidenced-based data on methods of treating and preventing delirium in the critical care units.

Crit Care Clin 33 (2017) xiii–xv
http://dx.doi.org/10.1016/j.ccc.2017.04.001
0749-0704/17/© 2017 Published by Elsevier Inc.

criticalcare.theclinics.com

Drs Rasimas and Sinclair (U of Minnesota) take us through a thorough description of the most common toxidromes likely to be faced by critically ill individuals, either because some form of poisoning got the patient to the ICU or because of the toxic effects of medical treatment. They do a masterful job discussing the interaction between toxicity, neuronal function, and mental status alteration, while guiding us through a maze of potentially deadly consequences of drug toxicity and how to help our patients survive them.

Drs Tetrault and Donroe (Yale) review the epidemiology of substance abuse and how it may contribute and/or complicate the treatment of the patient's underlying medical condition. Their article discusses both iatrogenic substances of abuse, in which doctors are partly complicit, and street drugs, such as cocaine, amphetamines, MDMA, synthetic cannabinoids, and bath salts, and their complications and provide clinical recommendations regarding the treatment of related conditions.

Dr Maldonado (Stanford) discusses the second most common substance use problem in the United States, alcohol use disorder, with an emphasis on the various withdrawal syndromes that may adversely affect the delivery of care in the critical care setting. Many clinicians have faced the problem of an agitated, withdrawing patient who is either requesting "more valium" or experiencing respiratory depression due to the central nervous system depressant effect of benzodiazepines. He discusses tools for the prediction of patients at risk for complicated alcohol withdrawal. He then provides a roadmap for the use of a Benzodiazepine-sparing protocol, designed to tackle the neurobiology of alcohol withdrawal, while avoiding the complications of conventional treatment approaches.

Dr Sher (Stanford) discusses the highly emotionally charged topic of lung disease and its relationship to psychopathology. Psychiatric conditions are prevalent among patients suffering from chronic lung disease, with rates of depression and anxiety significantly higher than the general population. She then provides a framework for the management of these psychiatric syndromes in the context of the highly emotionally charged setting of the critical care unit.

Similarly, Dr Shapiro (Columbia U) summarizes the specific psychiatric challenges experienced by patients with heart disease in acute, intensive, and critical care. He focuses on the strong emotional reactions experienced by patients admitted to cardiac critical care, including patient's psychological reactions to the various assistive technologies, such as mechanical ventilation, ventricular-assist devices, and defibrillation, ending with a discussion of the various psychiatric scenarios clinicians are likely to encounter in this setting.

Dr Garcia (Stanford) addresses the emotional and difficult topic of suicide, including predisposing factors leading to it and its neurobiology, and discusses the complexities of the assessment and management of suicide and its aftermath. Different from many other topics in this issue, this is one possible exception when the patient involuntarily ends up in the ICU, because he survived an attempt at ending his life.

The various conditions leading to an acute care admission and the environment and procedures performed in a critical care unit may render patients, their family members, and the staff liable to suffer any number of anxiety symptoms. Drs Bienvenu and Gerstenblith (Johns Hopkins) focus on one form of psychiatric morbidity in critical illness survivors, PTSD, which affects nearly 20% of critical illness survivors. They discuss the risk factors, treatment modalities, and what ICU personnel can do to prevent this disorder.

The ICU team plays an integral part in the medical journeys of transplant recipients. The critical care unit serves as the threshold between the failed organ and their new life. The ICU is the place where they wait for a new organ or die waiting for one. Drs Sher (Stanford) and Zimbrean (Yale) discuss the most up-to-date information on the psychosocial aspects of transplant patients in the critical care setting, including pretransplant evaluation, psychological considerations of assist devices in the ICU, peritransplantation neuropsychiatric syndromes, and relevant aspects of their psychopharmacology, including potential drug-drug interactions.

Drs Munjal and Ferrando (New York Medical College) and Dr Freyberg (Columbia) provide a detailed review of a select number of infectious agents with predilection to the central nervous system, which may lead to or complicate the assessment and management of ICU patients. In particular, they focus on HIV/AIDS, herpes encephalitis, pediatric acute-onset neuropsychiatric syndrome or childhood acute neuropsychiatric symptoms (formerly known as PANDAS), neurocysticercosis, neurosyphilis, Lyme disease, and Creutzfeldt-Jakob disease. In the process, they discuss their neuropsychiatric manifestations, diagnosis, and treatment.

Psychotropic agents are commonly used in the critical care setting, often serving as an indispensable adjunct to manage many neuropsychiatric and behavioral conditions, which present as a complication of medical treatment or represent part of the patient's substrate. In any case, psychoactive agents can present with any number of life-threatening situations, including serotonin syndrome, neuroleptic malignant syndrome and other forms of extrapyramidal syndromes, cardiac dysfunction, endocrine disturbances, discontinuation syndromes, and others. Drs Lahijani (Stanford) and Harris (Rush) discuss the most likely presentation, diagnostic techniques, and state-of-the-art management tips for each of these conditions.

We finish with a discussion of palliative and end-of-life care. This is a core component of critical care medicine and addresses the multiple domains of suffering that patients, families, and medical personnel experience. Dr Harman (Stanford) discusses the characteristically comprehensive approach of the palliative medicine specialist, with their unique role as consultants and their emphasis on patient/family-centered care. Often addressing and bridging complex ethical and end-of-life issues, her discussion provides a great conclusion to our attempt to integrate psychiatry and high-tech medicine in one comprehensive issue.

I am immensely honored for the opportunity to work with such a wonderful group of dedicated professionals and humbled by the passion, dedication, skill, and wisdom each of my colleagues brings with their contribution to the field of medicine and patient care.

José R. Maldonado, MD, FAPM, FACFE
Psychosomatic Medicine Service
Emergency Psychiatry Service
Stanford University School of Medicine
401 Quarry Road, Office #2317
Stanford, CA 94305, USA

E-mail address:
jrm@stanford.edu

Neurobehavioral Management of Traumatic Brain Injury in the Critical Care Setting: An Update

Earl De Guzman, MD, Andrea Ament, MD*

KEYWORDS

- Traumatic brain injury • Post-traumatic amnesia • Post-traumatic encephalopathy

KEY POINTS

- Traumatic brain injury (TBI) is an alteration in brain function, or other evidence of brain pathology, caused by an external force.
- TBI is a major cause of disability and mortality worldwide.
- Post-traumatic amnesia (PTA), or the interval from injury until the patient is oriented and able to form and later recall new memories, is an important index of TBI severity and functional outcome.

INTRODUCTION

Critical care in the early post-traumatic brain injury (TBI) involves stabilizing hemodynamics and systemic oxygenation with the goal of preventing secondary brain injury.[1] However, neurobehavioral disturbances after injury may also manifest in the emergency department (ED) or intensive care unit (ICU).[2] Whereas previous authors have described a broad range of psychiatric disorders after TBI, including depression, mania, post-traumatic stress disorder, alcohol use disorder, and personality changes,[3] as well as cognitive, behavioral, and somatic complaints,[4,5] only few have discussed post-traumatic encephalopathy (PTE) and neurobehavioral presentations specifically in the critical care setting.[2,6] Thus, this article will discuss the updates in the epidemiology, definition and classification, pathophysiology, diagnosis, and

This article is an update of an article previously published in Critical Care Clinics, Volume 24, Issue 4, October 2008.

Disclosure: None.

Psychosomatic Medicine, Department of Psychiatry, Stanford University School of Medicine, 401 Quarry Road, Palo Alto, CA 94305, USA

* Corresponding author.

E-mail address: aament@stanford.edu

Crit Care Clin 33 (2017) 423–440
http://dx.doi.org/10.1016/j.ccc.2017.03.011
0749-0704/17/© 2017 Elsevier Inc. All rights reserved.

management of common acute neuropsychiatric sequelae of TBI that the critical care specialist may encounter.

Epidemiology

TBI is a major cause of disability and mortality worldwide affecting approximately 10 million people.[7,8] In the United States, approximately 1.7 million people sustain a TBI annually, with about 1.7 million ED visits, 275,000 hospitalizations, and 52,000 deaths.[9] From 2001 to 2010, while TBI-related ED visits increased by 70% and hospitalizations increased by 11%, death rates decreased by 7%.[10] Whereas the increased proportion of individuals with TBI in well-developed areas such as Europe, Japan, and the United States tended to be elderly and suffer falls (leading cause of deaths of persons 65 and above) and contusion injuries,[10–12] the incidence of TBI in middle and low-income nations was attributable to lower standards of motor vehicle and traffic safety regulations.[13] A large, statewide population-based survey found that up to 42.5% of participants reported at least 1 TBI episode during their lifetime.[14] However, there is variability in the incidence reporting of TBI, owing to differences among multiple epidemiologic studies with different inclusion criteria, definition and classification standards, neuroimaging, and under-reporting or lack of recognition.[12] Once thought of as a silent epidemic, TBI, particularly its mild form, is estimated to be greater in incidence compared with previous studies.[15,16]

Mild TBI and concussion account for over 80% of cases.[17–19] The most common causes of TBI were falls (about 40%), unintentional blunt trauma (about 15%), and motor vehicle accidents (about 14%), although the latter represents the largest percentage of TBI-related deaths.[9,10] Men tended to have higher rates of TBI deaths and hospitalizations compared with women, with rates higher for those aged 65 and older.[10] Among the US military, more than 300,000 service members have been diagnosed with TBI, of whom 80% had concussions, likely reflective of "signature injuries" suffered from improvised explosive devices used during Operation Enduring Freedom (OEF) and Operation Iraqi Freedom (OIF) compared with penetrating injuries sustained during the Vietnam War and earlier campaigns.[20–23]

Those who suffer from severe TBI have a lower life expectancy than the general population, facing prolonged hospitalization and rehabilitation in addition to long-term affective, behavioral, cognitive, and physical disorders that impact disruptions in interpersonal relationships, independence, and work.[24] Moreover, severe TBI incurs significant socioeconomic consequences, with direct and indirect medical costs estimated at $60 billion in 2000, with costs for disability and productivity greatly outweighing those for medical care and rehabilitation.[24,25]

DEFINITION

TBI is an alteration in brain function, or other evidence of brain pathology, caused by an external force, and alteration in brain function is further defined as one of the following clinical signs: any period of loss of consciousness (LOC), any loss of memory for events immediately before (retrograde amnesia) or after the injury (post-traumatic amnesia [PTA]), neurologic deficits, and alteration in mental state at the time of injury (eg, confusion or disorientation).[26]

CLASSIFICATION

TBI is often categorized as mild, moderate, or severe using the Glasgow Coma Scale (GCS) during the acute phase of injury, assessing 3 components: eye opening, verbal response ('T' to denote intubation), and motor response. A GCS score of 13 to

15 characterizes mild TBI; a score of 9 to 12 represents moderate TBI; and a score of 3 to 8, represents severe TBI.[27,28] Although helpful during early management and prognosis, particularly with detecting subtle neurologic changes over time in the critical care setting,[29] other indicators such as post-traumatic amnesia are more helpful in late outcome predictions of TBI.[30]

Post-traumatic amnesia (PTA), or the interval from injury until the patient is oriented and able to form and later recall new memories, is an important index of TBI severity and functional outcome. PTA extending more than 24 hours falls within at least the moderate–severe range.[27,31] PTA was found to be associated with predicting long-term global outcome on the Glasgow Outcome Scale (GOS) and predicting long-term functional disability.[32,33] A more sensitive reorganization of Russel & Smith's PTA classification for TBI,[31] defining PTA 0 to 14 (moderate TBI), 15 to 28 (moderately severe TBI) and 29 to 70 (severe TBI), showed that 67% of those patients with moderate TBI returned to productivity within 1 year.[33]

There are particular limitations with reliability of using single indicators of TBI severity. For instance, a patient given opiate or sedating medications or who sustained organ failure associated with polytrauma may be misclassified as TBI.[34–37] GCS scores between 13 and 15 but with abnormal neuroimaging may also resemble those with moderate TBI.[38] In response to such limitations, other classification systems have incorporated multiple indicators rather than individual indicators alone: GCS, PTA, LOC, altered mental state, neuroimaging, and presence of skull fractures.[18,34]

Classifying TBI according to its severity may help inform the critical care specialist with acute medical treatment decisions, determination of neurorehabilitation needs, and prognosis.[36,39,40] However, understanding the underlying and unique neuropathologic changes of TBI further informs the critical care specialist in making meaningful comparisons among different sets of patients,[41,42] particularly those who develop neurobehavioral changes depending on the neurocircuitry and mechanism of TBI involved.[6]

PATHOPHYSIOLOGY

Treatment for TBI implies a fundamental understanding of the biomechanical and neurochemical changes when physical forces impact brain damage.

Closed head injuries (CHIs) occur either with direct contact with a blunt object or from a blast injury through shock wave pressures,[43] with concussions as the most common type of TBI. In CHI, 2 mechanisms occur: (1) impact, whereby an immediate force is applied to the skull, causing the brain to abut the frontal and temporal fossae of the skull; and (2) impulse, whereby a force indirectly impacts the brain.[44,45] Translational (linear) and rotational (angular) forces, with acceleration and deceleration, act near or far from the brain's center of gravity, and this combination of impact and acceleration/deceleration represents the most common form of TBI.[46,47] These forces create pulses of increased intracranial pressure gradients, causing varying degrees of straining and shearing, ultimately causing focal or diffuse axonal injury.[48,49] Rotational acceleration is more likely than translational acceleration to be the primary cause of CHI, and those injuries affecting the lateral and coronal planes appear to be more severe with worse outcomes.[50–52] Other authors have found increased stress and strain along multifocal sites along the bottom sulci of the frontal, temporal, and parietal cortices,[53] in addition to the corpus callosum, subcortical white matter, fornices, brainstem, and cerebellum.[41,54] After axonal injury, microtubule instability and disruption cause axonal varicosities to form, resulting in ineffective axonal transport.[55,56] Disruption of axonal membranes via neurofilament compaction triggers a cascade of calcium-mediated events, including activation of calpains and caspases and cleavage of spectrin and neurofilament side arms.[57] This ultimately leads to axonal swelling and disconnection.[58]

Injury to the gray and white matter areas affects imbalance of excitatory and inhibitory functioning.[59] Excess neuroexcitation and ionic flux are features of TBI that often reflect severity of injury. In the acute phase of brain injury, high levels of glutamate, an excitatory neurotransmitter, are observed through various mechanisms:

Exocytosis from presynaptic nerve terminals of depolarized neurons
Extravasation through and impaired reuptake from damaged membranes of glial and astrocytic cells
Leakage through the disrupted blood brain barrier
Disrupted glutamate transporters[60–62]

This acute increase in glutamate then releases intracellular calcium, which in turn activates calcium-mediated proteases, generation of reactive oxygen species, and mitochondrial impairment. Whereas intracellular calcium release results in apoptosis, excessive glutamate results in necrosis.[41,43] Neuroinflammatory factors are further implicated in TBI through an array of immune reactions, with the added vulnerability of changes in the blood–brain barrier.[63] These include inflammatory cytokines, chemokines, reactive oxygen and nitrogen species, and the complement system, all of which ultimately lead to the development of cerebral edema and increased intracranial pressure.[41,43] Cerebral edema is a common secondary brain injury and frequent cause of death among those with severe TBI.[64]

Penetrating TBI is characterized by direct intrusion of an object, such as a projectile, that passes through the cranium, brain tissue, and blood vessels.[43] The initial contact of a projectile creates a shock wave, followed by kinetic energy and depression of the surrounding medium directly in front of the projectile, then a compression wave with formation of a cavity through cycles of stretching and collapse of the surrounding tissue that in turn dampens the kinetic energy.[65] Most penetrating injuries are caused by firearms with various wound types: penetrating, perforating, tangential, ricochet, and careening.[66] As the cerebrovascular system is affected, the rupture of blood vessels and disruption of the blood brain barrier are characterized by hemorrhaging along the epidural, subdual, subarachnoid, or intracerebral/intraventricular spaces; pseudoaneurysms and traumatic cerebral vasospasm may also ensue.[43] This releases cytotoxic metabolites that further cause secondary injuries with increased cerebral edema, increased intracranial pressure, and resultant ischemia and necrosis through a cascade of neuroinflammatory factors.[48] Whereas vascular complications occur in early phase (<1 week), nonvascular complications occur later (>1 week) and include infection, hydrocephalus, cerebrospinal fluid leaks, and foreign body migration.[66]

Once thought to be shell shock,[67] TBI has undergone a reconceptualization over the past few decades in understanding brain damage that may even occur from a blast wave alone.[68] Although primary blast injuries render gas-containing organs as particularly vulnerable, blast-related TBI may even occur in the absence of secondary or tertiary mechanisms.[69] Blast-related TBI is a distinct type of brain injury, encountered among combat soldiers in warfare and among civilians in terrorist attacks, that occurs through the following mechanisms: primary, secondary, tertiary, quaternary, and quinary.[48,70] Primary blast injury is caused by direct exposure to the pressure of the blast wave itself. Secondary blast involves contact or penetrating trauma sustained when an object is propelled by a blast, striking the body. Tertiary blast injury describes the event wherein the body is propelled in motion, striking the ground, structure, or object in the environment. Quaternary blast injury results from exposure to burns or toxins from the explosion, crush injuries, or exacerbation of pre-existing medical conditions. Lastly, quinary blast injury refers to the hyperinflammatory response to exposure to toxins released by the exposure.[48,65,71] However, 3 mechanisms have been proposed that may explain concussion in primary blast-related TBI: acceleration, direct cranial injury, and thoracic.[70] As discussed previously, linear and rotational accelerations of the brain may occur as a result of a blast wave, causing axonal injury.[72,73] In contrast to coup-contre-coup injury from inertial effects from blunt trauma, direct cranial injury results from a pressure transient, either through direct transmission or pressure wave from the bulk motion of the skull.[72] When a blast wave applies pressure on the thorax, there may be a subsequent surge in blood volume, which then leads to increased intracranial pressure enough to damage the blood–brain barrier with resulting capillary hemorrhaging. Moreover, a vagal-mediated response may occur after high transient pressure waves are transmitted from the thorax to the brain through soft tissue or vascular involvement and without bulk motion of the skull.[72,74]

NEUROANATOMICAL CIRCUITRY

Understanding TBI further at the neuroanatomical and circuitry level enables the provider to understand and appreciate the potential functional systems involved that may explain particular neuropsychiatric presentations. For instance, the orbitofrontal frontal cortex (OFC) plays an important role in self-regulation of behavior according to social cues, feedback, and situations.[75] Behavioral disinhibition and impulsivity are prototypical symptoms of OFC lesions, but may include antisocial rigid behavior,[76,77] pathologic gambling,[78] obsessive–compulsive behaviors,[79] and hoarding.[80] In contrast, executive functioning, mediated by the dorsolateral prefrontal cortex (DLPFC), is involved in modulating response inhibition, interference control, set shifting, and working memory.[81] The anterior cingulate circuit is involved in both motivational and mood regulation, and thus may explain its pathology in those with decreased motivation and akinetic mutism.[82] Whereas the first 3 circuits are involved in social comportment, executive functioning and motivation, the medial temporal region modulates emotional memory with new learning according to ongoing environmental stimuli.[6] Damage to any one of these circuits in TBI represents potential mechanisms through which different neuropsychiatric symptoms arise.

NEUROBEHAVIORAL SYMPTOMS

Neuropsychiatric sequelae of TBI can range from mild deficits to chronic vegetative states.[83] Although life-threatening physical injuries caused byTBI are most acutely addressed in the critical care setting, several neurobehavioral syndromes have important implications on both the short-term management of the acutely ill, and the long-term recovery of individuals with TBI.

Risk factors for head injury include alcohol/drug use, lower socioeconomic status, and underlying psychiatric and/or cognitive disorders.[84,85] Furthermore, risk factors for neuropsychiatric symptoms after TBI include increasing age, vasculopathic risk factors (eg, hypertension, arteriosclerosis, diabetes), and alcoholism, which have been proposed to negatively affect central nervous system repair.[86]

Conceptualization of neuropsychiatric symptoms of traumatic brain injury can be divided into 2 categories: acute/severe (requiring immediate management in the ICU/hospital), versus more chronic conditions that require treatment well after the acute stabilization of physical injuries in the inpatient setting. Acute and severe neuropsychiatric complications of TBI include coma, vegetative states, agitation, delirium, and a variety of emotional disturbances. More chronic neuropsychiatric sequelae include depression, anxiety, post-traumatic stress disorder (PTSD) aggression, psychosis, mania, memory disturbances, personality changes, substance abuse, and sleep disturbances[87] (**Boxes 1** and **2**).

Acute Phase

Emergency and critical care management of TBI includes severity scoring with GCS classification, necessary clinical evaluation (including neurologic examination), close monitoring of vital signs and laboratory findings, airway management, and oxygenation. Depending on the GCS and level of consciousness of the patient, a psychiatric and cognitive screening is performed also. The time when a comatose patient regains consciousness (or is in the process of doing so, making the transition from a state of coma, through stupor, to eventual awakeness) is the time at which delirium most often occurs.[6] Delirium is defined an acute disturbance in attention, awareness, and cognition (including memory deficit, disorientation, language, perception) that tends to fluctuate in severity during the course of the day.[88] The syndrome of delirium in post-TBI patients can encompass hypoactive to hyperactive, and mixed states in between. In the critical care management of TBI, post-traumatic agitation as it occurs within the setting of delirium often requires pharmacologic management, as it tends to be (in terms of neuropsychiatric symptoms), most disruptive to recovery in that acute setting. There have been some alternate descriptions of post-TBI mental status changes, including post-traumatic amnesia and post-traumatic confusional state, both of which are thought to be consistent with delirium,[89] which is reported to occur in up to 70% of patients with severe TBI.[90] For reference, delirium is common in the general hospital (up to 20%), and very common in the ICU (up to 80%).[91] The median duration of delirium has been reported to be 43 days for TBI patients with severe injuries.[92]

A classification has been proposed which describes 4 different stages of post-traumatic encephalopathy, which is defined as "the clinical manifestations of brain dysfunction that develop immediately following application of an external physical

---

Box 1
Overlap of different proposed classifications of post-TBI neurobehavioral syndromes

1. Post-traumatic coma
   a. Coma
   b. Persistent vegetative state
   c. Unconscious
   d. GCS less than 8

2. Post-traumatic delirium
   a. Delirium
   b. Agitation
   c. Aggression
   d. Alteration in arousal/attention

3. Post-traumatic amnesia
   a. Cognitive impairment

4. Post-traumatic dysexecutive syndrome
   a. Cognitive impairment
   b. Mood disturbances
   c. Aggression
   d. Behavioral dyscontrol disorder

Box 2
Neurobehavioral symptoms of traumatic brain injury

1. Acute, severe, ICU/inpatient management
   a. Coma
   b. Vegetative state
   c. Delirium

2. Chronic, long-term management
   a. Depression
   b. Anxiety
   c. Aggression
   d. Psychosis
   e. Memory disturbances
   f. Personality change
   g. Substance abuse
   h. Sleep Disturbance
   i. PTSD
   j. Mania
   k. Behavioral dyscontrol disorder

---

force to the brain".[93] This term specifically denotes brain dysfunction that is specifically induced *by* neuro-trauma. Post-traumatic encephalopathy includes post-traumatic coma, post-traumatic delirium, post-traumatic amnesia, and post-traumatic dysexecutive syndrome. **Box 1** outlines how this particular classification overlaps with the individually described post-TBI neuropsychiatric syndromes.

POST-TRAUMATIC BRAIN INJURY SYNDROMES

Long-term psychiatric complications of TBI interfere with quality of life, rehabilitation efforts, overall level of function, and independence.[94] These post-TBI syndromes are briefly discussed for overview, but in-depth study is outside the scope of this article.

Cognitive Deficits in Traumatic Brain Injury

Cognitive deficits occur in up to 80% of patients with significant TBI.[95] There are a wide range of cognitive deficits in TBI, including loss of memory (verbal and nonverbal skills), disturbance in executive functioning, impairment of arousal, impairment of concentration, impairment of attention, impairment of judgment, and impulse control.[1] Cognitive deficits after TBI have been described in 4 groups, corresponding to phases of TBI.[96] Shortly after injury there is the period of coma and loss of consciousness, as described previously. This then transitions to a period of post-traumatic delirium,[1] involving the cognitive and behavioral abnormalities of agitation, confusion, and disorientation that was described previously. During the next 6 to 12 months is a period of the most rapid recovery of cognitive function, and followed by a plateauing of recovery, which tapers off around 2 years after the injury. The fourth and final phase is characterized by a variety of possible cognitive deficits that persist for the remainder of the patient's lifetime. This final phase has been described as dementia due to head trauma[97] and permanent cognitive syndrome, and includes problems with speed of information processing, attention and vigilance, short- and long-term memory deficits, verbal and nonverbal deficits, problems with executive functioning, and mental flexibility.[1] Pathogenesis of post-TBI cognitive impairment has been attributed in part due to decreased levels of choline acetyltransferase, thereby reducing brain acetylcholine levels.[98]

Psychosis

There are limited and conflicting data on the incidence and risk factors for post-traumatic psychosis (which is distinguished from acute delusions or hallucinations seen in post-TBI delirium). One study reported 20% of 40 TBI survivors developed psychosis after being followed for up to 15 years,[99] while another study reported up to 10%.[100] The delay of psychotic symptoms after TBI (up to 4 years) has made causality challenging.[100] Family history of psychosis and duration of loss of consciousness are thought to be risk factors for post-traumatic psychosis, along with language impairment and frontal and parietal lobe injury.[101] The first and second most common psychotic symptoms in TBI patients are persecutory delusions and auditory hallucinations, respectively.

Post-traumatic Stress Disorder

Post-traumatic stress disorder (PTSD) is not surprisingly common after TBI, as trauma is an inherent part of the injury. PTSD occurs in up to 27% of patients,[102] even when the traumatic event is associated with altered consciousness and amnesia. Acute stress disorder is a strong risk factor for subsequent development of PTSD; of patients who met criteria for acute stress disorder at 1 month after TBI, 82% developed PTSD at 6 months after injury.[103] Avoidant coping and the presence of anxiety were also found to be risk factors for development of PTSD.[104]

Post-traumatic Brain Injury Depression

Post-TBI depression has an incidence of 15% to 33% and a prevalence of 18% to 42%.[105] The challenge with diagnosis of depression in this population is challenging, as it is with any medical population, because neurovegetative symptoms of depression (ie, poor concentration, decreased energy, or insomnia) may occur in TBI patients independent of a mood disorder. It is well established that TBI patients with depression have worse functional and psychosocial outcomes.[106] Risk factors include stress, social isolation, and maladaptive coping styles.[107] Depressive symptoms such as fatigue, irritability, suicidal thoughts, anhedonia, amotivation, and insomnia can be seen for over 2 years after TBI.[108] With regards to suicidal ideation, risk is increased with frontal contusions.[109]

Post-traumatic Brain Injury Mania

Post-TBI mania occurs in less than 10% of patients.[110] However, there are otherwise little conclusive data regarding this diagnosis, as many symptoms of mania overlap with other post-TBI syndromes such as aggression.

Post-traumatic Brain Injury Aggression

Aggression after TBI, including agitation, disinhibition, lability, impulsivity, and personality changes occur in variable frequencies depending on criteria, ranging from 20% to 49%, and typically within the first year after injury.[111] Lack of a consensus definition of aggression and agitation is particularly problematic; there is significant overlap between aggression and personality/mood symptoms, and aggression may occur within multiple other syndromes.[25] Post-traumatic aggression excludes the agitation that is seen in hyperactive or mixed-type delirium. Risk factors for development of aggression include frontal lobe lesions, male gender, prior head injury, premorbid mood, substance or alcohol use disorder, premorbid aggressive behavior, low IQ, and low socioeconomic status.[112]

Behavioral Dyscontrol Disorder

In addition to the previously mentioned post-TBI syndromes, other categories have been described including anxiety, personality changes, apathy, and sleep disturbances. This highlights the fact that neuropsychiatric complications associated with TBI are numerous, complex, and often overlapping. Rao and Lyketsos in 2000 proposed a description, called behavioral dyscontrol disorder, with major and minor variants.[1] The major variant encompasses mood disturbance (ie, irritability, anger, or rage), cognitive impairment (attention, memory, executive function, judgment, distractibility, disorganization), and behavior disturbance (impulsivity, aggressivity, hyperactivity, hyperphagia). Pathophysiologically, disinhibition is a result of damage of orbital–frontal areas; dysexecutive symptoms are a result of frontal lobe dysfunction, and emotion/memory problems are a result of temporal lobe damage.[113]

TREATMENT
Introductory Remarks

Similar to pharmacologic treatments for delirium in the critical care setting, there are no US Food and Drug Administration (FDA)- approved medications for the treatment of acute neuropsychiatric symptoms related to TBI. Review of the evidence on pharmacologic management of TBI-related neuropsychiatric symptoms are confined to open-label case series, single case reports, and a handful of small double-blinded randomized controlled trials (RCTs). All discussed treatments are off-label. Additionally, when considering psycho-pharmacologic agents for treating patients with TBI, consideration must be taken regarding agents that might be harmful to this specific population (eg, benzodiazepines and antipsychotics).

Treatment of Post-traumatic Brain Injury Delirium

Treatment of post-TBI delirium includes standard treatment of delirium, including identifying and treating contributing medical factors including infection, dehydration, electrolyte disturbances, severe anemia, hypoxia, and hypotension, among others. Further review of a patient's medications should be made to eliminate any medications that are known to contribute to delirium, such as benzodiazepines, medications that are highly anticholinergic, and unnecessary or excessive opiate administration. Urine and stool output should be monitored, and pain should be treated. Psychosocial measures are crucial to the treatment of delirium, including regulating the sleep–wake cycle with adequate daylight, and keeping the patient awake during the day and asleep at night when possible. Frequent reorientation, sensory aids (hearing aids, glasses), and early mobilization with physical therapy and being out of bed may also be necessary.[114]

Several drug classes and agents have been used for post-traumatic delirium and agitation; however, validated controlled trials have still been limited. To the authors' knowledge, there are no established guidelines or algorithms for pharmacologic management. Due to the TBI patient's sensitivity to central nervous system (CNS)-acting medications, proposed guidelines have included the recommendations to start at low doses and titrate slowly, therapeutic trial of all medications, frequent reassessment of clinical condition, careful monitoring of drug–drug interactions, and augment when there is partial response.[115]

Antipsychotics

Antipsychotics are the mainstay of treatment for delirium in the general hospital and in the ICU. There has been some debate about whether typical antipsychotics may impair cognitive recovery in TBI patients, including an initial animal study showing impaired neuronal recovery after administration of haloperidol to rats.[116] The same study demonstrates that after discontinuation of treatment with haloperidol, cognitive recovery resumes a normal course compared with the nonhaldol group. This can be explained by the fact that antipsychotics do cause motor adverse effects, which are relieved after discontinuation. There may continue to be a benefit to treatment of post-traumatic delirium with antipsychotics given the significant repercussions of delirium in the ICU. Atypical antipsychotics are recommended for treatment of post-TBI delirium as they have fewer motor adverse effects, and have been shown to not cause impairment in cognitive performance after TBI in rats compared with a typical agent.[117] Chlorpromazine has been shown to provide neuroprotection against brain ischemia.[118]

Anticonvulsants

Anticonvulsants are used to treat multiple neuropsychiatric sequalae of TBI, including seizure disorder, mood lability, mania, impulsivity, and aggression. Case series report lower agitation and aggression with valproic acid in TBI patients,[119] and further case series report management of hyperactive delirium with valproic acid.[120] Doses are started at 250 mg twice daily and may be increased up to 2000 mg per day with careful monitoring of trough levels. Rare but serious adverse effects must be monitored including thrombocytopenia, agranulocytosis, transaminitis, and hyperammonemia. Another case report documents the use of lamotrigine for agitation following TBI.[121]

Alpha-2 Antagonists

Agents such as clonidine, guanfacine, and dexmedetomidine are used to decrease the adrenergic overdrive that is seen in patients with hyperactive delirium, and is common to post-traumatic patients with delirium and agitation in the ICU. Dexmedetomidine, a highly selective alpha-2 adrenergic receptor agonist, has been reported to be beneficial over propofol in achieving target Richmond Agitation-Sedation Scale in mechanically ventilated ICU patients with TBI.[122] It is becoming more commonly used in the ICU setting, and is a preferred continuous sedative agent as its use greatly reduces development of delirium over other traditional agents such as propofol.[123] With all 3 of these agents, blood pressure must be monitored, as their limiting adverse effect is hypotension.

Treatment of Post-traumatic Brain Injury Cognitive Deficits

Early cognitive and physical rehabilitation is crucial for post-traumatic cognitive recovery. This should be initiated in the ICU as soon as the patient is able to engage in even the most basic activity. Furthermore, even if a patient is unable to follow commands or to move on his or her own accord, even having the patient getting into a chair or performing passive range of movement is helpful for cognitive recovery. Beyond the ICU, long-term cognitive rehabilitation is important, particularly in the first 6 months after the injury.[124]

Dopaminergic Agents

TBI involves disturbances in dopamine transmission, which may persist for years after the injury.[125] Dopaminergic agents such as amantadine, bromocriptine, and levodopa are commonly used dopaminergic agents, and in TBI patients have been theorized to target the decreased frontal lobe dopamine activity. Amantadine enhances the release of dopamine, inhibits reuptake, and increases activity at the postsynaptic receptors. Amantadine has been shown to increase the rate of functional recovery during active treatment in patients with disruption of consciousness caused by TBI,[126] and appears to be an effective and safe means of reducing frequency and severity of irritability and aggression.[127] At doses of 200 to 400 mg/d, amantadine appears to safely improve arousal and cognition in patients with TBI.[128] Furthermore, there was a consistent trend toward more rapid functioning improvement on various neuropsychiatric and functional measures in patients with diffuse axonal injury-associated TBI when amantadine was starting within the first 3 months of injury.[129] Several case reports have documented amantadine's benefit for outcomes including mutism, impulsivity, aggression, information processing, apathy, inattention, short-term memory, planning, problem-solving, disinhibition, and poor motivation.[130] The authors propose starting amantadine dosing at 25 mg or 50 mg 3 times daily, with first dosing around 0500 and latest dosing around 1300, so not to potentiate insomnia or disrupt sleep. Amantadine is renally cleared, so close monitoring of renal function is necessary; potential risks include seizures (at accumulation of high doses) and activation/agitation.

Bromocriptine is a dopamine D_2 receptor agonist that may improve cognitive functions, although with data limited to 1 case report and 1 small RCT, which demonstrated that TBI patients treated with bromocriptine improved performance on executive function tasks.[131] Bromocriptine is dosed at 2.5 to 7.5 mg/d; it is contraindicated in patients with uncontrolled hypertension and hypersensitivity to ergot alkaloids. Adverse effects are generally mild but include dizziness, drowsiness, and gastrointestinal upset. Levodopa/carbidopa has been found to be helpful with TBI cognitive recovery; however, possible adverse effects of paranoia and hallucinations generally preclude its use in this population.

Psychostimulants

Psychostimulant medications are widely used in TBI patients to target those patients with poor arousal and attention. Traditional psychostimulants such as amphetamine and methylphenidate produce widespread CNS stimulation; they increase catecholamine activity by blocking the reuptake of dopamine and norepinephrine. Both agents are initiated at 2.5 mg (start low, go slow), and the first dose can be given early at 0600, with subsequent doses every 2 hours to monitor response, with last dose at 1300. Maximum dose for both drugs is 60 mg/d. Heart rate and blood pressure should be monitored in patients started on these agents. Modafinil is a CNS stimulant that acts on a number of pathways (monoamine, glutamate, gaba, orexin), and is selective to brain areas involved in regulation of sleep, wakefulness, and circadian rhythms; it is thought to stimulate these areas to regulate normal wakefulness. Modafinil can be initiated at 25 or 50 mg daily in the morning, with a maximum dose of 400 mg daily.

SUMMARY

Traumatic brain injury (TBI) is a major cause of morbidity and mortality, of which its neurobehavioral and neuropsychiatric sequelae may present potential diagnostic and treatment challenges for the critical care specialist. Understanding the varying degrees of potential phenotypic presentations and the different permutations of potential mechanistic, structural, functional, and neuropathological changes of TBI may better inform treatment within the critical care setting.

REFERENCES

1. Kinoshita K. Traumatic brain injury: pathophysiology for neurocritical care. J Intensive Care 2016;4:29.
2. Arciniegas DB, McAllister TW. Neurobehavioral management of traumatic brain injury in the critical care setting. Crit Care Clin 2008;24(4):737–65.
3. Schwarzbold M, Diaz A, Martins ET, et al. Psychiatric disorders and traumatic brain injury. Neuropsychiatr Dis Treat 2008;4(4):797–816.
4. Riggio S. Traumatic brain injury and its neurobehavioral sequelae. Neurol Clin 2011;29(1):35–47.
5. Warriner EM, Velikonja D. Psychiatric disturbances after traumatic brain injury: neurobehavioral and personality changes. Curr Psychiatry Rep 2006;8(1): 73–80.
6. McAllister TW. Neurobiological consequences of traumatic brain injury. Dialogues Clin Neurosci 2011;13(3):287–300.
7. Hyder AA, Wunderlich CA, Puvanachandra P, et al. The impact of traumatic brain injuries: a global perspective. NeuroRehabilitation 2007;22(5):341–53.
8. Stocchetti N, Zanier ER. Chronic impact of traumatic brain injury on outcome and quality of life: a narrative review. Crit Care 2016;20(1):148.
9. Faul M, Xu L, Wald MM, et al. Traumatic brain injury in the United States: emergency department visits, hospitalizations and deaths 2002–2006. Atlanta (GA): Centers for Disease Control and Prevention; National Center for Injury Prevention and Control; 2010.
10. Centers for Disease Control and Prevention. Traumatic brain injury in the United States: Fact sheet. 2016. Available at: http://www.cdc.gov/traumaticbraininjury/get_the_facts.html. Accessed November 12, 2016.
11. Harvey LA, Close JC. Traumatic brain injury in older adults: characteristics, causes and consequences. Injury 2012;43(11):1821–6.
12. Roozenbeek B, Maas AI, Menon DK. Changing patterns in the epidemiology of traumatic brain injury. Nat Rev Neurol 2013;9(4):231–6.
13. Maas AI, Stocchetti N, Bullock R. Moderate and severe traumatic brain injury in adults. Lancet Neurol 2008;7(8):728–41.
14. Whiteneck GG, Cuthbert JP, Corrigan JD, et al. Risk of negative outcomes after traumatic brain injury: a statewide population-based survey. J Head Trauma Rehabil 2016;31(1):E43–54.
15. Feigin VL, Theadom A, Barker-Collo S, et al. Incidence of traumatic brain injury in New Zealand: a population-based study. Lancet Neurol 2013;12(1):53–64.
16. Rusnak M. Traumatic brain injury: Giving voice to a silent epidemic. Nat Rev Neurol 2013;9(4):186–7.
17. Cassidy JD, Carroll LJ, Peloso PM, et al. Incidence, risk factors and prevention of mild traumatic brain injury: results of the WHO Collaborating Centre task force on mild traumatic brain injury. J Rehabil Med 2004;43(Suppl):28–60.
18. The Management of Concussion/mTBI Working Group. VA/DoD clinical practice guideline for management of concussion/mild traumatic brain injury. Washington, DC: Department of Veterans Affairs and Department of Defense; 2009.
19. McCrory P, Meeuwisse WH, Aubry M, et al. Consensus statement on concussion in sport: the 4th International Conference on concussion in sport held in Zurich, November 2012. Br J Sports Med 2013;47(5):250–8.
20. Helmick KM, Spells CA, Malik SZ, et al. Traumatic brain injury in the US military: epidemiology and key clinical and research programs. Brain Imaging Behav 2015;9(3):358–66.

21. Ling G, Bandak F, Armonda R, et al. Explosive blast neurotrauma. J Neurotrauma 2009;26(6):815–25.
22. Okie S. Traumatic brain injury in the war zone. N Engl J Med 2005;352(20): 2043–7.
23. Owens BD, Kragh JF, Wenke JC, et al. Combat wounds in Operation Iraqi Freedom and Operation Enduring Freedom. J Trauma 2008;64(2):295–9.
24. Rosenfeld JV, Maas AI, Bragge P, et al. Early management of severe traumatic brain injury. Lancet 2012;380(9847):1088–98.
25. Finkelstein E, Corso P, Miller T. The incidence and economic burden of injuries in the United States. New York: Oxford University Press; 2006.
26. Menon DK, Schwab K, Wright DW, et al. Position statement: definition of traumatic brain injury. Arch Phys Med Rehabil 2010;91(11):1637–40.
27. Kay T, Harrington DE, Adams R, et al. Definition of mild traumatic brain injury. J Head Trauma Rehabil 1993;8(3):86–7.
28. Teasdale G, Jennett B. Assessment of coma and impaired consciousness. A practical scale. Lancet 1974;2(7872):81–4.
29. Green SM. Cheerio, laddie! Bidding farewell to the Glasgow Coma Scale. Ann Emerg Med 2011;58(5):427–30.
30. Sherer M, Struchen MA, Yablon SA, et al. Comparison of indices of traumatic brain injury severity: Glasgow Coma Scale, length of coma and posttraumatic amnesia. J Neurol Neurosurg Psychiatry 2008;79(6):678–85.
31. Russell WR, Smith A. Post-traumatic amnesia in closed head injury. Arch Neurol 1961;5:16–29.
32. Brown AW, Malec JF, McClelland, et al. Clinical elements that predict outcome after traumatic brain injury: a prospective multicenter recursive partitioning (decision-tree) analysis. J Neurotrauma 2005;22(10):1040–51.
33. Nakase-Richardson R, Sherer M, Seel RT, et al. Utility of post-traumatic amnesia in predicting 1-year productivity following traumatic brain injury: comparison of the Russell and Mississippi PTA classification intervals. J Neurol Neurosurg Psychiatry 2011;82(5):494–9.
34. Malec JF, Brown AW, Leibson CL, et al. The Mayo classification system for traumatic brain injury severity. J Neurotrauma 2007;24(9):1417–24.
35. McCarter RJ, Walton NH, Moore C, et al. PTA testing, the Westmead post traumatic amnesia scale and opiate analgesia: a cautionary note. Brain Inj 2007; 21(13–14):1393–7.
36. Friedland DP. Improving the classification of traumatic brain injury: the Mayo classification system for traumatic brain injury severity. J Spine 2013;S4:5.
37. Ruff RM, Iverson GL, Barth JT, et al. Recommendations for diagnosing a mild traumatic brain injury: a National Academy of Neuropsychology education paper. Arch Clin Neuropsychol 2009;24(1):3–10.
38. van der Naalt J, Hew JM, van Zomeren AH, et al. Computed tomography and magnetic resonance imaging in mild to moderate head injury: early and late imaging related to outcome. Ann Neurol 1999;46(1):70–8.
39. National Institute for Clinical Excellence Head Injury. Triage, assessment, investigation and early management of head injury in infants, children and adults. Clinical Guideline 4. Developed by the National Collaborating Centre for Acute Care. London: NICE; 2003.
40. Friedland D, Hutchinson P. Classification of traumatic brain injury. Adv Clin Neurosci Rehabil 2013;4:12–3.
41. McGinn MJ, Povlishock JT. Pathophysiology of traumatic brain injury. Neurosurg Clin N Am 2016;27(4):397–407.

42. Saatman KE, Duhaime AC, Bullock R, et al. Classification of traumatic brain injury for targeted therapies. J Neurotrauma 2008;25(7):719–38.

43. de Lanerolle NC, Kim JH, Bandak FA. Neuropathology of traumatic brain injury: comparison of penetrating, nonpenetrating direct impact and explosive blast etiologies. Semin Neurol 2015;35(1):12–9.

44. Bigler ED. Traumatic brain injury and cognitive reserve. In: Stern Y, editor. Cognitive reserve: theory and applications. New York: Taylor and Francis; 2007. p. 85–116.

45. Shaw NA. The neurophysiology of concussion. Prog Neurobiol 2002;67: 281–344.

46. Kotapka MJ, Gennarelli TA, Graham DI, et al. Selective vulnerability of hippocampal neurons in acceleration-induced experimental head injury. J Neurotrauma 1991;8:247–58.

47. Adams JH, Graham DI, Murray LS, et al. Diffuse axonal injury due to nonmissile head injury in humans: an analysis of 45 cases. Ann Neurol 1982;12(6):557–63.

48. Bauer D, Tung ML, Tsao JW. Mechanisms in traumatic brain injury. Semin Neurol 2015;35(1):e14–22.

49. Young LA, Rule GT, Bocchieri RT, et al. Biophysical mechanisms of traumatic brain injuries. Semin Neurol 2015;35:5–11.

50. Gennarelli TA, Thibault LE, Adams JH, et al. Diffuse axonal injury and traumatic coma in the primate. Ann Neurol 1982;12:564–74.

51. Zhang L, Yang KH, King AI. A comparison of brain responses between frontal and lateral impacts by finite element modeling. J Neurotrauma 2001;18:21–30.

52. Zhang J, Yoganandan N, Pintar FA. Role of translational and rotational accelerations on brain strain in lateral head impact. Biomed Sci Instrum 2006;42:501–6.

53. Cloots RJH, Gervaise HMT, van Dommelen JAW, et al. Biomechanics of traumatic brain injury: Influences of the morphologic heterogeneities of the cerebral cortex. Ann Biomed Eng 2008;26(7):1203–15.

54. McKee AC, Daneshvar DH, Alvarez VE, et al. The neuropathology of sport. Acta Neuropathol 2014;127:29–51.

55. Christman CW, Grady MS, Walker SA, et al. Ultrastructural studies of diffuse axonal injury in humans. J Neurotrauma 1994;11:173–86.

56. Tang-Schomer MD, Johnson VE, Baas PW, et al. Partial interruption of axonal transport due to microtubule breakage accounts for the formation of periodic varicosities after traumatic axonal injury. Exp Neurol 2012;233:364–72.

57. Povlishock JT, Katz DI. Update of neuropathology and neurological recovery after traumatic brain injury. J Head Trauma Rehabil 2005;20(1):76–94.

58. Buki A, Povlishock JT. All roads lead to disconnection?-Traumatic axonal injury revisited. Acta Neurochir 2006;148:181–93 [discussion: 193–4].

59. Kasahara M, Menon DK, Salmond CH, et al. Traumatic brain injury alters the functional brain network mediating working memory. Brain Inj 2011;25:1170–87.

60. Bullock R, Zauner A, Woodward JJ, et al. Factors affecting excitatory amino acid release following severe human head injury. J Neurosurg 1998;89(4):507–18.

61. Rao V, Spiro J, Vaishnavi S, et al. Prevalence and types of sleep disturbances acutely after traumatic brain injury. Brain Inj 2008;22(5):381–6.

62. Yi JH, Hazell AS. Excitotoxic mechanisms and the role of astrocytic glutamate transporters in traumatic brain injury. Neurochem Int 2006;48(5):394–403.

63. Habgood MD, Bye N, Dziegielewska KM, et al. Changes in blood-brain barrier permeability to large and small molecules following traumatic brain injury in mice. Eur J Neurosci 2007;25:231–8.

64. Plesnila N. Decompression craniectomy after traumatic brain injury. Prog Brain Res 2007;161:393–400.
65. Risdall JE, Menon DK. Traumatic brain injury. Philos Trans R Soc Lond B Biol Sci 2011;366(1562):241–50.
66. Vakil MT, Singh AK. A review of penetrating brain trauma: epidemiology, pathophysiology, imaging assessment, complications and treatment. Emerg Radiol 2017;1–9 [Epub ahead of print].
67. Mott FW. Mental hygiene and shell shock during and after the war. Br Med J 1917;2:39–42.
68. Battacharjee Y. Shell shock revisited: solving the puzzle of blast trauma. Science 2008;319(5862):406–8.
69. Cernak I, Savic J, Ignjatovic D, et al. Blast injury from explosive munitions. J Trauma 1999;47(1):103–4.
70. Courtney A, Courtney M. The complexity of biomechanics causing primary blast-induced traumatic brain injury: a review of potential mechanisms. Front Neurol 2015;6:221.
71. Champion HR, Holcomb JB, Young LA. Injuries from explosions: physics, biophysics, pathology, and required research focus. J Trauma 1999;66(5): 1468–77.
72. Courtney MW, Courtney AC. Working toward exposure thresholds for blast-induced traumatic brain injury: thoracic and acceleration mechanisms. Neuroimage 2011;54(Suppl 1):S55–61.
73. Zhang L, Yang KH, King AI. A proposed injury threshold for mild traumatic brain injury. J Biomed Eng 2004;126(2):226–36.
74. Chen Y, Huang W. Non-impact, blast-induced mild TBI and PTSD: Concepts and caveats. Brain Inj 2011;25(7–8):641–50.
75. Rolls ET. The orbitofrontal cortex and reward. Cereb Cortex 2000;10:284–94.
76. Jonker FA, Jonker C, Scheltens P, et al. The role of the orbitofrontal cortex in cognition and behavior. Rev Neurosci 2014;26(1):1–11.
77. Umeda S, Mimura M, Kato M. Acquired personality traits of autism following damage to the medial prefrontal cortex. Soc Neurosci 2010;5:19–29.
78. Floris G, Cannas A, Melis M, et al. Pathological gambling, delusional parasitosis and adipsia as a post-haemorrhagic syndrome: a case report. Neurocase 2008; 14:385–9.
79. Ogai M, Iyo M, Mori N, et al. A right orbitofrontal region and OCD symptoms: a case report. Acta Psychiatr Scand 2005;111:74–6 [discussion: 76–7].
80. Volle E, Beato R, Levy R, et al. Forced collectionism after orbitofrontal damage. Neurology 2002;58:488–90.
81. Diamond A. Executive functions. Annu Rev Psychol 2013;64:136–68.
82. Kurukumbi M, Dang T, Crossley N, et al. Unique presentation of akinetic mutism and coexisting thyroid storm relating to stroke. Case Rep Neurol Med 2014; 2014:320565.
83. Rao V, Lyketsos C. Neuropsychiatric sequelae of traumatic brain injury. Psychosomatics 2000;41(2):95–103.
84. Ilie G, Boak A, Adlaf EM, et al. Prevalence and correlates of traumatic brain injuries among adolescents. JAMA 2013;309:2550.
85. Liao CC, Chiu WT, Yeh CC, et al. Risk and outcomes for traumatic brain injury in patients with mental disorders. J Neurol Neurosurg Psychiatry 2012;83:1186.
86. Lishman WA. Physiogenesis and psychogenesis in the post-concussional syndrome. Br J Psychiatry 1988;153:460–9.

87. Bhalerao SU, Geurtjens C, Thomas GR, et al. Understanding the neuropsychiatric consequences associated with significant traumatic brain injury. Brain Inj 2013;27(7–8):767–74.
88. American Psychiatric Association. Diagnostic and statistical manual of mental disorders. 5th edition. Arlington (VA): American Psychiatric Publishing; 2013.
89. Sherer M, Nakase-Thompson R, Yablon SA, et al. Multidimensional assessment of acute confusion after traumatic brain injury. Arch Phys Med Rehabil 2005;86:896–904.
90. Vaishnavi S, Rao V, Fann JR. Neuropsychiatric problems after traumatic brain injury: unraveling the silent epidemic. Psychosomatics 2009;50:198–205.
91. McEvoy JP. Organic brain syndromes. Ann Intern Med 1981;95:212–20.
92. Nakase-Thompson R, Sherer M, Yablon SA, et al. Acute confusion following traumatic brain injury. Brain Inj 2004;18:131–42.
93. Arciniegas DB. Neuropsychiatric distrubances in TBI rehabilitation. Dialogues Clin Neurosci 2011;13(3):325–45.
94. Nicholl J, LaFrance WC. Neuropsychiatric sequelae of traumatic brain injury. Semin Neurol 2009;29:247–55.
95. Barker-Collo S, Feigin VL. Memory deficit after traumatic brain injury: how big is the problem in New Zealand and what management strategies are available? N Z Med J 2008;121:2903–13.
96. Levin HS. Neurobehavioral sequelae of head injury. In: Cooper PR, editor. Head injury. 2nd edition. Baltimore (MD): Williams & Wilkins; 1987. p. 442–63.
97. Capruso DX, Levin HS. Neuropsychiatric aspects of head trauma. In: Kaplan HI, Saddock BJ, editors. Comprehensive textbook of psychiatry, vol. 1. Baltimore (MD): Williams & Wilkins; 1995. p. 207–20.
98. Murdoch I, Nicoll JA, Graham DI, et al. Nucleus basalis of Meynert pathology in the human brain after fatal head injury. J Neurotrauma 2002;19:279–84.
99. Thomsen IV. Late outcome of very severe blunt head trauma: a 10–15 year second follow-up. J Neurol Neurosurg Psychiatry 1984;47:260–8.
100. Davison K, Bagley CK. Schizophrenia-like psychosis associated with organic disorder of the CNS. Br J Psychiatry 1969;4(Suppl):113–84.
101. Sachdev P, Smith JS, Cathcart S. Schizophrenia-like psychosis following traumatic brain injury: a chart-based descriptive and case-control study. Psychol Med 2001;31:231–9.
102. Turnbull SJ, Campbell EA, Swann IJ. Post-traumatic stress disorder symptoms following a head injury: does amnesia for the event influence the development of symptoms? Brain Inj 2001;15(9):775–85.
103. Bryant RA, Harvey AG. Relationship between acute stress disorder and post-traumatic stress disorder following mild traumatic brain injury. Am J Psychiatry 1998;155:625–9.
104. Vasa RA, Grados M, Slomine B, et al. Neuroimaging correlates of anxiety after pediatric traumatic brain injury. Biol Psychiatry 2004;55:208–16.
105. Jorge RE, Robinson RG, Moser D, et al. Major depression following traumatic brain injury. Arch Gen Psychiatry 2004;61(1):42–50.
106. Rapoport MJ, McCullagh S, Streiner D, et al. The clinical significance of major depression following mild traumatic brain injury. Psychosomatics 2003;44:31–7.
107. Kim E, Lauterbach EC, Reeve A, et al. Neuropsychiatric complications of traumatic brain injury: a critical review of the literature (a report by the ANPA committee on research). J Neuropsychiatry Clin Neurosci 2007;19:106–27.
108. Van Zomeran AH. Residual complaints of patients two years after severe head injury. J Neurol Neurosurg Psychiatry 1985;48:21–8.

109. Yurgelun-Todd DA, Bueler CE, McGlade EC, et al. Neuroimaging correlates of traumatic brain injury and suicidal behavior. J Head Trauma Rehabil 2011;26: 276–89.
110. Shukla S, Cook BL, Mukherjee S, et al. Mania following head trauma. Am J Psychiatry 1987;144(1):93–6.
111. Rao V, Spiro JR, Handel S, et al. Clinical correlates of personality changes associated with traumatic brain injury. J Neuropsychiatry Clin Neurosci 2008;20(1): 118–9.
112. Wood R, Liossi C. Neuropsychological and neurobehavioral correlates of aggression following traumatic brain injury. J Neuropsychiatry Clin Neurosci 2006;18:3.
113. Duffy JD, Campbell JJ. The regional prefrontal syndromes: a theoretical and clinical overview. J Neuropsychiatry Clin Neurosci 1994;6:379–87.
114. Maldonado JR. Delirium in the acute care setting: characteristics, diagnosis and treatment. Crit Care Clin 2008;24:657–722.
115. Silver JM, Yudofsky SC. Psychopharmacology. In: Silver JM, Yudofsky SC, Hales RE, editors. Neuropsychiatry of Traumatic Brain Injury. 1st edition. Washington, DC: American Psychiatric Press; 1994. p. 631–70.
116. Feeney DM, Gonzalez A, Law WA. Amphetamine, Haloperidol, and experience interact to affect rate of recovery after motor cortex injury. Science 1982;217: 855–7.
117. Wilson MS, Gibson CJ, Hamm RJ. Haloperidol, but not olanzapine, impairs cognitive performance after traumatic brain injury in rats. Am J Phys Med Rehabil 2003;82:871–9.
118. Li HJ, Zhang YJ, Zhou L, et al. Chlorpromazine confers neuroprotection against brain ischemia by activating BKCa channel. Eur J Pharmacol 2014;735:38–43.
119. Wroblewski BA, Joseph AB, Kupfer J, et al. Effectiveness of valproic acid on destructive and aggressive behaviours in patients with acquired brain injury. Brain Inj 1997;11:37–47.
120. Sher Y, Miller AC, Lolak S, et al. Adjunctive valproic acid in management-refractory hyperactive delirium: a case series and rationale. J Neuropsychiatry Clin Neurosci 2015;27:365–70.
121. Whiting WL, Sullivan GA, Stewart JT. Lamotrigine treatment for agitation following traumatic brain injury. Psychosomatics 2016;57:330–3.
122. Pajoumand M, Kufera JA, Bonds BW, et al. Dexmedetomidine as an adjuct for sedation in patients with traumatic brain injury. J Trauma Acute Care Surg 2016;81:345–51.
123. Maldonado JR, Wysong A, van der Starre PJ, et al. Dexmedetomidine and the reduction of postoperative delirium after cardiac surgery. Psychosomatics 2009;50:206–17.
124. Lee HB, Lykestsos CG, Rao V. Pharmacologic management of the psychiatric aspects of traumatic brain injury. Int Rev Psychiatry 2003;15:359–70.
125. Vecht CJ, van Woekom TCAM, Teelken AW, et al. Homovanilic acid and 5-hydroxyindole acetic acid cerebrospinal fluid levels. Arch Neurol 1995;32:792–7.
126. Giacino JT, Whyte J, Bagiella E, et al. Placebo-controlled trial of amantadine for severe traumatic brain injury. Placebo-controlled trial of amantadine for severe traumatic brain injury. N Engl J Med 2012;366(9):819–26.
127. Hammond FM, Bickett AK, Norton JH, et al. Effectiveness of amantadine hydrochloride in the reduction of chronic traumatic brain injury irritability and aggression. J Head Trauma Rehabil 2014;29(5):391–9.

128. Sawyer E, Mauro LS, Ohlinger MJ. Amantadine enhancement of arousal and cognition after traumatic brain injury. Ann Pharmacother 2008;42(2):247–52.
129. Meythaler JM, Brunner RC, Johnson A, et al. Amantadine to improve neurore-covery in traumatic brain injury-associated diffuse axonal injury: a pilot double-blind randomized trial. J Head Trauma Rehabil 2002;17(4):300–13.
130. Lee HB, DeLoatch CJ, Cho S, et al. Detection and management of pre-existing cognitive impairment and associated behavioral symptoms in the intensive care unit. Crit Care Clin 2008;24(4):723–36.
131. McDowell S, Whyte J, D'Esposito M. Differential effect of a dopaminergic agent on prefrontal function in traumatic brain injury patients. Brain 1998;121:1155–64.

Detection and Management of Preexisting Cognitive Impairment in the Critical Care Unit

CrossMark

Mark A. Oldham, MD*, Walter Piddoubny, MD, Ryan Peterson, MD, Hochang B. Lee, MD

KEYWORDS

- Cognitive impairment • Dementia • Delirium • Neuropsychiatric symptoms
- Behavioral and psychological symptoms in dementia

KEY POINTS

- Older adults account for half of intensive care unit (ICU) admissions and ICU days, and older adults in the ICU have a 40% prevalence of preexisting cognitive impairment (PCI).
- PCI increases risk of ICU admission, in-hospital mortality, nosocomial infection, and delirium. It may also impact ICU utilization and care decisions, including medical decision-making surrogacy.
- More than half of PCI may remain unidentified without screening. Screening takes less than 5 minutes and ideally involves collateral informants (eg, using the Informant Questionnaire on Cognitive Decline in the Elderly).
- First-line management of neuropsychiatric symptoms associated with PCI should involve nonpharmacological interventions as feasible (eg, addressing sources of distress, healthy sleep-wake cycles, active caregiver involvement).
- Common neuropsychiatric symptoms of PCI include impulse dyscontrol, comportment (personality) change, affective dysregulation, motivational deficit, perceptual change/psychosis, and sundowning behavior (acronym: I CAMP at sundown).

IMPORTANCE OF PREEXISTING COGNITIVE IMPAIRMENT IN THE INTENSIVE CARE UNIT

Brain health among the critically ill has received increasing interest among clinicians and researchers alike for the past 2 decades, and older adults deserve particular attention because they represent the most cognitively vulnerable population. As of 2015, nearly 50 million adults in the United States were 65 and older, and by 2030,

This article is an update of an article previously published in Critical Care Clinics, Volume 24, Issue 4, October 2008.
Conflicts of Interest: The authors report no relevant conflicts of interest.
Department of Psychiatry, Yale School of Medicine, 20 York Street, Fitkin 615, New Haven, CT 06510, USA
* Corresponding author.
E-mail address: mark.oldham@yale.edu

older adults are projected to comprise one-fifth of the US adult population.[1] An estimated 5 million, or 1 in 10, older adults has Alzheimer disease (AD), the most common cause of dementia worldwide, and of these, more than half are undiagnosed.[2] An aging population with increasing burden of cognitive impairment has pressing relevance for intensive care, because older adults account for half of intensive care unit (ICU) admissions[3] and more than half of ICU hospital days.[4] Furthermore, despite marked regional differences in ICU admissions for older adults with advanced dementia, ICU utilization in the last 30 days of life has been increasing.[5]

In comparison with data on long-term cognitive impairment after critical care (see José R. Maldonado's article, "Acute Brain Failure: Pathophysiology, Diagnosis, Management and Sequelae of Delirium," in this issue), the role of preexisting cognitive impairment (PCI) in patients in the ICU has received significantly less attention. Nevertheless, dementia predicts nearly twice the rate of in-hospital mortality,[6] an effect attributed to greater rates of infection,[7] acute organ dysfunction, severe sepsis,[8] and lower use of life-support treatments.[9] Even mild cognitive impairment (MCI) increases the risk of ICU admission by 50%,[10] and predicts a greater than fivefold odds of developing delirium after elective coronary artery bypass grafting.[11] Moreover, among patients undergoing elective surgery requiring surgical ICU admission, cognitive impairment is associated with a higher postoperative complication rate, longer hospitalization, and higher rate of institutionalization on discharge.[12]

As proactive delirium detection and management are becoming standard of care in the ICU, the role of PCI among patients in the ICU, particularly among older adults, deserves similar attention. Here we discuss the critical role that cognitive impairment plays in ICU care and provide a review on detection and management of PCI in patients in the ICU.

DEFINITIONS

Cognition may be impaired in many ways, and due to a variety of not-uncommonly concurrent processes. *Delirium* is an acute state of confusion. Per the fifth edition of the *Diagnostic and Statistical Manual of Mental Disorders* (DSM-5), it is characterized by impaired awareness of one's surroundings, inattention, and at least 1 demonstrable cognitive deficit, which can include poor memory, disorientation, disorganized thinking, or executive dysfunction. Delirium represents a change from baseline cognition, and it cannot be better characterized as coma or a progressive neurocognitive or neurodegenerative disorder.[13]

DSM-5 reframed dementia as major neurocognitive disorder (NCD) in 2013. *Major NCD* represents a global decline in cognitive and general functioning from baseline and typically progresses over the course of months to years. The 6 cognitive domains included for NCD diagnosis include complex attention, executive function, learning and memory, language, perceptual motor, and social cognition. Only 1 domain must be "significantly" impaired to the extent this deficit interferes with independence in activities of daily living; NCD due to AD is an exception in that it requires impairment in at least 2 domains, 1 of which must be learning and memory.[13] Similarly, the National Institute on Aging and Alzheimer's Association (NIA-AA) published separate diagnostic criteria for all-cause dementia and dementia due to AD in 2011, which differ only slightly from those in the DSM-5 (**Box 1**).[14] The NIA-AA guidelines outline 5 cognitive domains, which exclude the DSM-5 domain of complex attention, and they require impairment in at least 2 domains for dementia of any cause. Worldwide, AD accounts for the vast majority of major NCD cases and may co-occur with ischemic cerebrovascular disease, cortical Lewy bodies, or other causes of neurocognitive decline.[15]

Box 1
National Institute on Aging–Alzheimer's Association diagnostic criteria of all-cause dementia

1. Interfere with the ability to function at work or at usual activities; and

2. Represent a decline from previous levels of functioning and performing; and

3. Are not explained by delirium or major psychiatric disorder;

4. Cognitive impairment is detected and diagnosed through a combination of
   a. history-taking from the patient and a knowledgeable informant; and
   b. An objective cognitive assessment, either a "bedside" mental status examination or neuropsychological testing. Neuropsychological testing should be performed when the routine history and bedside mental status examination cannot provide a confident diagnosis.

5. The cognitive or behavioral impairment involves a minimum of 2 of the following domains:
   a. Impaired ability to acquire and remember new information. Symptoms include repetitive questions or conversations, misplacing personal belongings, forgetting events or appointments, getting lost on a familiar route.
   b. Impaired reasoning and handling of complex tasks, poor judgment. Symptoms include poor understanding of safety risks, inability to manage finances, poor decision-making ability, inability to plan complex or sequential activities.
   c. Impaired visuospatial abilities. Symptoms include inability to recognize faces or common objects or to find objects in direct view despite good acuity, inability to operate simple implements, or orient clothing to the body.
   d. Impaired language functions (speaking, reading, writing). Symptoms include difficulty thinking of common words while speaking, hesitations; speech, spelling, and writing errors.
   e. Changes in personality, behavior, or comportment. Symptoms include uncharacteristic mood fluctuations, such as agitation, impaired motivation, initiative, apathy, loss of drive, social withdrawal, decreased interest in previous activities, loss of empathy, compulsive or obsessive behaviors, socially unacceptable behaviors.

Adapted from McKhann GM, Knopman DS, Chertkow H, et al. The diagnosis of dementia due to Alzheimer's disease: recommendations from the National Institute on Aging–Alzheimer's Association workgroups on diagnostic guidelines for Alzheimer's disease. Alzheimers Dement 2011;7:263–9.

Despite ongoing change of nomenclature, we use the more common term dementia throughout, in large part because previous studies have not used these updated terms and operationalized definitions.

Mild NCD was added to DSM-5 as an analog to the widely accepted construct of MCI, and its diagnostic criteria are substantially congruent with those for MCI.[13] Diagnosis of mild NCD (DSM-5) or MCI (NIA-AA, **Box 2**) are nearly identical: they each require a concern for cognitive decline (by patient, collateral informant, or clinician) and some degree of demonstrable cognitive impairment that does not substantially interfere with functional independence.[16] Mild NCD is on the spectrum with major NCD, and virtually all patients with major NCD will meet criteria for mild NCD beforehand. In fact, mild NCD is a strong risk factor for progressive neurocognitive decline: 1 in 10 will progress to major NCD each year,[17] and 15% to 25% of older adults in the United States have mild NCD.[18]

NCDs often present with *neuropsychiatric symptoms* (NPSs), which include decreased motivation, affective dysregulation, impulse dyscontrol, social inappropriateness, and abnormal perception or thought content.[19] These have also been called "behavioral and psychological symptoms of dementia." NPSs often represent a prodrome of a progressive neurocognitive disorder and can be identified early in the

---

Box 2

National Institute on Aging–Alzheimer's Association diagnostic criteria for all-cause mild cognitive impairment

1. Cognitive concern reflecting a change in cognition reported by patient or informant or clinician (ie, historical or observed evidence of decline over time)

2. Objective evidence of impairment in 1 or more cognitive domains (ie, formal or bedside testing to establish level of cognitive function in multiple domains)

3. Preservation of independence in functional abilities

4. Not demented

The criteria listed here pertain to all-cause mild cognitive impairment, although the article by Albert and colleagues[16] describes additional features unique to Alzheimer disease.

Adapted from Albert MS, DeKosky ST, Dickson D, et al. The diagnosis of mild cognitive impairment due to Alzheimer's disease: recommendations from the National Institute on Aging–Alzheimer's Association workgroups on diagnostic guidelines for Alzheimer's disease. Alzheimers Dement 2011;7:270–9.

---

course of the illness. In one study in which the Neuropsychiatric Inventory was administered to 1010 subjects with MCI, 59% were found to have significant NPS.[20] Not only are NPSs common in NCDs, they increase the risk of conversion to major NCD. Increasing awareness of their prevalence and clinical significance has led to recent conceptualization of a behavioral-variant construct of MCI known as *mild behavioral impairment*.[19] In the DSM-5, either mild or major NCD can be given the specifier "with behavioral disturbance."

PCI here describes the presence of clinically significant cognitive impairment before ICU admission and includes mild and major NCD. Because PCI excludes delirium and other cognitive impairment related to intensive care (such as chemical sedation), cognitive impairment identified in patients in the ICU requires arbitration by a collateral informant, a clinician who knows the patient's baseline cognitive status, or reference with cognitive evaluations completed before ICU admission. On the other hand, a patient whose cognition is fully intact while in the ICU cannot have PCI.

ROLE OF PREEXISTING COGNITIVE IMPAIRMENT IN INTENSIVE CARE UNIT UTILIZATION AND CARE DECISIONS

PCI and its identification have significant effects on utilization of critical care and associated decision making. The presence of MCI, itself, is a risk factor for ICU admission,[10] and individuals with PCI have shorter duration of survival after critical illness.[21] Furthermore, the diagnosis of PCI can significantly influence care utilization in the ICU and during end-of-life management. Interestingly, among patients admitted to acute care settings, patients with dementia had improved family-reported quality of end-of-life care compared with patients with end-stage kidney disease, cardiopulmonary failure, or frailty.[22] This discrepancy was attributed to increased likelihood of palliative care consultation and lower likelihood of death in the ICU among patients with dementia. Patients with advanced dementia who have health care surrogates who are educated on care options are less likely to receive nonbeneficial invasive treatments near end of life.[23] In addition, having an advanced directive has been associated with lower rate of ICU admission among patients with advanced dementia but not among patients with mild dementia or normal cognition.[24]

Identification of PCI before ICU admission may lead to patient-centered outcomes and reduce costs of care by shortened hospital and ICU lengths of stay. Proactive palliative care consultation for high-risk patients with dementia also may be considered.[25] Palliative care providers can help clarify goals of care, identify patient wishes, facilitate family discussions, shorten nonbeneficial stay in the ICU, and ultimately improve quality of life.[25] Identification of patients with PCI in the ICU also can facilitate more rapid referral to neuro-rehabilitative therapy post-ICU, as PCI is a risk factor for further cognitive decline.[26] Intensiveness of care always should be balanced with autonomy. When accounting for covariates, dementia status does not necessarily predict ICU outcomes[27]; however, not all older patients agree to ICU-level care. In a retrospective study of older adults referred for critical care, patients who declined this referral did not have a lower survival rate.[28] The question of ICU utilization among older adults with cognitive impairment vis-à-vis patient preference remains an area of active inquiry.

PCI also is important when considering surrogacy. Hospital inpatients with cognitive impairment may be less likely to agree to ICU treatment.[28] Unfortunately, though, when deciding whether to admit a patient to the ICU, emergency department (ED) physicians have been found to be less likely to ask a patient's preference if the patient had dementia.[29] Surrogates ought to be involved in medical decisions when a patient lacks capacity, but decision making should always seek to include a patient's wishes wherever possible. Again, regarding ICU admission, one study found that more than 75% of health care surrogates accepted ICU treatment for patients with advanced dementia, but 70% of surrogates' decisions were made independent of any previously expressed wishes of the patient.[30] Furthermore, rates of ICU admission in the last 30 days of life has increased over the past decade even though 90% of health care representatives for patients with dementia identify comfort as the goal of care.[31,32] The proportion of patients with dementia discharged to hospice after ICU admission also has risen dramatically, with most of these representing new referrals to hospice after ICU care. This may suggest that many such end-of-life care discussions are being initiated after admission to the ICU rather than before.[31]

DETECTION OF PREEXISTING COGNITIVE IMPAIRMENT IN THE INTENSIVE CARE UNIT

Cognitive impairment in acute medical settings, both preexisting and new-onset as seen in delirium, often goes undetected. For instance, failure to assess formally for cognitive impairment may miss up to 76% of patients with moderate cognitive impairment.[33] Nevertheless, detection of PCI by screening in the ICU is often complicated by the high prevalence of delirium, frequent inability of patients in the ICU to speak due to intubation and/or mechanical ventilation, and patient fatigue or distress. Ideally, each patient's cognitive status would be known reliably before ICU admission; however, this is seldom the case.

The 2 primary means of ascertaining cognitive status of patients in the ICU include previous medical documentation or bedside cognitive assessment in the ICU. Physicians may reasonably first turn to a patient's medical record, but cognitive impairment often goes unrecognized even in outpatient settings. According to one large study across southern California, 40% of patients who were cognitively impaired had not received a diagnosis of cognitive impairment; however, as expected, more severe baseline cognitive impairment was associated with higher likelihood of a diagnosis in the medical record.[34]

Two key pre-ICU care settings in which routine evaluation for cognitive impairment may be feasible include the ED and during outpatient preoperative assessments. Use of a quick cognitive screening instrument in these settings could meaningfully inform ICU care. In the ED, for instance, the Short Blessed Test (SBT), brief Alzheimer's Screen, and Ottawa 3DY each have been shown to be 95% sensitive in detecting patients who scored ≤23 on the Mini-Mental State Examination (MMSE), itself a not uncommon proxy for dementia, but among these the SBT had the greatest specificity at 65%.[35] Such bedside assessment for cognitive impairment is sure to identify previously undiagnosed patients.

Cognitive screening in the ICU can be performed at the bedside, but the high prevalence of delirium makes it difficult to know how much of the impairments detected is preexisting versus secondary to ongoing illness or iatrogenic factors. Despite the difficulty of differentiating PCI from delirium, PCI is among the strongest and most robust risk factors for developing delirium.[36] Assessment for PCI among patients in the ICU should start with a screen for delirium because delirium can be assessed rapidly with screening instruments such as the Confusion Assessment Method for the Intensive Care Unit (CAM-ICU) or the Intensive Care Delirium Screening Checklist (ICDSC).[37] If delirium is absent and patients can communicate, a brief cognitive screen such as the Mini-Cog can be used to assess for cognitive impairment. However, the prevalence of delirium in the ICU makes detection of PCI using this method feasible with only a portion of patients in the ICU.[38]

When a collateral informant is available, validated instruments such as the Informant Questionnaire on Cognitive Decline in the Elderly (IQCODE),[39] Modified Blessed Dementia Rating Scale (MBDRS),[40] or Ascertain Dementia 8-Item Informant Questionnaire (AD8)[41] can be used to assess for cognitive impairment. These assessments have been validated in both inpatient and outpatient settings and take less than 5 minutes to administer.

The IQCODE is a 16-item structured questionnaire completed by an informant who knows the patient well and assesses the patient's change in task performance over the previous 5 years. It has been used in hospital settings to identify older adults who are at risk for dementia and discriminates between patients with and without cognitive decline.[39] The MBDRS is an 11-item instrument that similarly discriminates between patients with and without dementia and correlates well with direct patient cognitive assessment; however, it is less sensitive than the IQCODE.[40] The most recent of the 3, the AD8, is an 8-item instrument that can identify patients with milder forms of dementia, including MCI.[41] Using a convenience sample of older adults in the ED, the AD8 identified previously undiagnosed cognitive impairment in 40% of cases, but in that study the primary barrier to its use was informant availability.[42]

PREVALENCE OF PREEXISTING COGNITIVE IMPAIRMENT IN THE INTENSIVE CARE UNIT

A PubMed search crossing terms related to cognitive impairment and critical care yielded 505 results. (Cognitive impairment terms included "*cognitive impair*," "*cognitive disorder*," "*cognitive decline," and "dement*." Terms related to the ICU included "intensive care," "critical care," "critical illness," and "ICU.") Forty-two references were not in English, and therefore were excluded, as were an additional 4 animal studies. Abstracts of the remaining 459 articles were reviewed for relevance. Of these, only 2 describe systematic detection of PCI among patients in the ICU,[43,44] both by the same research team.

Using the IQCODE and MBDRS as proxy-measures of PCI, Pisani and colleagues[43,44] found a 37% to 42% prevalence of PCI among patients in the ICU aged 65 and older. Attending and intern physicians alike were unaware of more than half of these cases of PCI.[44] Factors that predicted PCI included older age, female gender, being single, admission to ICU from nursing home, and greater illness severity on the APACHE II at time of admission.[44] Physicians were more likely to identify PCI in patients with more advanced cognitive impairment, limitations in activities of daily living, or who were admitted from a nursing home.[44] We are aware of no similar studies investigating PCI prevalence among patients in the ICU younger than 65.

RELATIONSHIP BETWEEN PREEXISTING COGNITIVE IMPAIRMENT AND DELIRIUM

Neurocognitive impairment is common in the ICU, but differentiating delirium from PCI is important in particular because delirium identification allows for prompt evaluation for causes. Clinical features that suggest delirium rather than PCI include acute onset, daily fluctuation in psychomotor activity and thought clarity, inattention, altered level of consciousness, and, in retrospect, symptom resolution.[45] However, dementia with Lewy bodies in particular, and most forms of advanced dementia can present with inattention and daily fluctuation, including sundowning behavior. Both delirium and PCI may present with perceptual disturbances, amnesia, disorganized thoughts, and emotional distress.

Neither of the 2 most commonly used delirium screening instruments for the ICU (ie, CAM-ICU or ICDSC) provide information on the patient's baseline cognitive status. As mentioned previously, caregiver collateral should be obtained to ascertain if cognitive decline is preexisting, as this may help differentiate delirium from dementia.[46] Simply inquiring about a history of dementia is insufficient. In a surgical ICU study investigating delirium and dementia (n = 114), only 3 surrogates (2.6%) reported a patient history of dementia; however, 21 (18%) patients were identified as cognitively impaired based on IQCODE assessment.[47]

DELIRIUM SUPERIMPOSED ON DEMENTIA

The prevalence of delirium superimposed on dementia (DSD) ranges from 22% to 89% among hospitalized community patients 65 and older with dementia.[48] Identifying delirium in patients with dementia has important prognostic value: it predicts a higher mortality rate, increased length of stay, and poorer function at discharge.[48] When DSD occurs, it not only speaks to marked cognitive vulnerability, but also predicts cognitive decline. In the year following an episode of delirium, the rate of cognitive decline for patients with AD proceeds at a rate 2.2 times that of patients with AD who did not develop delirium. A more rapid rate of cognitive decline has been documented for at least the next 5 years in these patients with AD who develop delirium.[49]

Unfortunately, no specific diagnostic criteria for identifying DSD exist.[50] This may explain in part why DSD is significantly underrecognized when compared with delirium in patients without dementia and why even experts may struggle to make the diagnosis. In an international survey of delirium specialists (n = 205), only one-third of responders said it was always possible to distinguish DSD from dementia alone, and the consensus was that delirium becomes more difficult to identify as the severity of dementia advances.[50]

When delirium occurs in dementia, the symptoms of delirium can obfuscate the underlying dementia. For instance, in a delirium phenomenology study using the Memorial Delirium Assessment Scale, no significant differences in severity of hallucinations, delusions, psychomotor behavior, and sleep-wake cycles were found between delirious patients with or without dementia; however, significant differences in severity were seen in impairments of arousal, awareness, and multiple cognitive domains.[51]

In a systematic review of clinical tools to detect DSD, Morandi and colleagues[52] found preliminary evidence to support the use of the Confusion Assessment Method

(CAM), CAM-ICU, and electroencephalography, but this evidence was limited by the fact that only 50 individuals across the 9 included studies had DSD. In 1 study comparing patients with delirium, dementia, DSD, and controls (n = 140), subjects with delirium or DSD had comparable scores on the Revised Delirium Ratings Scale (DRS-R98) and Cognitive Test for Delirium, which were greater than in dementia or control groups.[45] Inattention and disorientation were more common in subjects with delirium than in subjects with dementia alone. Forward spatial span was disproportionately impaired in delirium groups and may serve as a tool to differentiate delirium, including DSD, from dementia.

MANAGEMENT OF NEUROPSYCHIATRIC SYMPTOMS ASSOCIATED WITH PREEXISTING COGNITIVE IMPAIRMENT

NPSs include aggression, agitation, apathy, depression, disinhibition, psychosis, and sleep disturbances.[53] Although the most common cause of NPSs in the ICU is delirium, they may also accompany PCI. In fact, NPSs may occur in up to 98% of individuals with dementia in the course of their illness and can have devastating consequences.[53] For instance, delusions in AD significantly impair functioning compared with patients with AD without delusions[54]; apathy and nighttime behavioral disturbances predict shorter survival,[55] and affective symptoms and agitation/aggression predict earlier progression to severe dementia and death.[56]

NPSs may be seen in 35% to 75% of patients with MCI, and their presence is a risk factor for progression to dementia.[57] Not surprisingly patients with MCI and NPSs have significantly greater decline in global, cognitive, and functional scores compared with those without NPSs.[20] The converse is also true: NPSs among older adults may herald the development of MCI. For instance, a cohort of community-dwelling older adults with agitation, apathy, anxiety, irritability, and depression were at increased risk of developing MCI versus those without NPSs.[58]

NONPHARMACOLOGIC MANAGEMENT

Nonpharmacologic interventions always should be first line in managing NPSs associated with PCI.[59] These include titrating stimulation level to the patient (prevent overstimulation and understimulation), removing access to dangerous items such as sharps, creating daily routine, facilitating daily activity as feasible, and the active involvement and education of caregivers.[60] Where a specific cause can be identified, such as pain, unfamiliarity with an upcoming procedure or intervention, or sensory impairment, these deserve prompt attention, as this often obviates the need for further treatment. Involvement of family and loved ones should be solicited actively for patient comfort. Where nonpharmacologic management is insufficient or infeasible in the ICU, pharmacologic interventions can be considered.

We discuss management of 6 common domains of NPSs associated with PCI in the following sections[19] and propose the mnemonic "I CAMP at sundown" to help the reader recall them. As a caveat, with the exception of dextromethorphan/quinidine (Nudexta) for pseudobulbar affect (PBA), no medication is approved by the Food and Drug Administration for NPSs associated with cognitive impairment, and all neuroleptics carry a black box warning for "increased mortality in elderly patients with dementia-related psychosis." As with all medical decisions, the risks and benefits of these agents should be discussed with patients and, where appropriate, their families and/or health care surrogate. Interested readers are referred to the recent American Psychiatric Association Practice Guideline on the use of antipsychotics to treat agitation or psychosis in patients with dementia.[61]

IMPULSE DYSCONTROL AND AGITATION

Agitation, which broadly describes emotional distress, excessive motor activity, verbal/physical aggression, and other behaviors,[62] occurs in a quarter of patients with AD (**Table 1**).[63] It may occur in response to various stressors, including pain, discomfort, medical illness, delirium, substance withdrawal or intoxication, psychiatric disorders, sensory impairment, or environmental stimuli. Management of agitation is often divided into (1) emergent, which requires prompt intervention for deescalation and very often rapid tranquilization, such as with neuroleptics, sedatives, opioids, or combinations thereof; and (2) nonemergent, in which medications may be more safely deferred to allow for nonpharmacologic interventions.

Pharmacologic interventions for agitation have largely consisted of typical and atypical neuroleptics, although data on their efficacy are conflicting. A 2-decades-old meta-analysis of randomized, placebo-controlled trials (RCTs) of typical neuroleptics in agitated patients with dementia demonstrated efficacy versus placebo ($P = .004$) with comparable efficacy across agents.[64] A more recent review of 2 meta-analyses and 2 RCTs of typical neuroleptics was unable to find improvements in NPSs except for slight improvement in aggression with haloperidol at dosages up to 3.5 mg/d.[65] Similarly, a review by Ballard and Howard[66] concluded that risperidone and haloperidol, both up to 2 mg, significantly improve aggression associated with cognitive impairment. Haloperidol has the notable advantage of being available for oral, intramuscular, and intravenous administration.

The Clinical Antipsychotic Trials of Intervention Effectiveness–Alzheimer Disease (CATIE-AD) effectiveness study (n = 421) represents the strongest ecological evidence to date for the use of the atypical neuroleptics olanzapine, risperidone, and quetiapine in AD.[67] Although none of the agents used in CATIE-AD improved the specific domain of agitation relative to placebo, both olanzapine and risperidone demonstrated significant improvements in hostile suspiciousness and overall improvements in NPSs as measured by the Neuropsychiatric Inventory.[68]

Antidepressants offer a safer and better-tolerated approach for long-term management of agitation[69]; however, their utility in the ICU may be limited, as they are available only in oral preparations and are not effective rapidly. Benzodiazepines are often best avoided in older adults, particularly in PCI, because of risk of precipitating delirium and causing paradoxic agitation. Their primary ICU applications in patients with PCI are for sedation or in combination with neuroleptics to treat acute, severe agitation. Data for mood stabilizers are limited. Only 1 of 5 studies of valproic acid or carbamazepine included in a review of their efficacy found statistically significant improvement; thus, their use for this purpose should be refrained to agitation where first-line interventions are contraindicated or ineffective.[70] Similarly, cholinesterase inhibitors and memantine have limited data in support of their use for agitation.[65]

COMPORTMENT/PERSONALITY CHANGE

Inappropriate social behavior in the ICU may be a presenting feature of delirium, in particular in response to the disinhibiting effect of GABA-ergic agents (eg, benzodiazepines, propofol). More so than in other types of cognitive impairment, frontotemporal dementia is associated with impaired self-awareness as well as personality changes, including dominance, submissiveness, or cold heartedness.[71] Poor insight can present with behavioral disinhibition or sexual inappropriateness, which can be embarrassing for patients, families, and caregivers alike. Antipsychotics, antidepressants, cholinesterase inhibitors, anticonvulsants, beta-blockers, and antiandrogens have all been reported to be effective for sexual inappropriateness in case reports and

Table 1
Medications commonly used off label for impulse dysregulation/agitation and affective dysregulation associated with preexisting cognitive impairment[a]

Medication	Formulations	Starting Dosage	Common Daily Dosage	Adverse Events	Comments
Neuroleptics					
Risperidone	Oral, ODT,[b] IM depot	0.25–0.5 mg	2 mg	EPS Elevated prolactin QTc prolongation	Limited sedation
Quetiapine	Oral	12.5–25 mg	100–200 mg	Sedation Orthostatic hypotension QTc prolongation	Very limited EPS Mood-stabilizing property
Olanzapine	Oral, ODT,[b] IM,[c] IM depot	2.5–5 mg	5–10 mg	EPS Sedation Orthostatic hypotension QTc prolongation	Mood-stabilizing property
Aripiprazole	Oral, ODT,[b] depot	2–5 mg	5–10 mg	Akathisia	72-h half-life Rare QTc prolongation
Haloperidol	Oral, IV,[d] IM, IM depot	0.5–1 mg	2–5 mg	EPS QTc prolongation[d]	Only neuroleptic available IV
Antidepressants (SSRIs/SNRIs)[e]					
Sertraline	Oral	25 mg	100–150 mg	GI upset Akathisia Hyponatremia Discontinuation syndrome Mild QTc prolongation Increased risk of bleeding	Weak 2D6 and 3A4 inhibition
Citalopram	Oral	10 mg	20–40 mg	Same as sertraline	Limited drug interactions

Escitalopram	Oral	5 mg	10–20 mg	Same as sertraline	Limited drug interactions
Venlafaxine	Oral	37.5 mg	75–150 mg	Same as sertraline	Rare diastolic hypertension; Pronounced discontinuation syndrome
Duloxetine	Oral	30 mg	60 mg	Same as sertraline; Rare risk of hepatotoxicity	Treats neuropathic pain
Mirtazapine	Oral, ODT	7.5 mg qhs	7.5–30 mg qhs	Sedation[f]; Weight gain[f]	Mild antiemetic property[f]
NMDA-receptor antagonist					
Dextromethorphan/ quinidine	Oral	20/10 mg	20/10 mg twice daily	QTc prolongation; Potent 2D6 inhibition	Low risk of cinchonism (quinidine toxicity)

Abbreviations: EPS, extrapyramidal symptoms (in the acute setting this includes dystonia and akathisia); GI, gastrointestinal; IM, intramuscular injection; IV, intravenous; ODT, orally disintegrating tablet; qhs, at bedtime; SNRI, serotonin-norepinephrine reuptake inhibitor; SSRI, selective serotonin reuptake inhibitor.

[a] With the exception of dextromethorphan/quinidine (Nudexta) for pseudobulbar affect, no medication is approved by the Food and Drug Administration for NPSs associated with cognitive impairment, and all neuroleptics carry a black box warning for "increased mortality in elderly patients with dementia-related psychosis."

[b] ODT may be helpful to mitigate against medication "cheeking."

[c] IM neuroleptics may be immediate-release (eg, olanzapine or haloperidol) or depot formulations (eg, risperidone [Risperdal Consta] or haloperidol [Haldol decanoate]). Depot formulations generally should not be initiated in the ICU. Immediate-release IM olanzapine never should be used with benzodiazepines, given the risk of fatal cardiorespiratory suppression.

[d] IV haloperidol carries an additional warning by the Food and Drug Administration for potential cardiac arrhythmias; oral haloperidol, on the other hand, is less likely to prolong QTc versus most other neuroleptics.

[e] SSRIs may paradoxically worsen anxiety on starting, and GI upset not uncommonly limits rapid titration. In general, paroxetine is ill-suited for patients with PCI due to its anticholinergic effects, 2D6 inhibition, and penchant for causing weight gain. The long half-life of fluoxetine and its active metabolite norfluoxetine along with 2D6 and 3A4 inhibition generally make it unsuitable for medically ill patients.

[f] These side effects are often used for therapeutic purpose in the medically ill.

case series, but RCTs are lacking. Pharmacotherapy is often best initiated based on the presence of other symptoms (eg, neuroleptics for agitation, selective serotonin reuptake inhibitors for obsessions, mood stabilizers for mania) (see agents in **Table 1**).[72]

AFFECTIVE DYSREGULATION

Depression is commonly comorbid with dementia, with prevalence ranging from 5% to 44% in AD depending on definition and often presents with associated features of agitation, anxiety, anhedonia, apathy, and irritability (see **Table 1**).[73] Treating depression, irritability, and anxiety in dementia is often more challenging than treating depression alone. A recent meta-analysis of antidepressants to treat depression in dementia yielded inconclusive results.[74] The investigators found a trend toward higher odds of response (odds ratio [OR] 2.12 [0.95–4.70], 6 trials) and remission (OR 1.97 [0.85–4.55], 5 trials), but neither of these reached statistical significance ($P = .07$ and 0.11, respectively). Unfortunately, each of the trials included in this meta-analysis were underpowered. Further evidence of potential efficacy of antidepressants in this patient population is derived from a double-blind RCT in which nursing home residents with dementia and NPSs (but no formal depressive disorder) were randomized to discontinue antidepressants.[75] Residents randomized to discontinue medication experienced significant worsening of depression but not total NPS score. Therefore, at the least, patients with PCI on an antidepressant at the time of ICU admission are often best continued on these agents unless contraindicated or administration is infeasible.

PBA describes disinhibition of emotion in which a person experiences pathologic crying or laughter out of proportion to emotional context, and it may be seen in a range of conditions causing intracranial pathology, including, for instance, AD, vascular neurocognitive disorder, multiple sclerosis, or traumatic brain injury. Serotonergic antidepressants are often first line for this condition based on case series, but clinical effects require weeks for effect, making their use in the ICU less feasible.[76] The combination agent dextromethorphan/quinidine (Nudexta) was recently approved to treat PBA, but ICU physicians should be aware that quinidine is a potent p450 2D6 inhibitor and thus liable to interact with other medications.

MOTIVATIONAL DEFICIT

Apathy, which is defined as the lack of goal-directed behavior (avolition), cognition, or emotion, is the most common NPS present throughout all stages of AD (**Table 2**).[53] Cholinesterase inhibitors are approved for the treatment of AD and/or Parkinson dementia and are commonly used off-label for apathy. A systematic review of donepezil for the treatment of apathy found that 4 of the 6 included studies demonstrated a statistically significant reduction in symptoms[77]; however, there is no clear evidence demonstrating superiority of one cholinesterase inhibitor over another.[78] Bupropion may be considered off-label to treat apathy, given its activating effects and mild dopaminergic activity.

Stimulants have long been used to treat apathy, particularly among the medically ill. Their rapid effect is well suited for hospitalized patients. In a randomized, placebo-controlled crossover trial of patients with AD, methylphenidate improved apathy relative to placebo; however, stimulant treatment was associated with a higher rate of adverse events, including delusions, agitation, irritability, and insomnia.[79] The role of antidepressants in apathy remains unclear: a review of 3 citalopram studies and a crossover study of trazodone was unable to find statistical evidence for apathy improvement with these agents.[78] Despite the 2 studies suggesting that haloperidol

Table 2
Medications commonly used off label for motivational deficit associated with preexisting cognitive impairment

Medication	Formulations	Starting Dosage	Common Daily Dosage	Adverse Events	Comments
Cognitive enhancers					
Donepezil	Oral, ODT	5 mg (for 4–6 wk before titration)	10 mg	Parasympathetic activation[a] Diarrhea Rare risk of seizures Vivid dreams	
Rivastigmine	Oral (also TD patch)	1.5 mg BID (increase by 1.5 mg BID no sooner than every 2 wk)	3–6 mg BID	Same as donepezil	Bypasses phase I metabolism
Galantamine	Oral	4 mg BID (increase by 4 mg BID no sooner than every 4 wk)	8–16 mg BID	Same as donepezil	
Activating antidepressant					
Bupropion	Oral	100–150 mg	150–300 mg	Lowers seizure threshold (>400 mg/d) Insomnia	Available in daily, twice-daily, and thrice-daily formulations
Psychostimulants[b]					
Methylphenidate	Oral	5 mg BID	10–20 mg qAM and noon	Insomnia Psychosis Agitation Anorexia	
Amphetamine	Oral	5 mg BID	10–20 mg qAM and noon	Same as methylphenidate	

Abbreviations: BID, twice daily; ODT, orally disintegrating tablet; qAM, each morning; TD, transdermal.
[a] Parasympathetic activation characterized by salivation, lacrimation, urination, defecation, gastrointestinal upset, emesis, and miosis (commonly known by the acronym SLUDGEM).
[b] There are more than 20 preparations of psychostimulants, but the immediate-release agents methylphenidate and mixed amphetamine salts are often most easily used in the hospital. They can be titrated by 5 mg BID each day to effect. Although they may have an anorectic effect, they may paradoxically activate an avolitional or aspontaneous patient to eat.

and loxapine enhance social interest, 10 of 14 studies of typical neuroleptics included in a recent review found no improvement in apathy. Preliminary evidence from retrospective and open-label studies with clozapine and risperidone suggest a potential application for atypical neuroleptics,[78] but in the CATIE-AD trial, olanzapine was associated with significant worsening of withdrawn depression and risperidone with a trend toward worsening.[68]

PERCEPTUAL CHANGE AND PSYCHOTIC SYMPTOMS

Perceptual disturbances in the ICU can occur due to delirium, underlying psychotic or affective disorders, cognitive impairment, or even visual impairment (ie, Charles Bonnet syndrome) (see neuroleptics in **Table 1**). Delusions are more common than hallucinations in dementia (25% vs 15% prevalence, respectively), and are typically seen earlier in the course of vascular neurocognitive disorders than in AD.[63] Common delusional themes in dementia include theft, jealousy, persecution, and misidentification, each of which can place a significant burden on caregivers, jeopardize independence in the community, and lead to conflict with treatment teams and medical recommendations. Visual hallucinations are more frequently encountered in Parkinson disease, dementia with Lewy bodies, and other alpha-synucleinopathies (60%–80% prevalence) than in other types of dementia, such as AD.[80] The most commonly occurring visual hallucinations are of anonymous people, followed by friends and family members, as well as children and babies.

Antipsychotics are frequently used in the management of dementia-related perceptual disturbances and psychotic symptoms. In the CATIE-AD effectiveness trial, only risperidone demonstrated statistically significant improvements in the psychosis factor relative to placebo, whereas olanzapine and quetiapine were not found to be effective.[68] Both olanzapine and risperidone, though, improved hostile suspiciousness. One double-blind RCT of olanzapine for the treatment of hallucinations and delusions in AD found clinical response at 7.5 mg/d.[81]

SUNDOWNING BEHAVIOR

Originally called nocturnal delirium, sundowning behavior describes a range of NPSs occurring in the late evening and overnight and may be seen in dementia or delirium.[82] Diversity across definitions has led to varied prevalence rates ranging from 2.4% to 66.0% and confounds data on outcome studies. Sundowning is thought to occur with degradation of the neurohumoral circadian system and has been associated with pathologic changes in the suprachiasmatic nucleus, the body's "master clock," in dementia.[83] Nonpharmacologic interventions emphasizing good sleep hygiene (eg, avoiding/clustering overnight interruptions, quiet and dark at night with consideration of eye masks and earplugs, and ample light and behavioral activation during the day) are often adequate treatment. Evidence supports the use of melatonin from 2 to 3 mg in the evening,[82] but morning light therapy and environment-wide lighting interventions may have a promising future as well.[84] Where sundowning is associated with psychosis or frank agitation, scheduling a sedating neuroleptic, such as quetiapine, at least an hour before the NPS presents also may be effective.

SUMMARY

An aging population means that an increasing number of patients with PCI will require acute medical care, including the ICU, and the sweeping majority of these will be older adults. Proactively identifying cognitive impairment allows for risk stratification, and patient preference should be included wherever possible in care decisions. PCI is a risk factor for delirium, and differentiating these two clinically often requires knowledge of a patient's baseline cognitive and functional status. First-line management of NPSs associated with PCI should always involve nonpharmacologic interventions. Where these are insufficient, psychotropics may be considered, although evidence in support of their efficacy is generally limited. In the end, early identification and management of PCI and its associated NPSs is critical to improve care delivery and clinical outcomes in this vulnerable population.

REFERENCES

1. US Census Bureau. 2014 National population projects: Summary Tables Available at: https://www.census.gov/population/projections/data/national/2014/summarytables.html. Accessed March 27, 2017.
2. Alzheimer's Association. 2013 Alzheimer's disease facts and figures. Alzheimers Demen 2013;9:208–45.
3. Chelluri L, Pinsky MR, Donahoe MP, et al. Long-term outcome of critically ill elderly patients requiring intensive care. JAMA 1993;269:3119–23.
4. Angus DC, Kelley MA, Schmitz RJ, et al. Caring for the critically ill patient. Current and projected workforce requirements for care of the critically ill and patients with pulmonary disease: can we meet the requirements of an aging population? JAMA 2000;284:2762–70.
5. Fulton AT, Gozalo P, Mitchell SL, et al. Intensive care utilization among nursing home residents with advanced cognitive and severe functional impairment. J Palliat Med 2014;17:313–7.
6. Marengoni A, Corrao S, Nobili A, et al. In-hospital death according to dementia diagnosis in acutely ill elderly patients: the REPOSI study. Int J Geriatr Psychiatry 2011;26:930–6.
7. Sampson EL, Blanchard MR, Jones L, et al. Dementia in the acute hospital: prospective cohort study of prevalence and mortality. Br J Psychiatry 2009;195:61–6.
8. Shen HN, Lu CL, Li CY. Dementia increases the risks of acute organ dysfunction, severe sepsis and mortality in hospitalized older patients: a national population-based study. PLoS One 2012;7:e42751.
9. Richardson SS, Sullivan G, Hill A, et al. Use of aggressive medical treatments near the end of life: differences between patients with and without dementia. Health Serv Res 2006;42:27–36.
10. Teeters DA, Moua T, Li G, et al. Mild cognitive impairment and risk of critical illness. Crit Care Med 2016;44:2045–51.
11. Oldham MA, Hawkins KA, Yuh DD, et al. Cognitive and functional status predictors of delirium and delirium severity after coronary artery bypass graft surgery: an interim analysis of the Neuropsychiatric Outcomes after Heart Surgery study. Int Psychogeriatr 2015;27:1929–38.
12. Robinson TN, Wu DS, Pointer LF, et al. Preoperative cognitive dysfunction is related to adverse postoperative outcomes in the elderly. J Am Coll Surg 2012; 215:12–7 [discussion: 7–8].
13. American Psychiatric Association. Diagnostic and Statistical Manual of Mental Disorders. Washington, DC: American Psychiatric Publishing; 2013.
14. McKhann GM, Knopman DS, Chertkow H, et al. The diagnosis of dementia due to Alzheimer's disease: recommendations from the National Institute on Aging-Alzheimer's Association workgroups on diagnostic guidelines for Alzheimer's disease. Alzheimers Dement 2011;7:263–9.

15. Schneider JA, Aggarwal NT, Barnes L, et al. The neuropathology of older persons with and without dementia from community versus clinic cohorts. J Alzheimers Dis 2009;18:691–701.

16. Albert MS, DeKosky ST, Dickson D, et al. The diagnosis of mild cognitive impairment due to Alzheimer's disease: recommendations from the National Institute on Aging-Alzheimer's Association workgroups on diagnostic guidelines for Alzheimer's disease. Alzheimers Dement 2011;7:270–9.

17. Summers MJ, Saunders NL. Neuropsychological measures predict decline to Alzheimer's dementia from mild cognitive impairment. Neuropsychology 2012; 26:498–508.

18. Petersen RC, Caracciolo B, Brayne C, et al. Mild cognitive impairment: a concept in evolution. J Intern Med 2014;275:214–28.

19. Ismail Z, Smith EE, Geda Y, et al. Neuropsychiatric symptoms as early manifestations of emergent dementia: provisional diagnostic criteria for mild behavioral impairment. Alzheimers Dement 2016;12:195–202.

20. Feldman H, Scheltens P, Scarpini E, et al. Behavioral symptoms in mild cognitive impairment. Neurology 2004;62:1199–201.

21. Iwashyna TJ, Ely EW, Smith DM, et al. Long-term cognitive impairment and functional disability among survivors of severe sepsis. JAMA 2010;304:1787–94.

22. Wachterman MW, Pilver C, Smith D, et al. Quality of end-of-life care provided to patients with different serious illnesses. JAMA Intern Med 2016;176:1095–102.

23. Mitchell SL, Teno JM, Intrator O, et al. Decisions to forgo hospitalization in advanced dementia: a nationwide study. J Am Geriatr Soc 2007;55:432–8.

24. Nicholas LH, Ynum JP, Iwashyna TJ, et al. Advance directives and nursing home stays associated with less aggressive end-of-life care for patients with severe dementia. Health Aff (Millwood) 2014;33:667–74.

25. Campbell ML, Guzman JA. A proactive approach to improve end-of-life care in a medical intensive care unit for patients with terminal dementia. Crit Care Med 2004;32:1839–43.

26. Baumbach P, Meissner W, Guenther A, et al. Perceived cognitive impairments after critical illness: a longitudinal study in survivors and family member controls. Acta Anaesthesiol Scand 2016;60:1121–30.

27. Pisani MA, Redlich CA, McNicoll L, et al. Short-term outcomes in older intensive care unit patients with dementia. Crit Care Med 2005;33:1371–6.

28. Kim J, Choi SM, Park YS, et al. Factors influencing the initiation of intensive care in elderly patients and their families: a retrospective cohort study. Palliat Med 2016; 30:789–99.

29. Le Guen J, Boumendil A, Guidet B, et al. Are elderly patients' opinions sought before admission to an intensive care unit? Results of the ICE-CUB study. Age Ageing 2016;45:303–9.

30. Cogen R, Patterson B, Chavin S, et al. Surrogate decision-maker preferences for medical care of severely demented nursing home patients. Arch Intern Med 1992;152:1885–8.

31. Oud L. Evolving patterns of intensive care unit use during end-of-life hospitalization in elderly adults with dementia in Texas: a population-based study. J Am Geriatr Soc 2016;64:679–80.

32. Teno JM, Gozalo PL, Bynum JP, et al. Change in end-of-life care for Medicare beneficiaries: site of death, place of care, and health care transitions in 2000, 2005, and 2009. JAMA 2013;309:470–7.

33. Ketterer MW, Alaali Y, Yessayan L, et al. "Alert and oriented x 3?" Correlates of mini-cog performance in a post/nondelirious intensive care unit sample. Psychosomatics 2016;57:194–9.
34. Chodosh J, Petitti DB, Elliott M, et al. Physician recognition of cognitive impairment: evaluating the need for improvement. J Am Geriatr Soc 2004;52:1051–9.
35. Carpenter CR, Bassett ER, Fischer GM, et al. Four sensitive screening tools to detect cognitive dysfunction in geriatric emergency department patients: brief Alzheimer's Screen, Short Blessed Test, Ottawa 3DY, and the caregiver-completed AD8. Acad Emerg Med 2011;18:374–84.
36. Inouye SK, Westendorp RG, Saczynski JS. Delirium in elderly people. Lancet 2014;383:911–22.
37. Gusmao-Flores D, Salluh JI, Chalhub RÁ, et al. The confusion assessment method for the intensive care unit (CAM-ICU) and intensive care delirium screening checklist (ICDSC) for the diagnosis of delirium: a systematic review and meta-analysis of clinical studies. Crit Care 2012;16:R115.
38. DiLibero J, O'Donoghue SC, DeSanto-Madeya S, et al. An innovative approach to improving the accuracy of delirium assessments using the confusion assessment method for the intensive care unit. Dimens Crit Care Nurs 2016;35:74–80.
39. Jorm AF. A short form of the informant questionnaire on cognitive decline in the elderly (IQCODE): development and cross-validation. Psychol Med 1994;24:145–53.
40. McLoughlin DM, Cooney C, Holmes C, et al. Carer informants for dementia sufferers: carer awareness of cognitive impairment in an elderly community-resident sample. Age Ageing 1996;25:367–71.
41. Galvin JE, Roe CM, Powlishta KK, et al. The AD8: a brief informant interview to detect dementia. Neurology 2005;65:559–64.
42. Dyer AH, Nabeel S, Briggs R, et al. Cognitive assessment of older adults at the acute care interface: the informant history. Postgrad Med J 2016;92:255–9.
43. Pisani MA, Inouye SK, McNicoll L, et al. Screening for preexisting cognitive impairment in older intensive care unit patients: use of proxy assessment. J Am Geriatr Soc 2003;51:689–93.
44. Pisani MA, Redlich C, McNicoll L, et al. Underrecognition of preexisting cognitive impairment by physicians in older ICU patients. Chest 2003;124:2267–74.
45. Meagher DJ, Leonard M, Donnelly S, et al. A comparison of neuropsychiatric and cognitive profiles in delirium, dementia, comorbid delirium-dementia and cognitively intact controls. J Neurol Neurosurg Psychiatr 2010;81:876–81.
46. Morandi A, Davis D, Taylor JK, et al. Consensus and variations in opinions on delirium care: a survey of European delirium specialists. Int Psychogeriatr 2013;25:2067–75.
47. Balas MC, Deutschman CS, Sullivan-Marx EM, et al. Delirium in older patients in surgical intensive care units. J Nurs Scholarsh 2007;39:147–54.
48. Fick DM, Agostini JV, Inouye SK. Delirium superimposed on dementia: a systematic review. J Am Geriatr Soc 2002;50:1723–32.
49. Gross AL, Jones RN, Habtemariam DA, et al. Delirium and long-term cognitive trajectory among persons with dementia. Arch Intern Med 2012;172:1324–31.
50. Richardson S, Teodorczuk A, Bellelli G, et al. Delirium superimposed on dementia: a survey of delirium specialists shows a lack of consensus in clinical practice and research studies. Int Psychogeriatr 2016;28:853–61.
51. Boettger S, Passik S, Breitbart W. Delirium superimposed on dementia versus delirium in the absence of dementia: phenomenological differences. Palliat Support Care 2009;7:495–500.

52. Morandi A, McCurley J, Vasilevskis EE, et al. Tools to detect delirium superimposed on dementia: a systematic review. J Am Geriatr Soc 2012;60:2005–13.

53. Lyketsos CG, Carrillo MC, Ryan JM, et al. Neuropsychiatric symptoms in Alzheimer's disease. Alzheimers Dement 2011;7:532–9.

54. Fischer CE, Ismail Z, Schweizer TA. Delusions increase functional impairment in Alzheimer's disease. Dement Geriatr Cogn Disord 2012;33:393–9.

55. Spalletta G, Long JD, Robinson RG, et al. Longitudinal neuropsychiatric predictors of death in Alzheimer's disease. J Alzheimers Dis 2015;48:627–36.

56. Peters ME, Schwartz S, Han D, et al. Neuropsychiatric symptoms as predictors of progression to severe Alzheimer's dementia and death: the Cache County Dementia Progression Study. Am J Psychiatry 2015;172:460–5.

57. Apostolova LG, Cummings JL. Neuropsychiatric manifestations in mild cognitive impairment: a systematic review of the literature. Dement Geriatr Cogn Disord 2008;25:115–26.

58. Geda YE, Roberts RO, Mielke MM, et al. Baseline neuropsychiatric symptoms and the risk of incident mild cognitive impairment: a population-based study. Am J Psychiatry 2014;171:572–81.

59. Kales HC, Gitlin LN, Lyketsos CG. Assessment and management of behavioral and psychological symptoms of dementia. BMJ 2015;350:h369.

60. Brodaty H, Arasaratnam C. Meta-analysis of nonpharmacological interventions for neuropsychiatric symptoms of dementia. Am J Psychiatry 2012;169:946–53.

61. Reus VI, Fochtmann LJ, Eyler AE, et al. The American Psychiatric Association practice guideline on the use of antipsychotics to treat agitation or psychosis in patients with dementia. Am J Psychiatry 2016;173:543–6.

62. Cummings J, Mintzer J, Brodaty H, et al. Agitation in cognitive disorders: International Psychogeriatric Association provisional consensus clinical and research definition. Int Psychogeriatr 2015;27:7–17.

63. Lyketsos CG, Mintzer J, Brodaty H, et al. Mental and behavioral disturbances in dementia: findings from the Cache County study on memory in aging. Am J Psychiatry 2000;157:708–14.

64. Schneider LS, Pollock VE, Lyness SA. A metaanalysis of controlled trials of neuroleptic treatment in dementia. J Am Geriatr Soc 1990;38:553–63.

65. Sink KM, Holden KF, Yaffe K. Pharmacological treatment of neuropsychiatric symptoms of dementia: a review of the evidence. JAMA 2005;293:596–608.

66. Ballard C, Howard R. Neuroleptic drugs in dementia: benefits and harm. Nat Rev Neurosci 2006;7:492–500.

67. Schneider LS, Tariot PN, Dagerman KS, et al. Effectiveness of atypical antipsychotic drugs in patients with Alzheimer's disease. N Engl J Med 2006;355:1525–38.

68. Sultzer DL, Davis SM, Tariot PN, et al. Clinical symptom responses to atypical antipsychotic medications in Alzheimer's disease: phase 1 outcomes from the CATIE-AD effectiveness trial. Am J Psychiatry 2008;165:844–54.

69. Seitz DP, Adunuri N, Gill SS, et al. Antidepressants for agitation and psychosis in dementia. Cochrane Database Syst Rev 2011;(2):CD008191.

70. Konovalov S, Muralee S, Tampi RR. Anticonvulsants for the treatment of behavioral and psychological symptoms of dementia: a literature review. Int Psychogeriatr 2008;20:293–308.

71. Rankin KP, Baldwin E, Pace-Savitsky C, et al. Self awareness and personality change in dementia. J Neurol Neurosurg Psychiatr 2005;76:632–9.

72. Tucker I. Management of inappropriate sexual behaviors in dementia: a literature review. Int Psychogeriatr 2010;22:683–92.

73. Vilalta-Franch J, Garre-Olmo J, López-Pousa S, et al. Comparison of different clinical diagnostic criteria for depression in Alzheimer disease. Am J Geriatr Psychiatry 2006;14:589–97.
74. Nelson JC, Devanand DP. A systematic review and meta-analysis of placebo-controlled antidepressant studies in people with depression and dementia. J Am Geriatr Soc 2011;59:577–85.
75. Bergh S, Selbaek G, Engedal K. Discontinuation of antidepressants in people with dementia and neuropsychiatric symptoms (DESEP study): double blind, randomised, parallel group, placebo controlled trial. BMJ 2012;344:e1566.
76. Ahmed A, Simmons Z. Pseudobulbar affect: prevalence and management. Ther Clin Risk Manag 2013;9:483–9.
77. Drijgers RL, Aalten P, Winogrodzka A, et al. Pharmacological treatment of apathy in neurodegenerative diseases: a systematic review. Dement Geriatr Cogn Disord 2009;28:13–22.
78. Berman K, Brodaty H, Withall A, et al. Pharmacologic treatment of apathy in dementia. Am J Geriatr Psychiatry 2012;20:104–22.
79. Herrmann N, Rothenburg LS, Black SE, et al. Methylphenidate for the treatment of apathy in Alzheimer disease: prediction of response using dextroamphetamine challenge. J Clin Psychopharmacol 2008;28:296–301.
80. Mosimann UP, Rowan EN, Partington CE, et al. Characteristics of visual hallucinations in Parkinson disease dementia and dementia with Lewy bodies. Am J Geriatr Psychiatry 2006;14:153–60.
81. De Deyn PP, Carrasco MM, Deberdt W, et al. Olanzapine versus placebo in the treatment of psychosis with or without associated behavioral disturbances in patients with Alzheimer's disease. Int J Geriatr Psychiatry 2004;19:115–26.
82. Cipriana G, Lucetti C, Carlesi C, et al. Sundown syndrome and dementia. Eur Geriatr Med 2015;6:375–80.
83. Stopa EG, Volicer L, Kuo-Leblanc V, et al. Pathologic evaluation of the human suprachiasmatic nucleus in severe dementia. J Neuropathol Exp Neurol 1999;58:29–39.
84. Hanford N, Figueiro M. Light therapy and Alzheimer's disease and related dementia: past, present, and future. J Alzheimers Dis 2013;33:913–22.

Acute Brain Failure

Pathophysiology, Diagnosis, Management, and Sequelae of Delirium

José R. Maldonado, MD*

KEYWORDS

- Delirium • Acute brain failure • Encephalopathy • Post-operative delirium
- ICU-psychosis • Neurotransmitter dysfunction • Network dysregulation
- Systems integration failure hypothesis

KEY POINTS

- Delirium is a neurobehavioral syndrome caused by the transient disruption of normal neuronal activity secondary to systemic disturbances.
- It is the most common neuropsychiatric syndrome found in the general hospital setting.
- In addition to causing distress to patients, families, and medical caregivers, the development of delirium has been associated with increased morbidity and mortality, increased cost of care, increased hospital-acquired complications, poor functional and cognitive recovery, decreased quality of life, prolonged hospital stays, and increased placement in specialized intermediate and long-term care facilities.

EPIDEMIOLOGY OF DELIRIUM

Delirium is the most common neuropsychiatric syndrome found in the acute care setting, with a prevalence ranging from 10% in general medicine to 85% in advanced cancer and critical care (**Table 1**).[1–14] One study found that 89% of survivors of stupor or coma progressed to delirium.[15]

Risk Factors for Delirium

A systematic review among intensive care unit (ICU) patients revealed the following: age, dementia, hypertension, pre-ICU emergency surgery or trauma, Acute Physiology and Chronic Health Evaluation (APACHE) II score, mechanical ventilation, metabolic acidosis, delirium on the prior day, and coma as strong risk factors for delirium; whereas multiple organ failure was a moderate risk factor.[16,17] For every year after age 50, the chance of delirium increases by 10%.

Psychosomatic Medicine Service, Emergency Psychiatry Service, Department of Psychiatry and Behavioral Sciences, Stanford University School of Medicine, 401 Quarry Road, Suite 2317, Stanford, CA 94305-5718, USA
* Emergency Psychiatry Service, Stanford University School of Medicine, Stanford, CA.
E-mail address: jrm@stanford.edu

Crit Care Clin 33 (2017) 461–519
http://dx.doi.org/10.1016/j.ccc.2017.03.013
0749-0704/17/© 2017 Elsevier Inc. All rights reserved.

Table 1
A comparison of the incidence of psychiatric disorder in the general population and delirium among medically ill patients

Selected Medical Populations	Incidence of Delirium (%)
Medical Services	
At admission to inpatient medicine ward	10–31
New delirium: general medicine wards	3–29
HIV-AIDS	20–40
Poststroke	13–48
Medical: ICU	60–87
Sepsis	9–71
CCU	26
Surgical Services	
General surgical wards	11–46
Postoperative delirium	4.7–74
Post-CABG	13–32
Vascular surgery	22
Abdominal aneurysm repair	33
Orthopedic surgery	12–41
Postorthotopic liver transplant	45.2
Postcardiotomy	32–67
Critical Care Setting	
Coronary care units	26
Medical ICU	60–87
ARDS	70–73
Survivors of stupor or coma	Up to 89
Elderly	
In nursing homes	15–70
Delirium present at hospital admission	10.5–39
In-hospital delirium	15–31
Frail-elderly patients	Up to 60
Postsurgery	20–65
In Cancer Patients	
General prevalence	25–40
Hospitalized cancer patients	25–50
BMT	73
Terminally ill cancer patients	45–88

Abbreviations: AIDS, acquired immunodeficiency syndrome; ARDS, acute respiratory distress syndrome; BMT, bone marrow transplantation; CABG, coronary artery bypass grafting surgery; CCU, cardiac care unit; HIV, human immunodeficiency virus; ICU, intensive care unit.

The mnemonic END ACUTE BRAIN FAILURE encapsulates the many risk factors known to contribute to the development of delirium (**Table 2**).

Neuropathogenesis of Delirium

The various precipitants of delirium have been extensively reviewed elsewhere and are not fully discussed here (**Fig. 1**).[18] Whatever the proximate underlying cause, delirium is a neurobehavioral syndrome caused by an alteration in neurotransmitter synthesis, function,

Table 2
END ACUTE BRAIN FAILURE: predisposing and precipitating risk factors for delirium

Risk Factors	Examples
Electrolyte imbalance & dehydration	Electrolyte disturbances (eg, hyperammonemia, hypercalcemia, hypokalemia or hyperkalemia, hypomagnesemia, hyponatremia or hypernatremia)
Neurologic disorder & injury	All neurologic disorders: CNS malignancies, abscesses, CVA, intracranial bleed, meningitis, encephalitis, neoplasms, vasculitis, MS, epilepsy, Parkinson disease, NPH, TBI, DAI, paraneoplastic syndrome Of the various forms of sensory impairment, only visual impairment has been shown to contribute to delirium Visual impairment can increase the risk of delirium 3.5-fold
Deficiencies (nutritional)	Nutritional deficiencies (eg, malnutrition, low serum protein or albumin, low caloric intake, failure to thrive), malabsorption disorders (eg, celiac disease), and hypovitaminosis: specifically deficiencies in cobalamin (B12), folate (B9), niacin (B3, leading to pellagra), thiamine (B1, leading to beriberi & Wernicke disorder)
Age & gender	Age >65 y & gender male > female Old age is likely a contributor due to increased number of medical comorbidities: ↑ overall frailty, ↓ volume of ACH producing cells, ↓ cerebral oxidative metabolism, ↑ cognitive deficits, ↑ risk of dementia, ↑ age-related cerebral changes in stress-regulating neurotransmitter, intracellular signal transduction systems, chronic neurodegeneration with an increased production of inflammatory mediators, including cytokines and acute phase proteins
Cognition	Baseline cognitive deficits, even subtle ones, have been associated with an increased the risk of developing delirium The presence of dementia more than doubles the risk for postoperative delirium
U-Tox (intoxication & withdrawal)	Substance abuse: acute illicit substance intoxication (eg, cocaine, PCP, LSD, hallucinogens) and substance withdrawal, particularly abstinence syndromes from CNS-dep agents (eg, alcohol, benzodiazepines, muscle relaxants, opioids)
Trauma	Physical trauma & injury: heat stroke, hyperthermia, hypothermia, severe burns, surgical procedures
Endocrine disturbance	Endocrinopathies such as hyperadrenal or hypoadrenal corticoid, hyperglycemia or hypoglycemia, hyperthyroidism or hypothyroidism
Behavioral, psychiatric	Certain psychiatric diagnoses, including undue emotional distress, a history of alcohol and other substance abuse, and depression, schizophrenia, and bipolar disorder
Rx & other toxins	Several pharmacological agents have been identified as highly deliriogenic, including prescribed agents (eg, narcotics, GABA-ergic agents, steroids, sympathomimetics, dopamine agonists, immunosuppressant agents, some antiviral agents) & various OTC agents (eg, antihistaminic and anticholinergic substances), and polypharmacy Also consider the toxic effects of pharmacologic agents (eg, serotonin syndrome, neuroleptic malignant syndrome, anticholinergic states) and the deleterious effects of toxic levels of various therapeutic substances (eg, lithium, VPA, carbamazepine, immunosuppressant agents) Various toxins, including carbon dioxide & monoxide poisoning, solvents, heavy metals (eg, lead, manganese, mercury), insecticides, pesticides, poisons, biotoxins (animal poison), can also manifest with delirium

(continued on next page)

Table 2 (continued)	
Risk Factors	**Examples**
Anemia, anoxia, hypoxia, & low perfusion states	Any state that may contribute to decreased oxygenation (eg, pulmonary or cardiac failure, hypotension, anemia, hypoperfusion, intraoperative complications, hypoxia, anoxia, carbon monoxide poisoning, shock)
Infections	Pneumonia, urinary tract infections, sepsis, encephalitis, meningitis, HIV/AIDS
Noxious stimuli (pain)	Data suggest that pain and medications used for the treatment of pain have been associated with the development of delirium Studies have demonstrated that the presence of postoperative pain is an independent predictor of delirium after surgery On the other hand, the use of opioid agents has been implicated in the development of delirium
Failure (organ)	End organ failure (eg, hepatic, cardiac, renal failure) may lead to a delirious state
APACHE score (severity of illness)	Evidence shows that the probability of transitioning to delirium increases dramatically for each additional point in the APACHE II severity of illness score
Isolation & immobility	Social isolation, decreased intellectual stimulation, physical immobility, and increased functional dependence (eg, requiring assistance for self-care and/or mobility)
Light, sleep, & circadian rhythm	Sleep deprivation, sleep disorders (eg, obstructive sleep apnea, narcolepsy), & disturbances in sleep-wake cycle
Uremia & other metabolic disorders	Acidosis, alkalosis, hyperammonemia, hypersensitivity reactions, glucose, acid-base disturbances
Restraints	The use of restraints, including endotracheal tubes (ventilator), soft and leather restraints, intravenous lines, bladder catheters, and intermittent pneumatic leg compression devices, casts, and traction devices all have been associated with an increased incidence of delirium
Emergence delirium	Emergence from medication-induced sedation, coma, or paralysis, which may be associated with CNS-dep withdrawal, opioid withdrawal, REM-rebound, sleep deprivation

Abbreviations: Ach, acetylcholine; APACHE, acute physiology and chronic health evaluation; CNS, central nervous system; CVA, cerebrovascular accident; DAI, diffuse axonal injury; GABA, gamma-Aminobutyric acid; LSD, Lysergic acid diethylamide; MS, multiple sclerosis; NPH, normal pressure hydrocephalus; OTC, over-the-counter; PCP, phencyclidine; REM, rapid eye movement; Rx, pharmacological agents; U-tox, urine toxicology test.

and/or availability, and a dysregulation of neuronal activity secondary to systemic disturbances that mediates the complex neurocognitive changes phenotypic manifestations.

Although many neurotransmitter systems have been implicated, the most commonly described changes associated with the development of delirium include deficiencies in acetylcholine (ACH) and/or melatonin (MEL) availability; excess in dopamine (DA), norepinephrine (NE), and/or glutamate (GLU) release; and variable alterations (eg, either a decreased or increased activity, depending on delirium presentation and cause) in 5-hydroxytryptamine or serotonin (5HT), histamine (His), and/or gamma-amino butyric acid (GABA) (**Table 3**).

A newly proposed theory, the Systems Integration Failure Hypothesis (SIFH), attempts to integrate and make sense of all previously described theories.[18] The SIFH

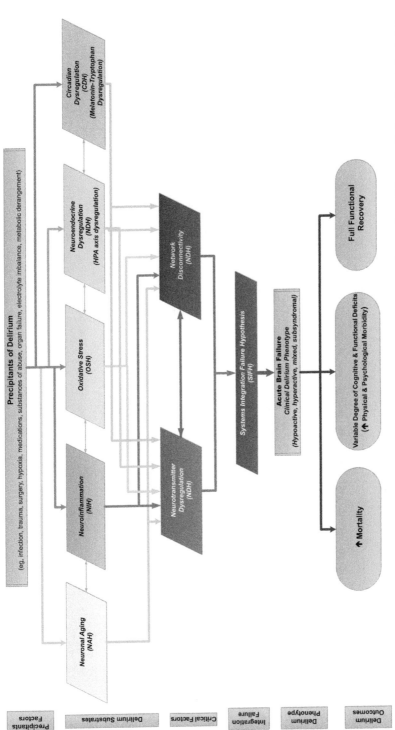

Fig. 1. Pathophysiology of delirium. (*Data from* Maldonado J. Delirium pathophysiology: current understanding of the neurobiology of acute brain failure. Int J Geriatr Psychiatry, in press.)

Table 3
Theorized neurochemical mechanisms associated with conditions leading to delirium

Delirium Source	ACH	DA	GLU	GABA	5HT	NE	Trp	MEL	Phe	His	Cytok	HPA Axis	Cort	NMDA activity	RBF Δ	Inflam	EEG
Anoxia or hypoxia	↓	↑	↑	↑	↓	↓	⇔	↓	↑	↑↓	↑↓	↑↓	↑	↑	↑↓	↑↓	↓
Aging	↓	↓	↓	↑	↓	↓	↑	↓	↑	↓	↑↓	↑↓	↑	↑	↑	↑	↓
TBI	↑	↑	↑	↑	↑	↑	↓	↑	↑	↑	↑↓	↑	↑	↑	↑	↑↓	↓
CVA	↓	↑	↑	↑	↑	↑	↓	↑	↑	↑	↑↓	↑	↑	↑	↑↓	↑↓	↓
Hepatic encephalopathy	⇔	↓	↑↑	↑	↑	↑	↑	↑	↑	↑	↑↓	↑↓	↑	↑	↑↓	↑	↓
Sleep deprivation	↓	↑↓	↑	↑	↑	↑	↑	↑↓	↑	↑	↑	↑	↑	↑	↑↓	↑↓	↓
Trauma, Sx, & Postoperative	↓	↑	↑	↑	↑	↑	↓	↓	↑	↑	↑↓	↑↑	↑	↑	→	↑	→
ETOH & CNS-Dep withdrawal	↑	↑	↓	↓	↑	↑	↓	↓	↓	↑	↑	↑↑	↑	↑	↑↓	↑	↑
Infection or sepsis	↓	↑	↓	↑	↓	↑	?	→	?	↑	↑	↑↓	↑	↑↓	↑↓	↑↓	↓
Dehydration & electrolyte imbalance	⇔	↑	↑	↓	↑	↑	↓	↓	↓	↑	↑	↑↓	↑	↑	→	↑↑	↑↓
Medical illness	↓	↑	↑	↑↓	↓	↑	↑	↓	↑	↑	↓	→	↑	↑	↑↓	↑↓	↑↓

Abbreviations: (—), likely not to be a contributing factor; ⇔, no significant changes; (⇊), likely a contributor, exact mechanism is unclear; ↑, likely to be increased or activated; ↓, likely to be decreased; Cort, cortisol; Cytok, cytokine; EEG, electroencephalograph; ETOH, alcohol; GABA, gamma-aminobutyric acid; His, histamine; HPA axis, hypothalamic-pituitary-adrenocortical axis; Inflam, inflammation; NMDA, N-methyl-D-aspartic acid; Phe, phenylalanine; RBF, regional blood flow; Sx, surgery; Trp, tryptophan.

Data from Maldonado JR. Neuropathogenesis of delirium: review of current etiologic theories and common pathways. Am J Geriatr Psychiatry 2013;21:1190–222; and Maldonado J. Delirium pathophysiology: current understanding of the neurobiology of acute brain failure. Int J Geriatr Psychiatry, in press.

proposes that the specific combination of neurotransmitter dysfunction and the variability in integration and appropriate processing of sensory information and motor responses, as well as the degree of breakdown in network connectivity within the brain, directly contributes to the delirium phenotype observed (see **Fig. 1**).

Clinical Presentation of Delirium

Delirium is an organic mental syndrome characterized by disturbance in attention (ie, reduced ability to direct, focus, sustain, and shift attention) and awareness, with impaired orientation to the environment (criterion A); with additional disturbances in cognition (eg, memory deficit, disorientation), language, visuospatial ability, or perception (eg, hallucinations or delusions; criterion C).[19]

The author suggests there are 5 core domains of delirium: (1) cognitive deficits (characterized by perceptual distortions, impairment in memory, abstract thinking and comprehension, executive dysfunction, and disorientation), (2) attentional deficits (characterized by disturbances in consciousness and a reduced ability to direct, focus, sustain and shift attention), (3) circadian rhythm dysregulation (characterized by fragmentation of the sleep–wake cycle), (4) emotional dysregulation (characterized by perplexity, fear, anxiety, irritability and/or anger), and (5) psychomotor dysregulation (which confers the various phenotypic presentations) (**Fig. 2**).

Delirium Phenotypes

The clinical features of delirium include a prodromal phase, usually marked by restlessness, anxiety, irritability, and sleep disturbances, which usually develop over a period of hours to days.

There are 5 delirium phenotypes: (1) the subsyndromal type (often under-recognized because it usually is associated with only partial diagnostic criteria); (2) the hypoactive

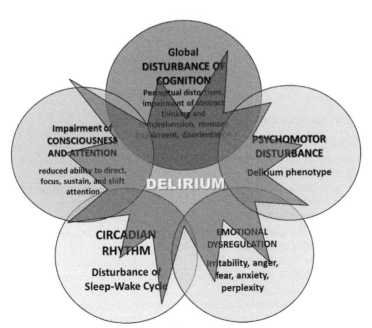

Fig. 2. Delirium core diagnostic characteristics.

delirium and its extreme, the catatonic subtype; (3) the hyperactive delirium and its extreme, the excited subtype; (4) and the mixed type, which often exhibits alternating characteristics of both hypoactive and hyperactive types, and likely gave rise to the classic description of delirium as waxing and waning in nature; and (5) the protracted or persistent type (**Fig. 3**). The progression or evolution of the syndrome can be best depicted in **Fig. 4**.

Subsyndromal delirium (SSD) represents an incomplete presentation of the diagnostic criteria, along with cognitive impairment. Available data suggest that medically ill patients with SSD experienced longer ICU length of stay and longer overall hospital stay, lower cognitive and functional outcomes, and increased postdischarge mortality.[20,21] In addition, patients with SSD have the same set of risk factors and experience similar outcomes as patients experiencing *Diagnostic and Statistical Manual of Mental Disorders* (DSM)-defined delirium.[22] Conversely, patients with no delirium are more likely to be discharged home and less likely to need convalescence or long-term care than those with SSD.[23]

Though the DSM suggests delirium is an acute and transient syndrome, chronic forms may be seen in several scenarios, such as those with baseline cognitive impairment or experiencing delirium as sequelae to new intracranial processes, or the effects of acute substance intoxication or withdrawal.

Diagnosing Delirium

Despite its high prevalence, delirium remains unrecognized by most ICU clinicians in as many as 66% to 84% of patients,[24,25] likely due to difficulty at making an accurate diagnosis at the extreme of symptom presentation (**Fig. 5**). Vigilance and a high level of suspicion may be the most important tools for the timely diagnosis of delirium, particularly in patients at higher risk, such as those in the ICU.

The DSM-5 (**Box 1**)[19] and the *International Statistical Classification of Diseases and Related Health Problems* (ICD-10)[26] (**Box 2**) are considered the diagnostic gold standards. There are many validated instruments to assist clinicians screen for the presence of delirium (**Box 3**), including an assessment for the re-emergence of pathologic primitive signs (**Box 4**). Newer surveillance and diagnostic tools include the Rapid Assessment Test for Delirium (4AT) (90% sensitive and 84% specific)[27] and the Stanford-Proxy Test for Delirium (S-PTD; 79% sensitivity and 90.8% specificity; using a cutoff score of 4).[28]

MANAGEMENT OF DELIRIUM

In general, the management of delirium includes the following steps: (1) knowledge and management of known delirium risk factors, (2) the implementation of prevention strategies (both pharmacologic and nonpharmacological) in an attempt to minimize the risk, (3) surveillance and accurate diagnosis of delirium (eg, hypoactive delirium vs depression, hyperactive delirium vs alcohol withdrawal or drug intoxication), (4) management of the behavioral and psychiatric manifestations and symptoms of delirium to prevent the patient from self-harm or harming of others, (5) identification of the etiologic causes of delirium, and (6) treatment of underlying medical problems. It is unclear whether (7) the pharmacologic manipulation to restore chemical balance and brain connectivity is of long-term usefulness and/or can mitigate the negative long-term effects of delirium.

A summary of the Stanford's Delirium Prevention and Management Model can be found in **Box 5**. The Stanford University ICU Delirium Management Protocol is shown in **Fig. 6**.

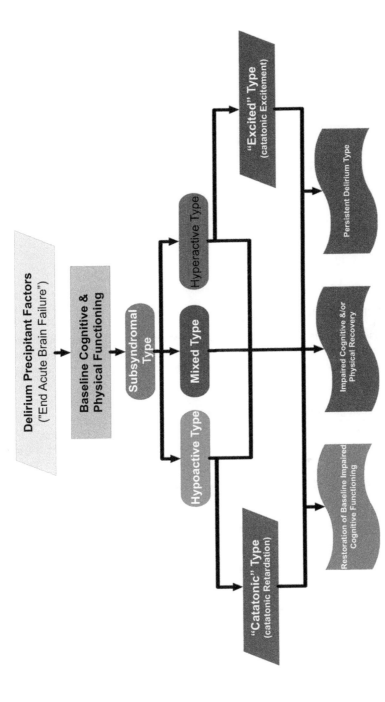

Fig. 3. Delirium phenotypes and clinical outcomes.

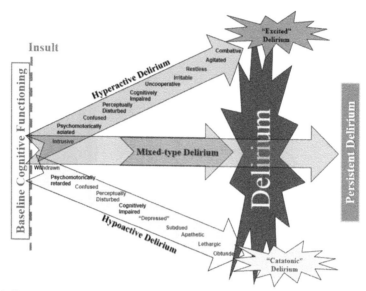

Fig. 4. Delirium phenotypes, symptom progression.

DELIRIUM PREVENTION STRATEGIES

Delirium has been listed as 1 of the 6 most common preventable conditions among hospitalized elderly patients.[58] Given the significant negative consequences of delirium, including worsening medical and cognitive outcomes, its prevention is of upmost importance.

Nonpharmacologic Management Strategies

The routine use of assessment scales or diagnostic interviews by properly trained personnel is paramount for the prevention and timely initiation of treatment. It is imperative to conduct a search for possible causes and conduct all appropriate diagnostic

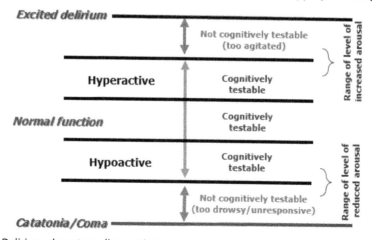

Fig. 5. Delirium phenotype diagnostic range.

Box 1
Diagnostic and Statistical Manual of Mental Disorders, 5th edition, diagnostic criteria for delirium

1. Disturbance in attention (ie, reduced ability to direct, focus, sustain, and shift attention) and awareness (reduced orientation to the environment).

2. The disturbance develops over a short period of time (usually hours to a few days), represents a change from baseline attention and awareness, and tends to fluctuate in severity during the course of a day.

3. An additional disturbance in cognition (eg, memory deficit, disorientation), language, visuospatial ability, or perception that is not better explained by a preexisting, established, or other evolving neurocognitive disorder.

4. The disturbances in Criteria 1 and 3 are not better explained by another preexisting, established, or evolving neurocognitive disorder and do not occur in the context of a severely reduced level of arousal, such as coma.

5. There is evidence from the history, physical examination, or laboratory findings that the disturbance is caused by the physiologic consequence of another medical condition, substance intoxication or withdrawal (ie, due to a drug of abuse or to a medication), or a toxin exposure, or is due to multiple causes.

Data from American Psychiatric Association. Diagnostic and statistical manual of mental disorders. 5th edition. Washington, DC: American Psychiatric Association; 2013.

---

tests. Correct malnutrition, dehydration, and electrolyte abnormalities as quickly and safely as possible. Conduct an inventory of all pharmacologic agents and discontinue any medication known to cause delirium or have high anticholinergic potential. Prompt restoration of a circadian rhythm should be attempted, preferably by

---

Box 2
International Statistical Classification of Diseases and Related Health Problems, 10th edition, diagnostic criteria for delirium

For a definite diagnosis, symptoms, mild or severe, should be present in each of the following areas:

1. Impairment of consciousness and attention (on a continuum from clouding to coma; reduced ability to direct, focus, sustain, and shift attention).

2. Global disturbance of cognition (perceptual distortions, illusions and hallucinations, most often visual; impairment of abstract thinking and comprehension, with or without transient delusions but typically with some degree of incoherence; impairment of immediate recall and of recent memory but with relatively intact remote memory; disorientation for time as well as, in more severe cases, for place and person).

3. Psychomotor disturbances (hypoactivity or hyperactivity and unpredictable shifts from 1 to the other, increased reaction time, increased or decreased flow of speech, enhanced startle reaction).

4. Disturbance of the sleep-wake cycle (insomnia or, in severe cases, total sleep loss or reversal of the sleep-wake cycle; daytime drowsiness; nocturnal worsening of symptoms; disturbing dreams or nightmares, which may continue as hallucinations after awakening).

5. Emotional disturbances, for example, depression, anxiety or fear, irritability, euphoria, apathy, or wondering perplexity.

Data from World Health Organization. The International Statistical Classification of Diseases and Related Health Problems (ICD-10): classification of mental and behavioural disorders. Geneva (Switzerland); World Health Organization: 1992.

Box 3
Objectives measures for the diagnosis of delirium (in order of development)

- DSM-II, gold standard[29]
  - Short Portable Mental Status Questionnaire (SPMSQ)[30]
- DSM-III gold standard[31]
  - Delirium Rating Scale (DRS)[32]
  - Confusion Assessment Method (CAM)[33]
  - Delirium Symptom Interview (DSI)[34]
- DSM-IV-TR, gold standard[35]
  - Delirium Assessment Scale (DAS)[36]
  - Cognitive Test for Delirium (CTD)[37]
  - Neelon and Champagne (NEECHAM) Confusion Scale[38]
  - Confusional State Evaluation (CSE)[39]
  - Memorial Delirium Assessment Scale (MDAS)[40]
  - Delirium Index (DI)[41]
  - Delirium Severity Scale (DSS)[42]
  - Confusion Assessment Method for the Intensive Care Unit (CAM-ICU)[10]
  - DRS, revised-98[43]
  - Delirium Detection Score (DDS)[44]
  - Delirium Detection Tool-Provisional (DDT-Pro) (Kean, Trzepacz and colleagues 2010)[205]
  - Brief Confusion Assessment Method (bCAM)[45]
  - 4AT[27]
- DSM-V (gold standard; APA 2014)
  - Stanford Proxy Test for Delirium (S-PTD)[28]

Tests for the Prediction of Delirium

- The Early Prediction (E-PRE-DELIRIC) model for delirium in ICU patients[46]
- Stanford's Algorithm for Predicting Delirium (SAPD)[47]

Brief Tests of Cognitive Functioning

- Mini-Mental State Examination (MMSE)[48]
- Modified Mini-Mental State Examination (3MS)[49]
- Trail-Making, A and B[50]

---

nonpharmacological means. Immobilizing lines and devices (eg, chest tubes, intravenous [IV] lines, bladder catheters) and physical restraints should be removed as early as possible. Correction of sensory deficits should be undertaken. Environmental isolation should be minimized, if possible. Family members and loved ones should be educated regarding the nature of delirium and how to assist in the patient's recovery, while encouraged to visit and provide a familiar and friendly environment, as well as provide appropriate orientation and stimulation.

A multicomponent approach, targeting identified, treatable, contributing factors may significantly decrease the risk of developing delirium, especially among populations at risk.[59,60] The awakening and breathing coordination, delirium prevention and management, and early physical mobility (ABCDE) bundle incorporates multidisciplinary measures to improve and/or preserve patients' function and neurocognitive status. Implementation of the ABCDE bundle was associated with a significant decrease in ICU delirium prevalence and the mean number of delirium days.[61]

The 2013 ICU pain, agitation, and delirium (PAD) guidelines were developed to provide a clear, evidence-based road map for clinicians to better manage PAD in critically ill patients. Strong evidence indicates that linking PAD management strategies with ventilator

---

Box 4
Primitive reflexes

These are clinical features that indicate brain dysfunction but that cannot be precisely localized or lateralized. When present, these signs suggest cortical disease, especially frontal cortex, resulting in disinhibition of usually extinguished or suppressed primitive reflexes. Their clinical significance is uncertain and is difficult to correlate with psychiatric illnesses and other behavior disorders, including delirium.

- Glabellar reflex: with the examiner's fingers outside of patient's visual field, tap the glabellar region at a rate of 1 tap per second. A pathologic response is either absence of blink, no habituation, or a shower of blinks. Normal response is blinking to the first few taps with rapid habituation.

- Rooting reflex: tested by stroking the corner of the patient's lips and drawing away. Pursing of the lips and movement of the lips or head toward the stroking is a positive response.

- Snout reflex: elicited by tapping the patient's upper lip with finger or percussion hammer causing the lips to purse and the mouth to pout.

- Suck reflex: tested by placing knuckles between the patient's lips. A positive response is puckering of the lips.

- Grasp reflex: elicited by stroking the patient's palm toward fingers or crosswise while the patient is distracted, causing the patient's hand to grasps the examiner's fingers.

- Palmomental reflex: test by scratching the base of the patient's thumb (noxious stimulus of thenar eminence). A positive response occurs when the ipsilateral lower lip and jaw move slightly downward, and does not extinguish with repeated stimulation.

- Babinski sign: downward (flexor response) movement of the great toe in response to plantar stimulation.

- Adventitious motor overflow: the examiner tests 1 hand for sequential finger movements, and the fingers of the other hand wiggle or tap. Also, test for choreiform movements.

- Double simultaneous stimulation discrimination: test with the patients eyes closed. The examiner simultaneously brushes a finger against 1 of the patient's cheeks and another finger against 1 of the patient's hands, asking the patient where he or she has been touched.

---

weaning, early mobility, and sleep hygiene in ICU patients resulted in significant synergistic benefits to patient care and reductions in costs.[62] Similarly, among mechanically ventilated subjects (n = 187), implementation of the ABCDE bundle was associated with earlier extubation, reduction in delirium odds, and increased odds of mobilizing out of bed.[63] **Table 4** contains a comprehensive review of all published data on the use of nonpharmacological approaches to the management of delirium.

Environmental Manipulations

Implementation of an environmental noise and light reduction program has been effective in reducing sleep deprivation and delirium.[71] A prospective, quality improvement project of medical ICU (MICU) patients incorporated evidence-based nonpharmacologic bundled interventions along with nursing education, resulting in significant reductions in the percentage of time spent delirious while reducing the risk of future delirium development.[72]

Physical and Occupational Therapy

Occupational therapy has been an effective, nonpharmacological intervention in decreasing the duration and incidence of delirium among nonventilated, elderly ICU

Box 5
Algorithm for the prevention and management of delirium

I. Recognition of patients at risk
  A. A particular patient's odds of developing delirium are associated with the interaction between the following conditions:
    1. Knowledge of a patient's characteristic (eg, patient's age, sex, baseline cognitive status, previous experiencing of delirium when exposed to medical illness or treatment)
    2. Predisposing and precipitating medical risk factors (END ACUTE BRAIN FAILURE)
    3. Consider the use of the Stanford's Algorithm for Predicting Delirium (SAPD)[47]
    4. Modifiable and nonmodifiable risk factors for that particular patient or patient population

Modifiable Factors	Nonmodifiable Factors
• Various pharmacologic agents, especially GABA-ergic and opioid agents, and medications with anticholinergic effects	• Older age
• Prolonged and/or uninterrupted sedation	• Baseline cognitive impairment
• Immobility	• Severity of underlying medical illness
• Acute substance intoxication	• Pre-existing mental disorders
• Substance withdrawal states	
• Use of physical restraints	
• Water and electrolyte imbalances	
• Nutritional deficiencies	
• Metabolic disturbances and endocrinopathies (primarily deficiency or excess of cortisol)	
• Poor oxygenation states (eg, hypoperfusion, hypoxemia, anemia)	
• Disruption of the sleep-wake cycle	
• Uncontrolled pain	
• Emergence delirium	

    5. Exposure to specific medical conditions and surgical procedures
  B. Obtaining the patient's baseline level of cognitive functioning using information from accessory sources (eg, Informant questionnaire on cognitive decline in the elderly [IQCODE])

II. Implementation of prevention strategies
  A. A key focus should be placed on prevention strategies, particularly in at-risk populations
  B. Minimize the use of pharmacologic agents that may contribute or worsen delirium
    1. If possible, avoid all pharmacologic agents with high deliriogenic potential or anticholinergic load
    2. If possible, avoid using GABA-ergic agents to control agitation
      a. Exceptions: cases of central nervous system-depressant withdrawal (ie, alcohol, benzodiazepines, barbiturates) or when more appropriate agents have failed and sedations are needed, benzodiazepine-sparing protocol to prevent patient harm
      b. An alternative is the use of the benzodiazepine-sparing protocol developed at Stanford University[51]
      c. Avoid the use of opioid agents for management of agitation
  C. Improve sleep-wake cycle and restore normal circadian rhythm
    1. Use nonpharmacological methods to promote a more natural sleep-wake cycle; that is, light control (ie, lights on and curtains drawn during the day, off at night) and noise control (ie, provide ear plugs and sleep masks, turn off TVs, and minimize night staff chatter)
    2. Provide as much natural light as possible during the daytime
  D. Implement early mobilization techniques, to include all of the following components
    1. Daily awakening protocols (sedation holiday)
    2. Remove intravenous (IV) lines, bladder catheters, physical restraints, and any other immobilizing apparatuses as early as possible
    3. Begin aggressive physical therapy (PT) and occupational therapy (OT) as soon as it is medically safe to do

4. In bedridden patients, this may be limited to daily passive range of motion
5. Once medically stable, get the patient up and moving as early as possible
6. Provide patients with any required sensory aids (ie, eyeglasses, hearing aids)
E. Provide adequate intellectual and environmental stimulation as early as possible
F. Adequately assess and treat pain
   1. Yet, avoid the use of opioid agents for behavioral control of agitation
   2. Rotate opioid agents from morphine to hydromorphone or fentanyl
G. For patients in the ICU, especially those on ventilation or IV sedation, consider
   1. Sedating to a prescribed or target sedation level (eg, RASS range between −2 to +1)
   2. Using the sedative agent with lowest deliriogenic potential
     a. Dexmedetomidine use is associated with the lowest incidence of delirium
     b. Propofol use is a good second choice, followed by midazolam
H. Reassess pain levels daily and titrate opioid agents to the lowest effective required to maintain adequate analgesia
   1. Hydromorphone is preferred as baseline agent of choice for pain management
   2. Limit the use of fentanyl for rapid initiation of analgesia and as rescue agent
   3. Avoid the use of opioid agents for sedation or management of agitation or delirium
I. Provide daily sedation holidays, if possible, this includes
   1. Interrupt sedative infusions daily until the patient is awake
   2. Restart sedation, if needed, at the lowest effective dose
   3. Reassess target sedation level (eg, RASS).
J. Use nonpharmacologic delirium prevention protocols. Three studies have demonstrated significant reduction in the incidence of delirium:
   1. The Hospital Elder Life Program (HELP), which has demonstrated a reduction in the occurrence of delirium from 50% (in the usual care group) to 32% (in the intervention group), in a cohort of hip fracture repair subjects. In this study, the length of stay did not significantly differ between intervention and usual-care groups.
   2. A study was done on the use of preemptive delirium expert consultants and implementation of nonpharmacological protocols after femoral neck fracture repair with a reduction in the incidence of delirium from 75.3% (in control group) down to 54.9% (in the intervention group), with a concomitant reduction in length of stay and postoperative complications.[70]
   3. A study was done on the use of artificial light therapy as a way to prevent alterations in circadian rhythm (ie, 5000 lux, at a distance from the light source of 100 cm) was found to be superior to natural lighting environment (control group) in preventing delirium after esophageal cancer surgery (16% vs 40%).[70]
K. Consider one of the following pharmacologic prevention strategies:
   1. Better anesthetic choices
     a. Alpha-2 agonist agents: The use of dexmedetomidine, instead of conventional GABA-ergic agents (ie, propofol, midazolam) has been demonstrated to lead to a significant reduction in the incidence of delirium in postoperative patients (3% vs 50%) when compared with midazolam and propofol[52]
     b. A systematic review and meta-analysis revealed that sedation with dexmedetomidine was associated with less delirium compared with sedation produced by conventional GABA-ergic agents (ie, midazolam, propofol; pooled risk ratio 0.39, 95% CI 0.16–0.95).[53]
   2. Dopamine antagonist agents
     a. Several studies have demonstrated the benefits of typical and second-generation antipsychotics (SGAs) in delirium prevention:
       i. Two recent meta-analyses of studies using dopamine antagonist agents for delirium prophylaxis found that pooled relative risk of published studies suggested a 50% reduction in the relative risk of delirium among those receiving antipsychotic medication compared with placebo ($P<.01$).[54,55]
       ii. A third meta-analysis demonstrated that both typical and second generation antipsychotics decreased delirium occurrence when compared with placebos.[53]
       iii. The studies suggest that perioperative use of prophylactic dopamine antagonist agents (both typical and second generation antipsychotics), when compared with placebo (PBO), may effectively reduce the overall risk of postoperative delirium, thereby potentially reducing mortality, disease burden, length of hospital stay, and associated health care costs.

3. Melatonin or melatonin-agonists
   a. Melatonin (eg, 3 mg every 2000) or melatonin agonists (eg, ramelteon 8 mg every 2000) to help promote a more natural sleep and prevention of all types of delirium
   b. If that is ineffective, consider trazodone (eg, 25–100 mg every 2000) or mirtazapine (eg, 3.75–7.5 mg every 2000)
4. Acetylcholinesterase inhibitors
   a. Early studies suggested that the use of rivastigmine was associated with a significantly lower incidence of delirium compared with controls, among patients with dementia (ie, 45.5 vs 88.9% and 40 vs 62%, respectively)
   b. Donepezil has also been described as effective
5. Ketamine use
   a. At least 1 study found that the use of ketamine may decrease the incidence of emergence agitation and delirium in pediatric subjects undergoing dental repair under general anesthesia

III. Enhanced surveillance, screening and early detection
   A. The most important aspect in this stage is surveillance
      1. Knowledge about the condition and presenting symptoms
      2. A high level of suspicion for patients at risk
   B. Be vigilant for the development of delirium in high risk groups
      1. Use a standardized surveillance tool (eg, CAM, CAM-ICU, Intensive Care Delirium Screening Checklist (ICDSC), 4-AT, MDAS, S-PTD)
      2. Use psychiatric consultants (ie, DSM-5 or ICD-10 criteria)
      3. Be particularly aware of the presence of hypoactive delirium and its different manifestations
   C. Use psychiatric consultants to help with assessment and design of the treatment plan, if available
   D. Train medical personnel at all levels regarding the prevalence and symptoms of delirium and its subsyndromal presentations, and on the use of screening tools

IV. Management of delirium
   A. Nonpharmacological treatment of all forms of delirium
      1. Identify and treat underlying medical causes
         a. Treatment or correction of underlying medical problems and potential reversible factors
         b. The definitive treatment of delirium is the accurate identification and timely treatment of its underlying causes
         c. Malnutrition, dehydration, and electrolyte abnormalities, if present, should be corrected as quickly and safely as possible
      2. Conduct an inventory of all pharmacologic agents administered to the patient
         a. Any medication or agent known to cause delirium or to have high anticholinergic potential should be discontinued, if possible, or a suitable alternative instituted
      3. Implement early mobilization techniques should include all of the following components
         a. Daily awakening protocols or sedation holiday
         b. Remove IV lines, bladder catheters, physical restraints and any other immobilizing apparatuses as early as possible
         c. Aggressive PT and OT as soon as medically safe
            i. In bedridden patients, this may be limited to daily passive range of motion
            ii. Once medically stable, get the patient up and moving as early as possible
         d. Provide patient with any required sensory aids (ie, eyeglasses, hearing aids)
         e. Promote as normal a circadian light rhythm as possible
            i. Better if this can be achieved by environmental manipulations, such as light control (ie, lights on and curtains drawn during the day, off at night) and noise control (ie, provide ear plugs, turn off television, and minimize night staff chatter)
            ii. Provide as much natural light as possible during the daytime
         f. Provide adequate intellectual and environmental stimulation as early as possible
            i. Minimize environmental isolation
      4. If possible, avoid using GABA-ergic agents to control agitation
         a. Exception: cases of CNS-depressant withdrawal (ie, alcohol, benzodiazepines, and barbiturates) or when more appropriate agents have failed and sedations are needed to prevent patient's harm

    b. An alternative is the use of the benzodiazepine-sparing protocol developed at Stanford University[51]

  5. Adequately assess and treat pain

    a. Yet, avoid the use of opioid agents for behavioral control of agitation

    b. Rotate opioid agents from morphine to hydromorphone or fentanyl

  6. The British National Institute for Health and Clinical Excellence (NICE) provided a set of guidelines for the prevention of delirium in elderly at-risk patients, mostly based on the correction of modifiable of factors and the implementation of the multicomponent intervention package[56] (full version of these recommendations available at http://guidance.nice.org.uk/CG103/Guidance/pdf/English)

B. For pharmacologic treatment of delirium (all types), consider using

  1. Dopamine antagonists to manage abnormally elevated levels of dopamine, and provide restoration of putative hippocampal functions (eg, short-term memory) and reversal of other regional brain disturbances (eg, agitation, psychosis, primitive reflexes), as well as to protect neurons against hypoxic stress and injury

    a. A systematic literature review of 28 delirium treatment studies with antipsychotic agents concluded (1) that around 75% of delirious patients who receive short-term treatment with low-dose antipsychotics experience clinical response, (2) that this response rates seem quite consistent across different patient groups and treatment settings, (3) that evidence does not indicate major differences in response rates between clinical subtypes of delirium, and (4) that there is no significant differences in efficacy for haloperidol versus atypical agent[57]

    b. The dose of dopamine antagonist use may depend on the type of delirium being treated

  2. Acetylcholinesterase inhibitor (eg, rivastigmine, donepezil) for patients with a history of recurrent delirium or delirium superimposed on known cognitive deficits

    a. Initial data seem rather promising but more recent studies have been unable to replicate original findings, probably because of the time needed to observe clinically significant effects. At least 1 study suggested an increased mortality associated with the use of these agents

    b. Physostigmine, a reversible acetylcholinesterase inhibitor, has been suggested as first-line treatment for the management of the central anticholinergic syndrome and antimuscarinic delirium

  3. Melatonin (eg, 6 mg every HS) or melatonin agonists (eg, ramelteon 8 mg every HS) to help promote a more natural sleep and management of all types of delirium

    a. If that is ineffective, consider trazodone (eg, 25–100 mg every HS) or mirtazapine (eg, 3.75–7.5 mg every HS)

C. Pharmacologic treatment of hyperactive delirium, consider the use of the following agents (in addition to IV-A)

  1. Dopamine antagonist agents to address DA excess (eg, haloperidol, risperidone, quetiapine, aripiprazole)

    a. Moderate-dose haloperidol (eg, 5–30 mg/24 h, in divided doses) is still considered the treatment of choice if the patient's cardiac condition allows it and there are no significant electrolyte abnormalities.

    b. No study has demonstrated any other agent to be clinically superior, or safer than haloperidol

    c. When the use of haloperidol is contraindicated or not desirable, atypical antipsychotics should be considered

      i. Better evidence for risperidone (as a nonsedating agent, T1/2 = 20 hours), quetiapine (for a sedating agent; T1/2 = 7 hours)

      ii. There are limited data for olanzapine (concerns include: sedation, anticholinergic potential and long T1/2 > 50 h), aripiprazole as nonsedating agent especially for cases of hypoactive delirium (slow onset of action, T1/2 = 75 hours), lurasidone as a sedating agent (T1/2 = 18 hours), and paliperidone as a sedating agent (T1/2 = 23 hours)

      iii. Avoid clozapine and ziprasidone

    Before using antipsychotic agents

      i. Obtain 12-lead electrocardiogram (ECG) and measure QTc

      ii. Check electrolytes, correct potassium (K) and magnesium (Mg), if needed

      iii. Carefully review the patient's medication list and identify any other agents with the ability to prolong QTc

        iv. If possible, avoid other medications known to increase QTc and/or inhibitors of CPY3A4

        v. Discontinue dopamine antagonist agents use if QTc increases to greater than 25% of baseline or greater than 500 msec

  2. Alpha-2 agonists (eg, dexmedetomidine, clonidine, guanfacine), for protection against the acute NE released secondary to hypoxia or ischemia, leads to further neuronal injury and the development of worsening of delirium

    a. Consider changing primary sedative agents from GABA-ergic agents (eg, propofol or midazolam) to an alpha-2 agent (eg, dexmedetomidine), starting at 0.4 mcg/kg/h, then, titrate dose every 20 minutes to targeted RASS goal

    b. In non-ICU patients, guanfacine is an excellent alternative (dose range from 0.5–3 mg/D in divided doses)

    c. Clonidine is also an alternative, especially to wean patients off dexmedetomidine but the main limiting factor is its hypotensive effect

  3. Anticonvulsant and other agents with glutamate antagonism or calcium channel (Ca2+) modulation (eg, valproic acid [VPA], gabapentin, amantadine, memantine)

    a. VPA (either by mouth or IV) is increasingly used in the management of agitated delirious patients who either are not responsive or cannot tolerate conventional treatment, yet there are very little data regarding its effectiveness, which is limited to case series; the author recommends its use for the management of hyperactive or agitated delirium not responding the use of dopamine antagonist agents and adequate sedation, agitation occurring in the context of weaning sedation, or agitation associated with alcohol withdrawal

    b. Carbamazepine (available by mouth and IV) and gabapentin (available by mouth only) may be of equal use, although there are scant research data available. Clinical data suggest effectiveness in the management of alcohol withdrawal; no parenteral form is available

  4. Consider the use of N-methyl-D-aspartic acid (NMDA)-receptor blocking agents, to minimize glutamate-induced neuronal injury (eg, amantadine, memantine), particularly in cases of traumatic brain injury (TBI) and cerebrovascular accident (CVA).

  5. Serotonin antagonist (eg, ondansetron 8 mg IV, every 8 hours PRN). Note: this agent may prolong QTc, be cautious when combining with other agents known to prolong QTc, such as amiodarone, haloperidol

D. Pharmacologic treatment of hypoactive delirium, consider the use of the following agents (in addition to IV-A)

  1. Evidence suggests that DA antagonists may still have a place given the excess DA theory. A systematic literature review of 28 delirium treatment studies with antipsychotic agents concluded (1) that around 75% of delirious patients who receive short-term treatment with low-dose antipsychotics experience clinical response, (2) that these response rates seem quite consistent across different patient groups and treatment settings, (3) that evidence does not indicate major differences in response rates between clinical subtypes of delirium (ie, hypoactive vs hyperactive), and (4) that there is no significant differences in efficacy for haloperidol versus atypical agents[57]

    a. If haloperidol is used, recommended doses are in the very-low range (ie, 0.25 to 1 mg/24 h); this is usually given as a single nighttime dose, just before sun down

    b. If an atypical is preferred, consider low doses of an agent with low sedation (ie, risperidone, <1 mg/24 h; aripiprazole, 2–10 mg/24 h)

  2. In cases of extreme psychomotor retardation or catatonic features, in the absence of agitation or psychosis, consider the use of psychostimulant agents (eg, methylphenidate, dextroamphetamine, modafinil)

  3. Consider the use of NMDA-receptor blocking agents, to minimize glutamate-induced neuronal injury (eg, amantadine, memantine, bromocriptine) and help manage extreme psychomotor retardation, particularly in cases of TBI and CVA.

Abbreviations: CPY3A4, cytochrome P450–3A4; HS, *hora somni*, every bedtime; PRN, pro re nata, or as needed; QTc, Corrected QT Interval; RASS, Richmond Agitation-Sedation Scale; T1/2, drug half-life.

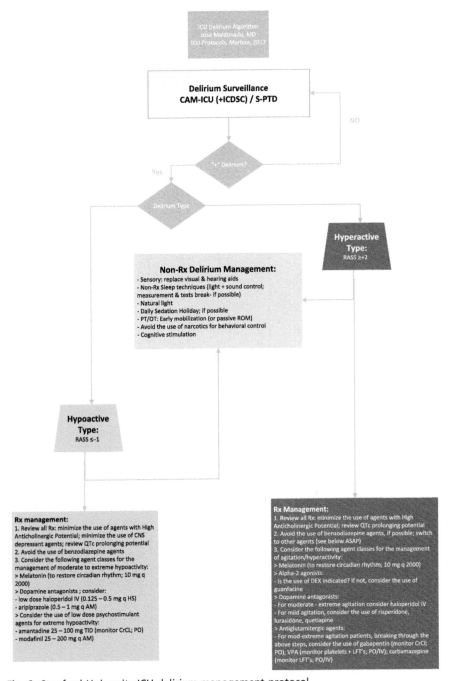

Fig. 6. Stanford University ICU delirium management protocol.

Table 4
Nonpharmacological prevention approaches

Study (n = 19)	Population	Intervention	Delirium Definition	Delirium Incidence (%)		P-Value
				Control	Intervention	
Schindler et al,[206] 1989 RCT, n = 33	CABG	NP: perioperative psychiatric intervention vs usual care	DSM-III	0 (0/17)	12.5 (2/16)	ns
Wanich et al,[207] 1992 NRCT, n = 235	Gen IM elderly subjects	NP: nursing intervention for elderly hospitalized subjects vs usual care	DSM-III	22 (22/100)	19 (26/135)	ns (P = .61)
Inouye et al,[64–69] 1999 NRCT, n = 852	Gen IM elderly subjects	NP: multicomponent intervention vs usual care	CAM	15 (64/426)	9.9 (42/426)	P = .02
Millisen et al,[208] 2001 NRCT, n = 120	Traumatic hip Fx Sx repair	NP: multicomponent vs usual care	CAM	23.3 (14/60)	20 (12/60)	P = .82
Marcantonio et al,[209] 2001 RCT, n = 126	Elderly subjects after hip Fx Sx	NP: multicomponent intervention vs usual care	CAM	50 (32/64)	32 (20/62)	P = .04
Tabet et al,[210] 2005 NRCT, n = 250	Gen IM elderly subjects	NP: staff education vs usual care	Single assessment psychiatrist	19.5 (25/128)	9.8 (12/122)	P = .034
Wong et al,[211] 2005 Pre-evaluation & postevaluation	Traumatic hip Fx Sx repair	NP: multicomponent vs usual care	CAM	35.7 (10/28)	12.7 (9/71)	P = .012

Study	Setting/Subjects	Intervention	Tool			P value
Vidan et al,[212] 2005 RCT, n = 319	Elderly subjects after hip Fx Sx	NP: multicomponent intervention vs usual care	CAM	45.2 (70/155)	61.7 (100/164)	P = .003 For ≥1 major complications
Lundström et al,[213] 2007 RCT, n = 199	Elderly subjects after hip Fx Sx	NP: multicomponent intervention vs usual care	OBSS	75.3 (73/97)	54.9 (56/102)	P = .003
Caplan et al,[214] 2007 Pre-evaluation & postevaluation, n = 37	Geriatric ward	NP: usual care vs volunteer-mediated intervention (Inouye style)	CAM	38.1 (8/21)	6.3 (1/16)	P = .032
Taguchi et al,[70] 2007 RCT, n = 11	Esophageal CA subjects	Normalization of natural circadian rhythm by of light therapy	NEECHAM scale	16	40	P = .42
Benedict et al,[215] 2009 NRCT, n = 65	Acute Care for Elders (ACE) units	NP: delirium prevention protocol vs usual care	Modified NEECHAM scale (3d average)	(3.24)	(3.76)	ns (P = .368)
Schweickert et al,[216] 2009 RCT, n = 104	MICU	Early exercise and mobilization (PT & OT) at daily sedation interruption vs sedation interruption	CAM-ICU	2 d	4 d	P = .02
Holroyd-Leduc et al,[217] 2010 NRCT, n = 134	Traumatic hip Fx Sx repair	NP: multicomponent delirium strategies	CAM	Preimplementation incidence 33 (23/70)	Postimplementation incidence 31 (20/64)	ns (P = .84)
Björkelund et al,[218] 2010 NRCT, n = 263	Elderly hip Fx Sx repair	NP: multicomponent delirium strategies	OBSS	34 (45/132)	22 (29/131)	P = .096

(continued on next page)

Table 4
(continued)

Study (n = 19)	Population	Intervention	Delirium Definition	Delirium Incidence (%)		
				Control	Intervention	P-Value
Colombo et al,[219] 2012 n = 314	All subjects admitted to mixed (med-surg) ICU over a year	NP: reorientation strategy + environmental, acoustic, and visual stimulation.	CAM-ICU	35.5 (60/170)	22 (31/144)	P = .020
Gagnon et al,[220] 2012 Randomized delirium prevention trial, n = 1516	Palliative care subjects, in 2 cancer centers	NP: multicomponent administered to subject and family education vs usual care	Confusion rating scale (CRS)	43.9 (370/842)	49.1 (330/674)	P = .045
Martinez et al,[221] 2012 n = 287	Older adults in gen medicine ward	Randomized to receive a multicomponent management protocol, delivered by family members (144 subjects) or standard management (143 subjects)	CAM	13.3 (19/143)	5.6 (8 kal/144)	P = .027

Abbreviations: CABG, coronary artery bypass grafting surgery; CAM, Confusion Assessment Method; CAM-ICU, Confusion Assessment Method for the ICU; IM, internal medicine; NEECHAM, NEECHAM Confusion Scale; NP, non-pharmacological; NRCT, non-randomized clinical trial; OBSS, Organic Brain Syndrome Scale; RCT, randomized clinical trial.

patients.[73] Even in patients unable to leave their beds, data suggest that range-of-motion exercises can prevent and shorten the duration of delirium among patients in the ICU who are 65 years and older.[74]

Light Therapy

Limited data suggest that therapeutic lighting might effectively reduce the incidence of delirium.[70]

PHARMACOLOGIC MANAGEMENT STRATEGIES

It cannot be overstated that the definitive treatment of delirium is the accurate identification and treatment of its underlying causes. Nevertheless, pharmacologic intervention often helps manage agitated or catatonic patients. A systematic review of ICU interventions concluded that pharmacologic interventions were associated with a reduction in delirium prevalence, length of stay, and duration of mechanical ventilation.[75]

Pharmacologic Prevention Options

Dopamine-antagonist agents

Antipsychotic agents have long been used for the treatment of delirium's behavioral manifestations. Space limitations prevent in-depth review of every published study. **Table 5** contains a comprehensive summary all published studies on the use of dopamine antagonist agents for the prevention of delirium.

In the ICU population, the use of low-dose risperidone was found to lower the incidence of postoperative delirium (POD).[76] Likewise, the use of low-dose olanzapine decreased the incidence of POD.[79] In a study of at-risk ICU subjects ($n = 177$) low-dose haloperidol was associated with lower delirium incidence, more delirium-free days, fewer ICU readmissions, and less frequent unplanned removal of tubes or lines compared with control group.[78]

Three meta-analyses concluded that perioperative use of prophylactic dopamine antagonist agents (both typical and second-generation antipsychotics [SGAs]), may effectively reduce the overall risk of POD, thereby potentially reducing mortality, disease burden, length of hospital stay, and associated health care costs.[53-55]

Alpha-2 agonists

The use of novel sedative agents may minimize delirium, in part by avoiding the use of more deliriogenic alternatives, such as GABA-ergic agents.[80] Studies have demonstrated that the choice of postoperative sedative may affect the incidence of delirium ($P<.01$): 3% for subjects on dexmedetomidine (DEX), 50% on propofol (PRO), or midazolam (MID) (**Fig. 7, Table 6**). Two subsequent double blind randomized placebo controlled trial (DBRPCT) confirmed DEX's delirium-sparing effects; achieving lower delirium incidence, a lower prevalence of coma, shorter intubation time, and more time within sedation goals.[81,82] Meta-analyses have found that the use of DEX is associated with significant reductions in the incidence of delirium, agitation and confusion.[53,83] **Table 7** contains a comprehensive summary all published studies on the use of alpha-2 adrenergic agonist agents for the prevention of delirium.

Glutamate antagonists and calcium channel modulators

Antiglutamatergic and calcium (Ca) channel blocking agents have been used in the prevention of delirium, including gabapentin, carbamazepine, and valproic acid (**Table 8**). Their deliriolytic effect is likely mediated via modulation of voltage-sensitive Ca2+ channels, N-methyl-D-aspartic acid (NMDA)-receptor antagonism, activation of spinal alpha-2 receptors, and attenuation of sodium (Na) dependent action potentials.

Table 5
Pharmacologic prevention of delirium: dopamine antagonist agents

Study (n = 10)	Population	Intervention	Delirium Definition	Delirium Incidence (%)			P-Value
				Control	Intervention		
Kaneko et al,[222] 1999 RPCT	Gastrointestinal surgery	Prophylaxis haloperidol vs PBO IV postoperatively for 5 d	DSM-III-R	32.5	10.5		P<.05
Kalisvaart et al,[223] 2005 DBRPCT, n = 430	Elderly hip-replacement Sx	PBO vs haloperidol 1.5 mg/d started preoperative, continued for up to 3 d postoperative	DSM-IV CAM DRS-R98	16.5 (36/216)	15.1 (32/212)		ns
Prakanrattana & Prapaitrakool,[76] 2007 DBRPCT, n = 126	Cardiac Sx under CPB	PBO vs sublingual risperidone immediately p-Sx	CAM	31.7 (20/63)	11.1 (7/63)		P = .009
Girard et al,[77] 2010* DBRPCT, n = 101	Med-surg ICU in mechanical ventilation	PBO vs haloperidol vs ziprasidone: days alive without delirium or coma, conducted in 6 tertiary medical centers.	CAM-ICU	12.5 (1.2–17.2) d	14.0 (6.0–18.0) d	15.0 (9.1–18.0) d	P = .66*
Larsen et al,[79] 2010 DBRPCT, n = 495	Elderly elective total joint-replacement	PBO vs 5 mg of orally disintegrating olanzapine 1 dose presurgery & 1 dose postsurgery	DSM-III-R	40.2 (82/204)	14.3 (28/196)		P<.001

Study	Population	Medication	Assessment tool			Findings	Significance
Wang et al,[224] 2012 RCT, n = 457	Elderly, noncardiac Sx	PBO vs HAL (0.5 mg bolus, followed by continuous infusion 0.1 mg/h × 12 h)	CAM	23.2	15.3		P = .031
Van den Boogaard et al,[78] 2013 Retrospective analysis, n = 177	ICU at risk for delirium	PBO vs HAL (1 mg/8 h) within 24 h of admission to ICU	CAM-ICU	75	65		P = .01
Hirota & Kishi,[54] 2013 Meta-analysis (RCTs), 6 studies, n = 1689	Various clinical settings	Meta-analysis of 6 studies (3 HAL, 1 olanzapine, 2 risperidone) using antipsychotic agent for delirium prophylaxis	Various tools			Sensitivity analysis showed that second-generation antipsychotics (SGAs) were superior to PBO (NNT = 4; P<.0001), whereas HAL failed to show superiority to PBO	P<.00001
Teslyar et al,[55] 2013 Meta-analysis (RCTs); 5 studies, n = 1491	Postoperative elderly subjects	Medication administered included haloperidol (3), risperidone (1), and olanzapine (1)	Various tools			The pooled relative risk of the 5 studies resulted in a 50% reduction in the relative risk of delirium among those receiving antipsychotic medication compared with placebo	P<.01
Neufeld et al,[225] 2016 Meta-analysis (RCTs); 19 studies, n = 140877	Prophylaxis (7) & treatment (12)	Various APA agents	Various tools			Antipsychotic use was not associated with change in delirium duration, severity, hospital or ICU length of stay, or mortality	(OR 0.56, 95% CI 0.23–1.34, I2 = 93%)

Abbreviations: APA, anti-psychotic agents; CAM, Confusion Assessment Method; DBPCT, double-blind, placebo clinical trial; DRS-R98, Delirium Rating Scale – revised 1998; DSM-III, Diagnostic and Statistical Manual of Mental Disorders, 3rd edition; DSM-IV, Diagnostic and Statistical Manual of Mental Disorders, 4th edition; NNT, number needed to treat; ns, sot significant; PBO, placebo; RPCT, randomized placebo clinical trial.

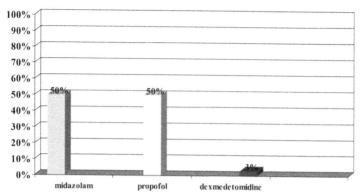

Fig. 7. DEX prophylaxis in postsurgical valve disease patients versus DEX, *P*<.01, adjusted for comparing multiple group means. (*Data from* Maldonado JR. Delirium in the acute care setting: characteristics, diagnosis and treatment. Crit Care Clin 2008;24(4):657–722.)

Ketamine

To date, there have been 2 studies using ketamine for delirium prevention.[85,86]

Melatonin and melatonin-agonists

The usefulness of melatonin and melatonin agonists in the prevention of POD has been documented.[87–90] Studies have found that subjects receiving melatonin experienced statistically significant lower incidence of medical delirium[91] and POD.[92] **Table 9** contains a comprehensive summary all published studies on the use of melatonin and agonist agents for the prevention of delirium.

Statins

The use of statins has been associated with associated with more delirium-free days and lower C-reactive protein (CRP), among critically ill patients,[95] and ICU patients with acute respiratory failure or shock.[96]

Acetylcholinesterase inhibitors

There have been at least 19 papers, mostly case reports, suggesting that acetylcholinesterase inhibitor agents may be effective in the prevention of delirium (**Table 10**).[97,98]

Pharmacologic Treatment Options

Among intubated delirious subjects, those treated with pharmacologic agents within 24 hours of the first positive delirium-screening test spent fewer days in physical restraints, less time receiving mechanical ventilation, and experienced shorter ICU and hospital length of stay (LOS) compared with controls (Michaud, Thomas and colleagues 2014).

Dopamine antagonists

The literature has long recognized IV neuroleptic agents as the recommended emergency treatment for agitated and mixed-type delirium.[64,100–104] **Table 11** contains a comprehensive summary all published studies on the use of dopamine antagonist agents for the treatment of delirium.

Safety concerns Despite the widespread use of IV-haloperidol and multiple reports describing its safety,[64,102,104,108–114] concerns about haloperidol's safety remain. These

Table 6
Selected postoperative outcome variables for cardiac patients with cardiopulmonary bypass by intervention group

	DEX (n = 30)	PRO (n = 30)	MID (n = 30)	Overall P-Value	Dex vs PRO	Dex vs MID
Delirium						
Incidence of Delirium (per protocol)	1/30 (3%)	15/30 (50%)	15/30 (50%)	<.001	<0.001	<0.001
Incidence of Delirium (ITT)	4/40 (10%)	16/36 (44%)	17/40 (44%)	<.001	0.001	0.002
Number of Days Delirious	2/216 (1%)	45/276 (16%)	75/259 (29%)	<.001	<0.001	<0.001
Average Length of Delirium[a] (d)	2.0 ± 0	3.0 ± 3.1	5.4 ± 6.6	.82	0.93	0.63
Time Variables						
ICU Length of Stay (d)	1.9 ± .9	3.0 ± 2.0	3.0 ± 3.0	.11	0.14	0.14
Hospital Length of Stay (d)	7.1 ± 1.9	8.2 ± 3.8	8.9 ± 4.7	.39	0.42	0.12
Intubation Time (h)	11.9 ± 4.5	11.1 ± 4.6	12.7 ± 8.5	.64	0.91	0.34
PRN Medications						
Fentanyl (mcg)	320 ± 355	364 ± 320	1088 ± 832	<.001	0.93	<0.001
Total Morphine Equivalents (mg)[b]	50.3 ± 38	51.6 ± 36	122.5 ± 84	<.001	0.99	<0.001
Antiemetic Use[c]	15/30 (50%)	17/30 (57%)	19/30 (63%)	.58	—	—
PRN Medications for the Management of Delirium[d]						
Lorazepam	1/30 (3%)	7/30 (23%)	6/30 (20%)	.07	0.06	0.11
Haloperidol	0/30	3/30 (10%)	2/30 (7%)	.23	0.07	0.15

Abbreviations: DEX, dexmedetomidine; ITT, intention-to treat; MID, midazolam; PRO, propofol.
[a] Of patients who developed delirium.
[b] Sum of average morphine equivalents (fentanyl, oxycodone, and hydrocodone) received in postoperative days 1 to 3.
[c] Number of patients who received dolasetron mesylate and/or promethazine HCl in postoperative days 1.
[d] Average amount over 3 days. None of these medications were given until a diagnosis of delirium was established.
Data from Maldonado JR. Delirium in the acute care setting: characteristics, diagnosis and treatment. Crit Care Clin 2008;24(4):657–722.

are mainly related to its effect on QTc prolongation, even though the risk of haloperidol inducing Torsade de pointes (TdP) is relatively low (0.27%).[115,116] Despite these concerns, multiple panels, task forces, expert panels, and various professional organizations (eg, American College of Critical Care Medicine, Society of Critical Care Medicine, American Psychiatric Association, National Institute for Health and Clinical Excellence) still recommend the use of IV haloperidol for the management of extreme agitation in the ICU.[117–122]

Antipsychotic alternatives to haloperidol

Due to stigma and fear of side effects, SGAs have been increasingly used for the management of psychiatric and behavioral symptoms among medically ill patients

Table 7
Pharmacologic management of delirium: centrally acting alpha-2-adrenergic receptors agonists

Study (n = 11)	Population	Intervention	Delirium Definition	Delirium Incidence (%)		P-Value
				Control	Intervention	
Berggren et al,[226] 1987 RCT, n = 57	Femoral Neck Fx repair	Epidural vs halothane anesthesia	DSM-III	38 (11/29)	50 (14/28)	ns
Williams-Ruso et al,[227] 1992 RCT, n = 60	B knee replacement Sx	Continuous epidural bupivacaine + fentanyl vs continuous IV fentanyl	DSM-III	44 (11/25)	38 (10/26)	ns (P = .69)
Aizawa et al,[228] 2002 OL, n = 42	Gastrointestinal surgery	Usual care vs BZDP administration to promote sleep p-Sx	DSM-IV	35	5	P = .023
Maldonado et al,[80] 2003; Maldonado et al,[229] 2009 RCT, n = 118	Cardiac valve Sx	Postoperative anesthesia w MID vs PROP vs DEX	DSM-IV DRS-R98	50 (15/30)	50 (15/30) 3 (1/30)	P<.001
Pandharipande et al,[81] 2007 (MENDS) DBRPCT, n = 106	Med-surg ICU in mechanical ventilation	DEX vs lorazepam (2 tertiary care centers), days alive w/o delirium or coma	CAM-ICU	3.0 d	7.0 d	P = .01
Reade et al,[84] 2009 R, OL pilot trial; n = 20	Tx-agitated ICU subjects	IV haloperidol 0.5–2 mg/h vs DEX 0.2–0.7 µg/kg/h	Intensive Care Delirium Screening Checklist (ICDSC)	42 h	20 h	P = .016
				Above numbers represent time to extubation		

Study	Population	Intervention	Assessment			P value
Hudetz et al,[85] 2009 DBRPCT, n = 58	Elective CABG or valve replacement/ repair w/ CPB	PBO vs IV ketamine (0.5 mg/kg) bolus during the induction of anesthesia	ICDSC	31 (9/29)	3 (1/29)	P = .01
Riker et al,[82] 2009 DBRPCT, n = 375	Med-surg ICU in mechanical ventilation	MID vs DEX; trial conducted in 68 centers in 5 countries	CAM-ICU	76.6 (93/122)	54 (32/244)	P<.001
Shehabi et al,[230] 2009 RCT, n = 306	Cardiac Sx	Morphine vs DEX	CAM-ICU	15	8.6	P = .088
Rubino et al,[231] 2010 DBRPCT, n = 30	Acute type-A aortic dissection repair	PBO vs clonidine IV on delirium neurologic outcome & respiratory function	Delirium Detection Score (DDS)	40	33	P = .705
				1.8 ± 0.8	0.6 ± 0.7	P = .001
Jakob et al,[232] 2012; RDBCT, n = 498	Adult ICU subjects mechanical ventilation	PROP vs DEX	CAM-ICU	29% (71/247)	18% (45/251)	P = .008

Abbreviations: BIS, Bispectral Index; BZDP, benzodiazepine; CAM, Confusion Assessment Method; CAM-ICU, Confusion Assessment Method for the ICU; DBPCT, double-blind, placebo clinical trial; DEX, dexmedetomidine; DRS-R98, Delirium Rating Scale – revised 1998; DSM-III, Diagnostic and Statistical Manual of Mental Disorders, 3rd edition; DSM-IV, Diagnostic and Statistical Manual of Mental Disorders, 4th edition; MDAS, Memorial Delirium Assessment Scale; MENDS, Maximizing Efficacy of Targeted Sedation and Reducing Neurologic Dysfunction trial; OL, open label; PBO, placebo; POD, post-operative day; PROP, propofol; RCT, randomized clinical trial; Tx, treatment.

Table 8
Delirium management: glutamate and calcium channel modulators

Drug	T ½	Product Availability	Bioavailability (%)	Metabolism	Protein Binding (%)	Mechanism Action
Lamotrigine	25 h	po	~ 100	Hepatic	55	• Stabilizes neuronal membranes • Inhibits voltage-sensitive Na+ channels and/or Ca+ channels → ↓ cortical GLU release • Ca+ channel blockers • Excitatory amino acid antagonists
Amantadine	17 ± 4 h	po	—	None Renal excretion	67	• NMDA-receptor antagonist • ↑ synthesis and release of dopamine
Memantine	60–80 h	po	100	Mostly unchanged renal excretion	45	• Noncompetitive NMDA-receptor antagonist • Blocks the effects of excessive levels of GLU • Some Ca+ channel blockade • 5HT antagonist
Gabapentin	5–7 h	po	60	None Renal excretion	<3	• Voltage-gated Ca+ channel blockade → ↓ cortical GLU release • NMDA antagonism • Activation of spinal alpha2-adrenergic receptors • Attenuation of Na+ dependent action potential
VPA	9–16 h	po or IV	90	Hepatic conjugation	90	• GABA transaminase inhibitor → ↑ GABA • Inhibits voltage-sensitive Na+ channels → ↓ cortical GLU release • ↓ release of the epileptogenic amino acid gamma-hydroxybutyric acid (GHB)

(eg, agitation, psychosis, delirium). Data on SGAs are limited to small case reports (see **Table 11**).

Head-to-head data comparing SGAs against haloperidol and other typical antipsychotics in the treatment of delirium are lacking. A Cochrane database review found no significant differences in SGA ability to lower delirium scores or incidence of adverse effects, confirming that low-dose haloperidol was effective in decreasing the degree and duration of POD, when compared with placebo.[123]

Risperidone is the most thoroughly studied SGA for the management of delirium, found to be approximately 80% to 85% effective, followed by olanzapine at approximately 70% to 76% effective.[124] Limited data suggest that quetiapine may also be a safe and effective alternative to high-potency antipsychotics.

A systematic literature review of delirium treatment with antipsychotic agents (n = 28 studies) concluded that (1) approximately 75% of delirious subjects who receive short-term treatment with low-dose antipsychotics experience a clinical response, (2) the response rate seems quite consistent across different subject groups and treatment settings, (3) the evidence does not indicate major differences in response rates between the various clinical subtypes of delirium (ie, hypoactive vs hyperactive), and (4) there are no significant differences in efficacy for haloperidol versus atypical agents.[57]

Dopamine antagonist agents: treatment recommendations When antipsychotic agents are needed, it is wise to review the patient's medication list and identify any other agents with the ability to prolong QTc. If possible, avoid other medications known to increase QTc and/or inhibitors of CPY3A4. Before and during the use of antipsychotic agents, obtain a 12-lead ECG (for QTc) and correct any electrolyte abnormalities (especially potassium + and magnesium +). Guidelines recommend discontinuing antipsychotic use if the QTc increases greater than 25% of baseline or greater than 500 msec.

When treating hypoactive delirium, the author recommends doses in the very low daily range (ie, haloperidol and risperidone in the 0.25–1 mg per 24 hours). Available data suggest that excess dopamine may occur in all delirium types, even hypoactive type. It also suggests that antipsychotics may help prevent and treat all forms of deliria, including hypoactive type. Medication is usually given as a single nighttime dose, before sundown. Sedating agents (eg, quetiapine, olanzapine) should be avoided. Reports have confirmed the usefulness of aripiprazole, particularly in hypoactive delirium.[106,107,125]

Alpha-2 agonists
A randomized, open-label trial for the treatment of agitated delirium found that DEX significantly shortened median time to extubation, decreased ICU length of stay, and cut in half the time PRO was needed compared with IV haloperidol.[84] An open-label, prospective trial of POD in cardiovascular subjects (n = 60), found that DEX was associated with shorter delirium duration, increased rates of spontaneous breathing, shorter ICU LOS, and better achieved targeted richmond agitation-sedation scale (RASS) compared with haloperidol (HAL).[126]

A systematic review of ICU studies confirmed that the use of DEX lowered delirium prevalence.[16] When compared with PRO, DEX-sedation reduced delirium incidence, delayed onset, and shortened duration of POD.[80,127,128] Despite its high cost, DEX use is associated with a mean savings of $4370 per subject due to reductions in ICU LOS.[129]

A retrospective ICU study of agitated POD among liver transplantation subjects found that DEX significantly decreased the ICU LOS and lowered MID requirements compared with HAL.[130] A meta-analysis of randomized controlled trials (RCTs; 8 studies, n = 969 adults after cardiac surgery) found that DEX was associated with a

Table 9
Delirium management: melatonin prevention and treatment

Study (n = 8)	Population	Intervention	Delirium Definition	Results
Bourne et al,[90] 2008 N = 24, DBPCT	s/p tracheostomy to assist weaning from vent	Melatonin 10 mg po at 2000	BIS	Melatonin associated with a 1-h increase in nocturnal sleep (P = .09) and a decrease in BIS AUC indicating better sleep Melatonin use was associated with increased nocturnal sleep efficiency
Al-Aama et al,[91] 2010 N = 145	≥65 y/o admitted through the emergency department to a medical unit	Randomized to MEL 0.5 mg vs PBO q HS × 14 d or D/H	CAM	Melatonin was associated with a lower risk of delirium (12.0% vs 31.0%, P = .014)
Sultan,[92] 2010 N = 300	≥65 y/o scheduled for hip arthroplasty under spinal anesthesia	Randomized to PBO Melatonin 5 mg MID 7.5 mg Clonidine 100 µg	—	Melatonin showed a statistically significant decrease in POD to 9.43% POD: PBO, 32.7%; MEL, 9.4% (P = .003); MID, 44 & (P = .245); CLO, 37.3% (P = .629) Melatonin was successful in treating 58.06% of subjects suffered POD

Study	Design/N	Subjects	Intervention	Diagnostic measure	Results
de Jonghe et al,[233] 2010 Review	Meta-analysis	—	—	—	9 papers, including 4 RCTs (n=243), and 5 case series (n = 87) were reviewed. 2 of the RCTs found a significant improvement on sundowning or agitated behavior. All 5 case series found an improvement
de Jonghe et al,[234] 2011 N = 452	≥65 y/o admitted for surgical repair of hip fracture	Randomized to: PBO, Melatonin 3 mg at 2100	CAM	Ongoing	
Kimura et al,[93] 2011 N = 3 (case report)	Subjects >59, medically ill	Open label; ramelteon 8 mg q HS	DSM-IV-TR MDAS-Jap	All 3 cases demonstrated significant improvement in delirium scores as measured by MDAS, with steady improvement over 7 d, ramelteon 8 mg at HS	
Furuya et al,[94] 2012 N = 5 (case report)	Elderly Hospitalized for delirium	Open label, ramelteon 8 mg	DSM-IV-TR	Successful treatment of 5 cases of delirium within 1 d, after ramelteon 8 mg at HS	
Hatta et al,[89] 2014 8 mg q 2000	N = 67, gen medicine & ICU	Randomized, PC trial, prophylaxis	DSM-IV-TR	Ramelteon associated w lower risk of delirium (3% vs 32%; $P = .003$), w relative risk of 0.09 (95% CI 0.01–0.69)	

Abbreviations: BIS, Bispectral Index; CAM, Confusion Assessment Method; DBPCT, double-blind, placebo clinical trial; DSM-IV, Diagnostic and Statistical Manual of Mental Disorders, 4th edition; MDAS, Memorial Delirium Assessment Scale; PBO, placebo; POD, post-operative day; RCT, randomized clinical trial; y/o, year-old.

Table 10
Acetylcholinesterase inhibitors in delirium prevention

Study (n = 7)	Population	Intervention	Delirium Definition	Delirium Incidence (%)		P-Value
				Control	Intervention	
Dautzenberg et al,[97] 2004 OL, retrospective review, n = 51	≥65 y/o hospitalized demented subjects	Subjects who used rivastigmine chronically with a randomly selected subgroup of all subjects not treated	Retrospective chart review of geriatric service consultations	88.9 (26/29)	45.5 (4/11)	P<.05
Moretti et al,[99] 2004 RCT, n = 230	≥65 y/o-o/p, w vascular dementia (24-mo follow-up)	Cardio aspirin vs rivastigmine po q D	CAM Behave-AD	62 (71/115)	40 (46/115)	P<.001
Liptzin et al,[235] 2005 DBRPCT, n = 80	Elderly elective total joint-replacement	PBO vs donepezil (14 d pre-Sx + 14 d post-Sx)	DSM-IV	17.1 (7/41)	20.5 (8/39)	Ns (P = .69)
Sampson et al,[236] 2007 DBRPCT, n = 33	Elderly elective hip replacement	PBO vs donepezil 5 mg immediately p-Sx + 3 d	DSI	35.7 (5/14)	9.5 (2/19)	P = .08
Oldenbeuving et al,[237] 2008 N = 26	Delirium p-CVA	Rivastigmine 3→12 mg/d; no PBO	DRS ≥12	In 16/17 (94%) delirium severity improved, mean decrease 14.8→8.5, mean duration 6.7 d, no side effects		
Gamberini et al,[238] 2009 DBRPCT, n = 120	Cardiac Sx under CPB	PBO vs po rivastigmine 1.5ª preoperative, until POD#6	CAM	30 (17/57)	32 (18/56)	ns (P = .8)
van Eijk et al,[239] 2012 DBRPCT, n = 109	>18 y/o in ICU	2-arms, both receiving haloperidol, 1 on PBO other on rivastigmine	CAM-ICU	3d	5d	P = .06

Abbreviations: BEHAVE-AD, Behavioral Pathology in Alzheimer's Disease Rating Scale; CAM, Confusion Assessment Method; CAM-ICU, Confusion Assessment Method for the ICU; CPB, cardio-pulmonary bypass machine; DBRPCT, double-blind, randomized, placebo clinical trial; OL, open label; PBO, placebo; p-CVA, after cerebro-vascular accident; RCT, randomized clinical trial.

ª Rivastigmine-treated subjects who experienced delirium had a shorter duration, lower use of benzodiazepine and neuroleptic for management of agitation, and improvement in all behavioral aspects measured by the BEHAVE-AD.

Table 11
Pharmacologic treatment of delirium: dopamine antagonist agents

Study (n = 32)	Population	Intervention	Delirium Definition	Results
Breitbart et al,[240] 1996 RCT, n = 30	AIDS, medical subjects	Haloperidol vs chlorpromazine vs lorazepam	DRS	Tx either HAL or CPM resulted in significant improvement in the symptoms of delirium, whereas no improvement was found in the LOR group Tx neuroleptic was associated with an extremely low prevalence of EPS, whereas all subjects receiving LOR developed treatment-limiting adverse effects
Sipahimalani et al,[241] 1998 OL, n = 22	Med-surg subjects	Haloperidol vs olanzapine	DRS	Improvement was similar in both groups (mean DRS + SD HAL = 11.1 ± 7.1; OLA = 10.3 ± 4.8; P = .760), with extrapyramidal symptoms found only in haloperidol subjects No side effects in olanzapine group
Schwartz et al,[242] 2000 Single-blind; n = 11	Med-surg subjects	Quetiapine vs haloperidol, retrospective chart review	DRS	Effectiveness of ≥50% in reducing DRS scores When compared with haloperidol, there was no difference in onset of symptom resolution, duration of treatment, and overall clinical improvement
Kim et al,[243] 2001 OL, n = 20	Med-surg subjects	Olanzapine po, variable dose	DRS	50% decrease in DRS scores (from pre of 20.0 ± 3.6, to post of 9.3 ± 4.6; $P<.01$) No side effects, including EPS
Breitbart et al,[105] 2002 OL, n = 79	Hospitalized cancer subjects	Olanzapine po, variable dose	MDAS	Olanzapine was effective in treating 76% of delirium subjects as evidenced by the MDAS, caused excessive sedation in 30% of subjects
Horikawa et al,[244] 2003 OL, n = 10	Med-surg subjects	Risperidone po	DSM-IV	At a low dose of 1.7 mg/d, on average, risperidone was effective in 80% of subjects and the effect appeared within a few days Most commonly cited adverse effects included sleepiness (30%) and mild drug-induced parkinsonism (10%)
Sasaki et al,[245] 2003 OL, n = 12	Med-surg subjects	Quetiapine po, flexible doses	DSM-IV	100% of subjects on quetiapine achieved resolution of delirium (mean on day 4.8 ± 3.5 d), no EPS reported
Kim et al,[246] 2003 OL, n = 12	Elderly medical in-subject	Quetiapine po, flexible doses	DSM-IV/DRS	100% of subjects on quetiapine achieved resolution of delirium by day 10 (mean on day 5.9 ± 2.2 d); no EPS reported Delirium Rating Scale scores along with scores of the MMSE and Clock Drawing Test continued to improve throughout the 3-mo study period

(continued on next page)

Table 11
(continued)

Study (n = 32)	Population	Intervention	Delirium Definition	Results
Liu et al,[247] 2004 Retrospective record review, n = 77	Med-surg subjects with hyperactive delirium	Risperidone (average dose 1.17 ± 0.76 mg/d) vs haloperidol (average dose 4.25 ± 2.62 mg/d)	DSM-IV	Subjects treated with haloperidol were younger than subjects treated with risperidone (P<.05) The mean hyperactive syndrome scale score was higher in the haloperidol than that of the risperidone group No significant difference in the efficacy or frequency of response rate between haloperidol and risperidone (100% vs 95%; P = ns) Subjects on risperidone experienced less EPS (7% vs 69%)
Mittal et al,[248] 2004 OL, n = 10	Subjects admitted to med-surg unit	Risperidone, 0.5 mg po BID, flexible PRNs	DSM-IV/DRS	Rapid resolution of delirium while receiving low-dose Risperidone (mean dose 0.75 mg/d); no EPS reported
Parellada et al,[249] 2004 OL	Prospective, multicenter, observational 7-d study	Risperidone po	DSM-IV DRS PANSS-P MMSE	Risperidone was administered at the time of diagnosis, and treatment was maintained according to clinical response Found a significant improvement in DRS scores in 90.6% of treated subjects and significantly improved all symptoms measured by the scales from baseline to day 7 (P<.0; only 3% side effects
Pae et al,[250] 2004 OL, n = 22	Med-surg subjects	Quetiapine po	DRS-R98 CGI-s	DRS-R98 and CGI-s scores were significantly reduced by 57.3% and 55.1%, respectively Quetiapine was effective and safe
Han et al,[251] 2004 DBRCT, n = 28	Med-surg subjects	Haloperidol vs risperidone, 7d medication trial	CAM DRS MDAS	Both groups showed significant improvement in baseline DRS and MDAS scores with either haloperidol (75%) or risperidone (42%, P<.05) There was no significant difference in improvement of DRS (P = .35) or MDAS (P = .51) scores, comparing haloperidol with risperidone subjects
Hu et al,[252] 2004 RPCT, n = 175	Med-surg elderly subjects	Haloperidol vs olanzapine vs placebo, 7d medication trial	DRS CGI	Tx groups showed a decrease in DRS scores by 7th day compared with baseline (P<.01) Decrease in DRS scores of treated subjects at day 7 (OLA 72.2%; HAL 70.4%) differed significantly from DRS scores of PBO subjects (29.7%; P<.01) but not from each other (P>.05)

Study	Population	Intervention	Delirium Index (DI)	Results
Skrobik et al,[253] 2004 OL-prospective RCT, n = 73	Critically ill med-surg subjects	Haloperidol (average 6.5 mg/d) vs olanzapine (average 4.5 mg/d)	Delirium Index (DI)	ICU DI Screening Checklist Scores were reduced in both groups compared with baseline (P<.05) but there was no significant difference in DIS scores between active Tx groups (P = .9). EPS were found in 13% of haloperidol subjects, 0% in olanzapine group
Toda et al,[254] 2005 n = 10	Elderly inpatient general medicine	Risperidone, OL, 0.5 mg oral sol; flexible titration, PRN	DSM-IV/DRS	Resolution reported in 7 subjects (mean dose 0.92 ± 0.47 mg/d). 1 nonresponder. 2 side effects requiring Tx discontinuation
Lee et al,[255] 2005 RCT, n = 40	Med-surg subjects	Amisulpride vs quetiapine	DRS-R98 CGI	After treatment, DRS-R98 scores were significantly decreased from the baseline in both treatment groups (P<.001) without group difference. Both atypical antipsychotics were generally well tolerated
Straker et al,[106] 2006 OL, n = 14	Medically ill subjects	Aripiprazole po was used in a flexible dosing range, from 5-15 mg/d	DSM-IV DRS-R98 CGI	50% of subjects had improved significantly by day 5, as indicated by a 50% reduction in DRS-R98 scores. 86% of subjects had a 50% reduction in their DRS-R98 scores by end of treatment. Mean CGI Severity scores at the beginning of treatment were 5.2, with a mean CGI improvement score after treatment of 2.1, indicating much improvement
Takeuchi et al,[256] 2007 OL, n = 38	Med-surg subjects	Perospirone, OL	DSM-IV/ DRS-R98	Perospirone was effective in 86.8% of subjects, within several days (5.1 ± 4.9 d). The initial dose was 6.5 ± 3.7 mg/d and maximum dose of perospirone was 10.0 ± 5.3 mg/d. There were no serious adverse effects
Maneeton et al,[257] 2007 OL, n = 17	Medically ill subjects	Quetiapine, flexible dosing	CAM/DRS, CGI	88% subjects responded. Mean (SDs) dose and duration (SD) of quetiapine treatment were 45.7 (28.7) mg/d and 6.5 (2.0) d, respectively. The DRS and CGI-S scores of days 2-7 were significantly lower than those of day 0 (P<.001) for all comparisons. Only 2 subjects were shown to have mild tremor
Reade et al,[84] 2009 OL-RCT	Med-surg ICU	Agitated delirium randomized to receive HAL 0.5–2 mg/h or DEX 0.2–0.7 µg/kg/h	ICDSC Time	DEX significantly shortened median time to extubation from 42.5 to 19.9 h (P = .016). Significantly decreased ICU length of stay, from 6.5 to 1.5 d (P = .004). Of subjects requiring ongoing sedation, it reduced the time PRO was required in half (79.5% vs 41.2%; P = .05)

(continued on next page)

Table 11
(continued)

Study (n = 32)	Population	Intervention	Delirium Definition	Results
Devlin et al,[258] 2010 DBRPCT, n = 36	MICU	PBO vs quetiapine (50 mg BID) Multicenter-3	ICDSC	Tx with QUE was associated with: a shorter time to first resolution of delirium ($P = .001$), a reduced duration of delirium ($P = .006$), less agitation ($P = .02$), greater chance to be discharged home vs long-term care facility ($P = .06$), and lower requirement of as-needed haloperidol ($P = .05$)
Girard et al,[77] 2010 DBRPCT, n = 101	Mechanically ventilated medical and surgical ICU subjects	PBO vs HAL vs ziprasidone	CAM-ICU	Subjects in the haloperidol group spent a similar number days alive without delirium or coma (14.0 d, range 6.0–18.0) as did those on ziprasidone (15.0 d, range 9.1–18.0) and PBO groups (12.5 d, range 1.2–17.2); $P = .66$
Kim et al,[259] 2010 SB-RCT, n = 32	Elderly, med-surg subjects	Risperidone vs olanzapine	DSM-IV/ DRS-R98	Significant within-group improvements in the DRS-R98 scores over time were observed at every time point in both treatment groups. The response rates did not differ significantly between the 2 groups (risperidone group, 64.7%; olanzapine group, 73.3%) and no difference in the safety profiles and side effects between groups
Tahir et al,[260] 2010 DBRCT, n = 42	Med-surg subjects	Quetiapine vs placebo	DSM-IV/ DRS-R98, CGI	Quetiapine has the potential to more quickly reduce the severity of noncognitive aspects of delirium. Study was underpowered for treatment comparisons
Grover et al,[261] 2011 Prospective, single blind, n = 64	Med-surg subjects	Haloperidol (0.25–10 mg) vs olanzapine (1.25–20 mg) vs risperidone (0.25–4 mg), flexible dosing	DSM-IV or DRS-R98	Subjects in all 3 groups experienced a significant reduction in DRS-R98 severity scores and a significant improvement in MMSE scores over the period of 6 d, with no difference between the treatment groups. Rate of side effects was also similar
Boettger & Breitbart,[107] 2011 OL, n = 21	Med-surg subjects at Cancer Center	Aripiprazole, flexible dosing	DSM-IV/MDAS	Subjects treated for delirium with aripiprazole (mean dose 18.3 mg, range of 5–30) experienced significant improvement and resolution of delirium. MDAS scores declining from a mean of 18.0 at baseline (T1) to mean of 10.8 at T2 and a mean of 8.3 at T3. There was a 100% resolution of hypoactive delirium vs 58.3% of hyperactive delirium

Study	Subjects	Intervention	Scale	Results
Hakim et al,[262] 2012 PCRCT	Subjects aged 65 y or older who experienced SSD after on-pump cardiac surgery	Randomized using a computer-generated list to receive placebo (n = 50) or 0.5 mg risperidone (n = 51) every 12 h by mouth	ICDSC	7 (13.7%) subjects in the risperidone group experienced delirium vs 17 (34%) in the placebo group (P = .031) Competing-risks regression analysis showed that failure to treat SSD with risperidone was an independent risk factor for delirium (P = .002) 2 (3.9%) subjects in the risperidone group experienced extrapyramidal manifestations vs 1 (2%) in the placebo group (P = 1.0)
Kishi et al,[263] 2012 OL, n = 29	Adult delirious cancer subjects	Risperidone, mean dosage, 1.4 ± 1.3 mg/d	DRS-R98	Entry DRS-R98 score = 19.8 ± 6.8; 7-d follow-up score = 14.3 ± 7.8 DRS-R98 scores improved in 79.3% of subjects (P<.001) 38% achieved remission (ie, DRS-R98 ≤10)
Tagarakis et al,[264] 2012 n = 80	POD after on-pump heart surgery	Ondansetron iv (8 mg) vs HAL IV (5 mg); pts evaluated before and 10 min after Rx administration	Self-developed rating scale: 0-4	Statistically significant improvement in the test score rating after the administration of both ondansetron (from 3.1 to 1.2, improvement 61.29%, P<.01) and haloperidol (from 3.1 to 1.3, ± percentage improvement 58.064%, P<.01)
Yoon et al,[265] 2013 Observational study; n = 80	Subjects with delirium at a tertiary level hospital	Assigned to receive either haloperidol (N = 23), risperidone (N = 21), olanzapine (N = 18), or quetiapine (N = 18)	Korean version of the Delirium Rating Scale-Revised-98 (DRS-K)	Haloperidol, risperidone, olanzapine, and quetiapine were equally efficacious and safe in the treatment of delirium The treatment response rate was lower in subjects >75 y than in subjects <75 y, especially for olanzapine
Maneeton et al,[266] 2013 DBRCT, n = 52	Medically ill subjects with delirium	25-100 mg/d of quetiapine (n = 24) or 0.5-2.0 mg/d of haloperidol (n = 28)	DRS-R98 and total sleep time	Means (standard deviation) of the DRS-R98 severity scores were not significantly different between the quetiapine and haloperidol groups (−22.9 [6.9] vs −21.7 [6.7]; P = .59) Concluding that low-dose quetiapine and haloperidol may be equally effective and safe for controlling delirium symptoms

Abbreviations: AIDS, acquired immunodeficiency syndrome; CAM-ICU, Confusion Assessment Method for the ICU; CGI, clinical global impression scale; CGI-s, clinical global impression scale-severity; CPM, chlorpromazine; DI, delirium index; DRS-R98, Delirium Rating Scale – revised 1998; DSM-IV, Diagnostic and Statistical Manual of Mental Disorders, 4th edition; EPS, extrapyramidal symptoms; HAL, haloperidol; ICDSC, Intensive Care Delirium Screening Checklist; LOR, lorazepam; MDAS, Memorial Delirium Assessment Scale; MMSE, mini mental status examination; OL, open label; OLA, olanzapine; PANSS-P, Positive and Negative Syndrome Scale; PBO, placebo; PCRCT, placebo-controlled, randomized clinical trial; PRN, as needed medication; RCT, randomized clinical trial.

lower risk of delirium, a shorter length of intubation but a higher incidence of brady-cardia compared with PRO.[131]

Glutamate antagonists and calcium channel modulators

Multiple agents can be used in the management of hyperactive or excited delirium, including lamotrigine, gabapentin, carbamazepine, and VPA (see **Table 8**). There are no RCTs available. Two case series suggest VPA is effective in managing delirium and decreasing time to extubation, even in cases in which other medications have failed, with minimal side effects.[132,133] As with any patient receiving VPA, closely monitor liver function tests, bilirubin, platelet count, and amylase. As in the case of SGAs, there are case reports on VPA-induced delirium.

Acetylcholinesterase inhibitors

All published data are limited to small series or case reports (n = 19) for the treatment of delirium in older persons.[97,98] **Box 6** lists published case reports suggesting a positive effect of acetylcholinesterase inhibitors in the treatment of delirium.

Physostigmine is a fast, short-acting acetylcholinesterase inhibitor that increases synaptic acetylcholine concentrations and can overcome the postsynaptic muscarinic receptor-blockade produced by anticholinergic agents. It can reverse both central and peripheral anticholinergic receptors, and has been successfully used to treat emergence delirium in both adults[138,149] and pediatric patients.[150]

Physostigmine should be considered when a delirious patient exhibits signs of a central anticholinergic state (eg, confusion, sinus tachycardia, markedly dilated and fixed pupils, dry mouth, hypoactive bowel sounds, dry and flushed skin) and/or when it is known that the patient's altered mental status is due to the use of known

---

Box 6
Case reports suggesting a positive effect of acetylcholinesterase inhibitors in the treatment of delirium

- Burt,[134] 2000
- Bruera et al,[135] 2003
- Dautzenberg et al,[97] 2004
- Fisher et al,[136] 2001
- Gleason,[137] 2003
- Hasse and Rundshagen,[138] 2007
- Hori et al,[139] 2003
- Kaufer et al,[140] 1998
- Kobayashi et al,[141] 2004
- Logan and Stewart,[142] 2007
- Moretti et al,[99] 2004
- Palmer,[143] 2004
- Rabinowitz,[144] 2002
- Weizberg et al,[145] 2006
- Wengel et al,[146,147] 1998
- Wengel et al,[148] 1999

anticholinergic substances, as in the case of medication overdose (whether accidental or intentional).[151–156] Other investigators have reported that, among subjects with suspected anticholinergic delirium, physostigmine controlled agitation and reversed delirium in 96% and 87% of cases, respectively,[157] with no significant side effects. An initial physostigmine dose of 1 to 2 mg (0.5 mg in children) given IV over 3 to 5 minutes is the recommended dose. If the response provides only an incomplete response, additional doses of 0.5 to 1.0 mg every 5 minutes may be given until delirium resolves or there are signs of cholinergic excess (eg, diaphoresis, salivation, vomiting, diarrhea). Absolute contraindications include a prolonged PR interval (>200 ms) or QRS complex (>100 ms and not related to bundle branch block) interval on ECG are for physostigmine use.

Serotonin antagonists
In a prospective study of ICU POD after coronary artery bypass graft surgery (n = 35), subjects were treated with a single dose (8 mg IV) of ondansetron with significant improvement in cognition and behavior, with no adverse events reported.[158]

Melatonin and melatonin agonists
Multiple case reports have documented the effectiveness of melatonin in treating severe POD unresponsive to conventional treatment (eg, antipsychotics or benzodiazepine agents),[87] demonstrating delirium resolution in 58% of subjects treated with melatonin.[92]

Similarly, there are 2 case reports of the successful use of ramelteon in the treatment of patients with delirium[93,94] (see **Table 9** for a summary of published case reports and studies on the use of melatonin for the treatment of delirium).

MANAGEMENT OF HYPOACTIVE DELIRIUM

Good, controlled studies on the management of hypoactive delirium are lacking. Similarly, given the mechanism of delirium development, there may be a rationale for the use of very low doses of nonsedating antipsychotic agents. The use of activating agents (eg, modafinil and psychostimulants) may help mobilize hypoactive patients, particularly to address extreme psychomotor retardation and extreme somnolence.

Some NMDA-receptor blocking agents, such as amantadine and memantine, can be used in the management of hypoactive delirium, especially when associated with intracranial insults, such as traumatic brain injury (TBI) and cerebrovascular accident (see **Table 8**). Studies have demonstrated that memantine may be effective in reducing the damage induced by acute ischemia or reperfusion (Yigit and colleagues, 2011), whereas amantadine has been shown to enhance cognitive recovery and minimize delirium after severe TBI in humans.[159] Furthermore, data suggest that amantadine use was an effective and safe means of reducing frequency and severity of irritability and aggression[160] and may accelerate the pace of functional recovery during active treatment in individuals with TBI.[159] In fact, studies suggest that amantadine use produced marked improvement in measures of arousal and cognition.[161,162] Finally, there are case reports suggesting that amantadine may be useful in the management of post-TBI amotivational syndrome.[163]

DELIRIUM MANAGEMENT: WHAT DOES AND WHAT DOES NOT WORK

Studies suggest that the implementation of a delirium protocol with pharmacologic and nonpharmacological interventions had an impact on ICU patients experiencing acute delirium by significantly increasing delirium-free days and reducing the ICU

LOS.[164] A systematic review revealed a statistically significant reduction in the incidence of ICU delirium and a reduced ICU length of stay with appropriate sleep intervention.[88]

Data suggest that the use of delirium prevention bundle interventions (ie, sedation cessation, pain management, sensory stimulation, early mobilization, and sleep promotion) was effective in reducing the incidence of delirium in critically ill medical-surgical patients.[165]

The implementation of an ICU analgesia, sedation, and delirium protocol has been associated with more RASS and CAM-ICU assessments per day than the baseline cohort, a reduction in hourly benzodiazepine dose, and a decreased delirium duration, as well as reductions in the median duration of mechanical ventilation, ICU stay, and length of hospitalization.[166]

A study designed to explore the effect of sedative administration for the prevention of delirium among ICU mechanically ventilated patients demonstrated that the incidence of delirium was significantly lowered in the simulated circadian clock group.[167] In the simulated circadian clock group, the incidence of delirium in the DEX group was significantly lower than that of the PRO group. Similarly, the duration of mechanical ventilation in the DEX group was significantly shorter than that of PRO group and the length of ICU stay was significantly shorter in the DEX versus PRO group. This study found that the use of DEX could reduce the incidence of delirium and improve the prognosis of patients compared with other sedative agents.

The Dexmedetomidine to Lessen ICU Agitation (DahLIA) study demonstrated that DEX increased ventilator-free hours at 7 days, reduced time to extubation, and accelerated resolution of delirium compared with placebo.[168] Among elderly patients admitted to the ICU after noncardiac surgery, the prophylactic use of low-dose DEX significantly decreased the occurrence of delirium (9% vs 23% in PBO) during the first 7 days after surgery.[169] A literature review found that the use of DEX for the prevention or treatment of ICU delirium in the elderly was associated with a reduction in delirium and decreased morbidity and mortality compared with benzodiazepines.[170]

A qualitative study using focus groups of doctors and nurses caring for patients with delirium in the ICU found that these professionals regarded patients with delirium with uncertainty and thought these patients were often underdiagnosed and poorly managed.[171] Doctors displayed discrepancies regarding pharmacologic prescriptions and decision-making, with choice of medication been determined by experience. Nurses thought that, for many doctors, delirium was not considered a matter of urgency in the ICU. Nurses also reported difficulties when applying restraint, managing sleep disorders, and providing early mobilization. Overall, participants thought that the lack of a delirium protocol generates conflicts regarding what type of care management to apply, especially during the night shift.

Although the ABCDE bundled approach to ICU care has been widely publicized and promoted by various medical and nursing professional organizations, a survey of attendees of the Michigan Health and Hospital Association's Keystone ICU collaborative annual meeting (76% response rate) found that only 12% reported having implemented routine spontaneous awakening trials and delirium assessments, as well as early mobility. Of these, 36% reported not having early mobility as an active goal in their units (nonmovers) and 52% reported attempts at early mobility without routine sedation interruption and delirium screening implementation.[172] In adjusted models, those who implemented exercise with sedation-interruption and delirium screening, were 3.5 times more likely to achieve higher levels of exercise in ventilated patients than those who implemented exercise without both sedation interruption and delirium screening (95% CI 1.4–8.6).

THE IMPACT OF DELIRIUM
Morbidity and Mortality Related to Delirium

Between 2000 and 2009, the number of ICU beds in the United States increased 15%, mirroring population growth.[173] Every year, 3.5 to 4 million patients survive critical care illness,[174,175] although studies suggest that up to 87% of critically ill patients develop delirium.[10] Patients who develop delirium fare much worse than their nondelirious counterparts when controlling for all other factors. Among medically ill inpatients, the development of delirium was associated with increased mortality at discharge and at 12 months, increased length of hospital stay, and institutionalization.[176] A systematic review found that delirium is associated with an increased risk of death compared with controls (38.0% vs 27.5%).[177]

Among mechanically ventilated ICU subjects (n = 275), delirium was associated with higher 6-month mortality rates, spending 10 days additional in-hospital days, fewer median days alive and without mechanical ventilation, and a higher incidence of cognitive impairment at hospital discharge compared with those without delirium.[178] Among elderly ICU subjects, the number of delirium days was significantly associated with time to death within 1-year post-ICU admission, after controlling all factors.[179] Among critically ill subjects, the presence of delirium at 24 hours from admission is an independent risk factor for increased in-hospital mortality.[180]

A meta-analysis of critically ill subjects (16 studies; n = 6410), found that subjects with delirium experienced higher mortality rates, had longer LOS in both the ICU and the general hospital, spent more time on mechanical ventilation, experienced a significantly higher rate (6 times) of complications, and were more likely to be placed at a long-term care facility rather than return home.[181]

Among coronary care unit patients, the occurrence of delirium was associated with an increased risk of in-hospital mortality and 1-year mortality.[114] A systematic review and meta-analysis revealed that delirious subjects experienced significantly higher mortality during admission and longer durations of mechanical ventilation and lengths of stay, in both the ICU and in hospital.[182] Among intubated ICU patients, delirium at the initiation of the weaning process was associated with more respiratory and neurologic complications, and a reduced probability of successful extubation.[183]

Among ICU patients with bloodstream infections, delirious patients (60% incidence) experienced a higher mortality, a lower proportion of return to functional baseline, and higher proportion of unfavorable outcome.[184] A study on weaning from mechanical ventilation and delirium (n = 393), revealed that 40.7% of subjects were diagnosed with delirium on the day of the first Spontaneous Breathing Trial, which was associated with difficult extubation and prolonged weaning (Jeon and colleagues, 2016).

Cognitive Sequelae

Among ICU subjects (n = 79), those who developed delirium experienced higher rates of cognitive impairment, and there was a positive association between severity of delirium scores and cognitive impairment at the time of hospital discharge.[9] Maldonado and colleagues[7] found that only 14% of subjects who developed ICU-delirium had returned to their baseline level of cognitive functioning by the time of discharge from the hospital. Although other investigators have found an even lower rate of recovery (4%) before discharge from the hospital, an additional 20.8% achieved resolution of symptoms by the third month, and an additional 17.7% by the sixth month after hospital discharge.[21]

Some investigators have estimated that about 40% of patients who experience delirium develop some form of chronic brain syndrome.[185,186] In some cases, the functional decline persisted longer than 6 months after hospital discharge.[187] Later studies found that cognitive deficits at hospital discharge were significantly associated with poor long-term cognitive functioning for up to 5 years after cardiac surgery.[188]

The occurrence of delirium among mechanically ventilated ICU patients was an independent predictor of worse scores on neuropsychological testing at follow-up, with cognitive impairment present in 79% and 71% of survivors at 3-month and 12-month follow-up, respectively, with 62% and 36% being severely impaired.[77] In addition, the investigators found that an increased delirium duration (from 1 to 5 days) was independently associated with a 7-point decline in cognitive battery mean scores at 12-month follow-up. Others have also found that longer duration of delirium was independently associated with worse global cognition and worse executive function at 3 and 12 months.[189]

A prospective 18-month follow-up study of ICU survivors (n = 1292) found that duration of delirium was significantly correlated to memory and naming impairments 18 months after discharge.[190] A study of critical care illness found that 81% and 72% of delirious patients experienced ongoing cognitive problems at 3 months and 12 months after release from the hospital, and that longer delirium duration was independently associated with increased odds of disability in activities of daily living and motor-sensory dysfunction in the following year.[191]

A systematic search found that patients who experienced delirium were at increased risk of dementia (62.5% vs 8.1%).[177] Even after adjusting for dementia severity, comorbidity, and demographic characteristics, patients who had developed delirium experienced greater cognitive deterioration in the year following hospitalization. With cognitive deterioration proceeding at twice the rate in the year after hospitalization compared with patients who did not develop delirium.[192]

The Vantaa 85+ study followed individuals 85 years and older (n = 553) for up to 10 years and found that delirium increased the risk of incident dementia and was associated with worsening dementia severity.[193] In fact, delirium was associated with the loss of 1.0 more Mini-Mental State Examination points per year (95% CI 0.11–1.89) compared with those with no history of delirium.

Studies have found a reciprocal relationship between cognitive deficits and dementia; that is, evidence suggests that the presence of baseline cognitive deficits, including dementia, lowers the threshold to develop delirium, whereas available data confirm that there is a significant acceleration in the slope of cognitive decline in patients with AD following an episode of delirium (Fong and colleagues, 2009).

Imaging studies have found a relationship between the occurrence of delirium and cerebral changes. Among ICU survivors with respiratory failure or shock, patients with longer delirium duration displayed greater evidence of brain atrophy as measured by a larger ventricle-to-brain ratio at the time of hospital discharge and at 3-month follow-up.[194] Similarly, longer delirium duration was also associated with smaller superior frontal lobe and hippocampal volumes at time of discharge ($P<.001$).

After ICU stay, fractional anisotropy was calculated using diffusion tensor imaging MRI. The imaging findings revealed that longer delirium duration (3 vs 0 days) was associated with lower fractional anisotropy in the genu ($P = .04$) and splenium ($P = .02$) of the corpus callosum, and in the anterior limb of the internal capsule ($P = .01$), at the time of hospital discharge and 3-month follow-up.[195] These associations persisted at 3 months for the genu ($P = .02$) and splenium of the corpus callosum ($P = .004$). Longitudinal follow-up revealed that white matter disruption was associated with worse cognitive scores up to 12 months later.

Behavioral Sequelae

An increasingly recognized consequence of delirium is the development of posttraumatic stress disorder (PTSD), likely associated with the dramatic and bizarre delusional thinking and hallucinations experienced during a delirious state and facilitated by a lack of factual recall of their ICU stay.[105,196–199] Among ICU patients, standardized interviews found that 73% of patients had delusional memories of their ICU experience at 2 weeks and that patients with no factual memories had the highest anxiety levels and PTSD symptoms after ICU discharge.[198]

A systematic review of studies (n = 26) in general ICU settings with mixed-diagnosis subjects found that the range of PTSD prevalence was 8% to 27%.[200] It identified several clinical (eg, use of benzodiazepines, duration of sedation, and mechanical ventilation) and psychological risk (ie, stress and fear experienced acutely in ICU, and frightening memories of the admission) factors for the development of PTSD.

Fiscal Impact

The economic impact of delirium is substantial, rivaling the health care costs of falls and diabetes mellitus. A retrospective study of medical and surgical subjects (n = 254) in a step-down critical care unit found that subjects who developed delirium used 22% of the total inpatient days and represented greater total costs per case ($63,900 vs $30,800).[7] Multiple studies have demonstrated that delirious subjects experienced prolonged hospital stays (average 5–10 days longer).[7,14,24,178,201,202] A systematic search found that subjects who experienced in-hospital delirium were at increased risk of institutionalization (33.4% vs 10.7%)[177] and had a greater need for placement in nursing homes or rehabilitation facilities.[24,203]

The national burden of delirium on the health care system has been estimated to range from $38 billion to $152 billion each year.[204]

SUMMARY

Delirium is a neurobehavioral syndrome caused by the transient disruption of normal neuronal activity secondary to systemic disturbances. It is also the most common neuropsychiatric syndrome found in the general hospital setting. In addition to causing distress to patients, families, and medical caregivers, the development of delirium has been associated with increased morbidity and mortality, increased cost of care, increased hospital-acquired complications, poor functional and cognitive recovery, decreased quality of life, prolonged hospital stays, and increased placement in specialized intermediate and long-term care facilities. What is clear from the evidence is that effective prevention and management strategies are needed in order better prevent delirium in the ICU and to decrease its economic burden and long-term physical, emotional, and cognitive effects. Given increasing evidence that delirium is not always reversible and the many sequelae associated with its development, physicians must do everything possible to prevents its occurrence or shorten its duration by recognizing its symptoms early, correcting underlying contributing causes, and using management strategies to improve functional outcomes.

REFERENCES

1. Bucht G, Gustafson Y, Sandberg O. Epidemiology of delirium. Dement Geriatr Cogn Disord 1999;10(5):315–8.
2. Fann JR. The epidemiology of delirium: a review of studies and methodological issues. Semin Clin Neuropsychiatry 2000;5(2):64–74.
3. Folstein MF, Bassett SS, Romanoski AJ, et al. The epidemiology of delirium in the community: the Eastern Baltimore Mental Health Survey. Int Psychogeriatr 1991; 3(2):169–76.

4. Levkoff S, Cleary P, Liptzin B, et al. Epidemiology of delirium: an overview of research issues and findings. Int Psychogeriatr 1991;3(2):149–67.
5. Schmidt LG, Grohmann R, Strauss A, et al. Epidemiology of toxic delirium due to psychotropic drugs in psychiatric hospitals. Compr Psychiatry 1987;28(3):242–9.
6. Vazquez F, O'Flaherty M, Michelangelo H, et al. Epidemiology of delirium in elderly inpatients. Medicina (B Aires) 2000;60(5 Pt 1):555–60 [in Spanish].
7. Maldonado JR, Dhami N, Wise L. Clinical implications of the recognition and management of delirium in general medical and surgical wards. Psychosomatics 2003;44(2):157–8.
8. Lahariya S, Grover S, Bagga S, et al. Phenomenology of delirium among patients admitted to a coronary care unit. Nord J Psychiatry 2016;70(8):626–32.
9. Sakuramoto H, Subrina J, Unoki T, et al. Severity of delirium in the ICU is associated with short term cognitive impairment. A prospective cohort study. Intensive Crit Care Nurs 2015;31(4):250–7.
10. Ely EW, Margolin R, Francis J, et al. Evaluation of delirium in critically ill patients: validation of the Confusion Assessment Method for the Intensive Care Unit (CAM-ICU). Crit Care Med 2001;29(7):1370–9.
11. Lin WL, Chan YF, Wang J. Factors associated with the development of delirium in elderly patients in intensive care units. J Nurs Res 2015;23(4):322–9.
12. Lawlor PG, Gagnon B, Mancini IL, et al. Occurrence, causes, and outcome of delirium in patients with advanced cancer: a prospective study. Arch Intern Med 2000;160(6):786–94.
13. Hughes CG, Pandharipande PP, Thompson JL, et al. Endothelial activation and blood-brain barrier injury as risk factors for delirium in critically ill patients. Crit Care Med 2016;44(9):e809–17.
14. Ely EW, Gautam S, Margolin R, et al. The impact of delirium in the intensive care unit on hospital length of stay. Intensive Care Med 2001;27(12):1892–900.
15. McNicoll L, Pisani MA, Zhang Y, et al. Delirium in the intensive care unit: occurrence and clinical course in older patients. J Am Geriatr Soc 2003;51(5):591–8.
16. Zaal IJ, Devlin JW, Peelen LM, et al. A systematic review of risk factors for delirium in the ICU. Crit Care Med 2015;43(1):40–7.
17. Bryczkowski SB, Lopreiato MC, Yonclas PP, et al. Risk factors for delirium in older trauma patients admitted to the surgical intensive care unit. J Trauma Acute Care Surg 2014;77(6):944–51.
18. Maldonado J. Delirium pathophysiology: current understanding of the neurobiology of acute brain failure. Int J Geriatr Psychiatry, in press.
19. American Psychiatric Association. Diagnostic and statistical manual of mental disorders. 5th edition. Washington, DC: American Psychiatric Association; 2013.
20. Levkoff SE, Liptzin B, Cleary PD, et al. Subsyndromal delirium. Am J Geriatr Psychiatry 1996;4(4):320–9.
21. Levkoff SE, Evans DA, Liptzin B, et al. Delirium. The occurrence and persistence of symptoms among elderly hospitalized patients. Arch Intern Med 1992;152(2):334–40.
22. Cole M, McCusker J, Dendukuri N, et al. The prognostic significance of subsyndromal delirium in elderly medical inpatients. J Am Geriatr Soc 2003;51(6):754–60.
23. Ouimet S, Kavanagh BP, Gottfried SB, et al. Incidence, risk factors and consequences of ICU delirium. Intensive Care Med 2007;33(1):66–73.
24. Francis J, Martin D, Kapoor WN. A prospective study of delirium in hospitalized elderly. JAMA 1990;263(8):1097–101.

25. Inouye SK. The dilemma of delirium: clinical and research controversies regarding diagnosis and evaluation of delirium in hospitalized elderly medical patients. Am J Med 1994;97(3):278–88.
26. World Health Organization. The international statistical classification of diseases and related health problems (ICD-10): classification of mental and behavioural disorders. Geneva (Switzerland): World Health Organization; 1992.
27. Bellelli G, Morandi A, Davis DH, et al. Validation of the 4AT, a new instrument for rapid delirium screening: a study in 234 hospitalised older people. Age Ageing 2014;43(4):496–502.
28. Maldonado J, Sher Y, Talley R, et al. The proxy test for delirium (PTD): a new tool for the screening of delirium based on DSM-5 and ICD-10 criteria. In Academy of Psychosomatic Medicine 2015 Annual Meeting. New Orleans, LA, November 13, 2015.
29. American Psychiatric Association. Diagnostic and statistical manual of mental disorders (DSM-II). Washington, DC: APPI; 1968.
30. Pfeiffer E. A short portable mental status questionnaire for the assessment of organic brain deficit in elderly patients. J Am Geriatr Soc 1975;23(10):433–41.
31. American Psychiatric Association. Diagnostic and statistical manual of mental disorders. 3rd edition. Washington, DC: American Psychiatric Association; 1987.
32. Trzepacz PT, Baker RW, Greenhouse J. A symptom rating scale for delirium. Psychiatry Res 1988;23(1):89–97.
33. Inouye S, van Dyck C, Alessi C, et al. Clarifying confusion: the confusion assessment method. A new method for detection of delirium. Ann Intern Med 1990; 113(12):941–8.
34. Albert MS, Levkoff SE, Reilly C, et al. The delirium symptom interview: an interview for the detection of delirium symptoms in hospitalized patients. J Geriatr Psychiatry Neurol 1992;5(1):14–21.
35. American Psychiatric Association. Diagnostic and statistical manual of mental disorders. 4th edition. Washington, DC: American Psychiatric Association; 1994.
36. O'keeffe S. Rating the severity of delirium: the delirium assessment scale. Int J Geriatr Psychiatry 1994;9(7):551–6.
37. Hart RP, Levenson JL, Sessler CN, et al. Validation of a cognitive test for delirium in medical ICU patients. Psychosomatics 1996;37(6):533–46.
38. Neelon VJ, Champagne MT, Carlson JR, et al. The NEECHAM Confusion Scale: construction, validation, and clinical testing. Nurs Res 1996;45(6):324–30.
39. Robertsson B, Karlsson I, Styrud E, et al. Confusional State Evaluation (CSE): an instrument for measuring severity of delirium in the elderly. Br J Psychiatry 1997; 170:565–70.
40. Breitbart W, Rosenfeld B, Roth A, et al. The Memorial Delirium Assessment Scale. J Pain Symptom Manage 1997;13(3):128–37.
41. McCusker J, Cole M, Bellavance F, et al. Reliability and validity of a new measure of severity of delirium. Int Psychogeriatr 1998;10(4):421–33.
42. Bettin KM, Maletta GJ, Dysken MW, et al. Measuring delirium severity in older general hospital inpatients without dementia. The Delirium Severity Scale. Am J Geriatr Psychiatry 1998;6(4):296–307.
43. Trzepacz PT, Mittal D, Torres R, et al. Validation of the Delirium Rating Scale-revised-98: comparison with the delirium rating scale and the cognitive test for delirium. J Neuropsychiatry Clin Neurosci 2001;13(2):229–42.
44. Otter H, Martin J, Basell K, et al. Validity and reliability of the DDS for severity of delirium in the ICU. Neurocrit Care 2005;2(2):150–8.

45. Han JH, Wilson A, Vasilevskis EE, et al. Diagnosing delirium in older emergency department patients: validity and reliability of the delirium triage screen and the brief confusion assessment method. Ann Emerg Med 2013;62(5):457–65.
46. Wassenaar A, van den Boogaard M, van Achterberg T, et al. Multinational development and validation of an early prediction model for delirium in ICU patients. Intensive Care Med 2015;41(6):1048–56.
47. Maldonado J, Sher Y, Garcia R, et al. Stanford's algorithm for predicting delirium (SAPD). Nashville (TN): American Delirium Society; 2017.
48. Folstein MF, Robins LN, Helzer JE. The Mini-Mental State Examination. Arch Gen Psychiatry 1983;40(7):812.
49. Bland RC, Newman SC. Mild dementia or cognitive impairment: the Modified Mini-Mental State examination (3MS) as a screen for dementia. Can J Psychiatry 2001;46(6):506–10.
50. O'Donnell WE, Reynolds DM, De Soto CB. Neuropsychological impairment scale (NIS): initial validation study using trailmaking test (A & B) and WAIS digit symbol (scaled score) in a mixed grouping of psychiatric, neurological, and normal patients. J Clin Psychol 1983;39(5):746–8.
51. Maldonado J. Novel algorithms for the prophylaxis & management of alcohol withdrawal syndromes – beyond benzodiazepines. Crit Care Clin, in press.
52. Maldonado J, van der Starre P, Wysong A, et al. Dexmedetomidine: can it reduce the incidence of ICU delirium in postcardiotomy patients? Psychosomatics 2004;45(2):173.
53. Zhang H, Lu Y, Liu M, et al. Strategies for prevention of postoperative delirium: a systematic review and meta-analysis of randomized trials. Crit Care 2013;17(2): R47.
54. Hirota T, Kishi T. Prophylactic antipsychotic use for postoperative delirium: a systematic review and meta-analysis. J Clin Psychiatry 2013;74(12):e1136–44.
55. Teslyar P, Stock VM, Wilk CM, et al. Prophylaxis with antipsychotic medication reduces the risk of post-operative delirium in elderly patients: a meta-analysis. Psychosomatics 2013;54(2):124–31.
56. O'Mahony R, Murthy L, Akunne A, et al, Guideline Development Group. Synopsis of the National Institute for Health and Clinical Excellence guideline for prevention of delirium. Ann Intern Med 2011;154(11):746–51.
57. Meagher DJ, McLoughlin L, Leonard M, et al. What do we really know about the treatment of delirium with antipsychotics? Ten key issues for delirium pharmacotherapy. Am J Geriatr Psychiatry 2013;21(12):1223–38.
58. Rothschild J, Leape L. The nature and extent of medical injury in older patients: executive summary. In Public Policy Institute, AARP. Washington, DC, May 2, 2000.
59. Inouye SK, Viscoli CM, Horwitz RI, et al. A predictive model for delirium in hospitalized elderly medical patients based on admission characteristics. Ann Intern Med 1993;119(6):474–81.
60. Inouye SK, Charpentier PA. Precipitating factors for delirium in hospitalized elderly persons. Predictive model and interrelationship with baseline vulnerability. JAMA 1996;275(11):852–7.
61. Bounds M, Kram S, Speroni KG, et al. Effect of ABCDE bundle implementation on prevalence of delirium in intensive care unit patients. Am J Crit Care 2016; 25(6):535–44.
62. Pandharipande PP, Patel MB, Barr J. Management of pain, agitation, and delirium in critically ill patients. Pol Arch Med Wewn 2014;124(3):114–23.

63. Balas MC, Vasilevskis EE, Olsen KM, et al. Effectiveness and safety of the awakening and breathing coordination, delirium monitoring/management, and early exercise/mobility bundle. Crit Care Med 2014;42(5):1024–36.
64. Inouye SK, Bogardus ST Jr, Charpentier PA, et al. A multicomponent intervention to prevent delirium in hospitalized older patients. N Engl J Med 1999;340(9): 669–76.
65. Maldonado JR. Delirium. In: Leigh H, Streltzer J, editors. Handbook of Consultation-Liaison psychiatry. 2nd edition. New York: Springer; 2014. p. 157–87.
66. Maldonado JR. Delirium: neurobiology, characteristics and management. In: Fogel B, Greenberg D, editors. Psychiatric care of the medical patient. New York: Oxford University Press; 2015. p. 823–907.
67. Maldonado JR, Dhami N. Recognition and management of delirium in the medical and surgical intensive care wards. J Psychosom Res 2003;55(2):150.
68. Pandharipande P, Shintani A, Peterson J, et al. Lorazepam is an independent risk factor for transitioning to delirium in intensive care unit patients. Anesthesiology 2006;104(1):21–6.
69. Richelson E. Receptor pharmacology of neuroleptics: relation to clinical effects. J Clin Psychiatry 1999;60(Suppl 10):5–14.
70. Taguchi T, Yano M, Kido Y. Influence of bright light therapy on postoperative patients: a pilot study. Intensive Crit Care Nurs 2007;23(5):289–97.
71. Patel J, Baldwin J, Bunting P, et al. The effect of a multicomponent multidisciplinary bundle of interventions on sleep and delirium in medical and surgical intensive care patients. Anaesthesia 2014;69(6):540–9.
72. Rivosecchi RM, Kane-Gill SL, Svec S, et al. The implementation of a nonpharmacologic protocol to prevent intensive care delirium. J Crit Care 2016;31(1): 206–11.
73. Álvarez EA, Garrido MA, Tobar EA, et al. Occupational therapy for delirium management in elderly patients without mechanical ventilation in an intensive care unit: a pilot randomized clinical trial. J Crit Care 2017;37:85–90.
74. Karadas C, Ozdemir L. The effect of range of motion exercises on delirium prevention among patients aged 65 and over in intensive care units. Geriatr Nurs 2016;37(3):180–5.
75. Serafim RB, Bozza FA, Soares M, et al. Pharmacologic prevention and treatment of delirium in intensive care patients: a systematic review. J Crit Care 2015; 30(4):799–807.
76. Prakanrattana U, Prapaitrakool S. Efficacy of risperidone for prevention of postoperative delirium in cardiac surgery. Anaesth Intensive Care 2007;35(5):714–9.
77. Girard TD, Jackson JC, Pandharipande PP, et al. Delirium as a predictor of longterm cognitive impairment in survivors of critical illness. Crit Care Med 2010; 38(7):1513–20.
78. van den Boogaard M, Schoonhoven L, van Achterberg T, et al. Haloperidol prophylaxis in critically ill patients with a high risk for delirium. Crit Care 2013;17(1): R9.
79. Larsen KA, Kelly SE, Stern TA, et al. Administration of olanzapine to prevent postoperative delirium in elderly joint-replacement patients: a randomized, controlled trial. Psychosomatics 2010;51(5):409–18.
80. Maldonado JR, van der Starre PJ, Block T, et al. Post-operative sedation and the incidence of delirium and cognitive deficits in cardiac surgery patients. Anesthesiology 2003;99:465.

81. Pandharipande PP, Pun BT, Herr DL, et al. Effect of sedation with dexmedetomidine vs lorazepam on acute brain dysfunction in mechanically ventilated patients: the MENDS randomized controlled trial. JAMA 2007;298(22):2644–53.
82. Riker RR, Shehabi Y, Bokesch PM, et al. Dexmedetomidine vs midazolam for sedation of critically ill patients: a randomized trial. JAMA 2009;301(5):489–99.
83. Pasin L, Landoni G, Nardelli P, et al. Dexmedetomidine reduces the risk of delirium, agitation and confusion in critically Ill patients: a meta-analysis of randomized controlled trials. J Cardiothorac Vasc Anesth 2014;28(6):1459–66.
84. Reade MC, O'Sullivan K, Bates S, et al. Dexmedetomidine vs. haloperidol in delirious, agitated, intubated patients: a randomised open-label trial. Crit Care 2009;13(3):R75.
85. Hudetz JA, Patterson KM, Iqbal Z, et al. Ketamine attenuates delirium after cardiac surgery with cardiopulmonary bypass. J Cardiothorac Vasc Anesth 2009;23(5):651–7.
86. Abu-Shahwan I. Effect of propofol on emergence behavior in children after sevoflurane general anesthesia. Paediatr Anaesth 2008;18(1):55–9.
87. Hanania M, Kitain E. Melatonin for treatment and prevention of postoperative delirium. Anesth Analg 2002;94(2):338–9. Table of contents.
88. Flannery AH, Oyler DR, Weinhouse GL. The impact of interventions to improve sleep on delirium in the ICU: a systematic review and research framework. Crit Care Med 2016;44(12):2231–40.
89. Hatta K, Kishi Y, Wada K, et al. Preventive effects of ramelteon on delirium: a randomized placebo-controlled trial. JAMA Psychiatry 2014;71(4):397–403.
90. Bourne RS, Mills GH, Minelli C. Melatonin therapy to improve nocturnal sleep in critically ill patients: encouraging results from a small randomised controlled trial. Crit Care 2008;12(2):R52.
91. Al-Aama T, Brymer C, Gutmanis I, et al. Melatonin decreases delirium in elderly patients: a randomized, placebo-controlled trial. Int J Geriatr Psychiatry 2011;26(7):687–94.
92. Sultan SS. Assessment of role of perioperative melatonin in prevention and treatment of postoperative delirium after hip arthroplasty under spinal anesthesia in the elderly. Saudi J Anaesth 2010;4(3):169–73.
93. Kimura R, Mori K, Kumazaki H, et al. Treatment of delirium with ramelteon: initial experience in three patients. Gen Hosp Psychiatry 2011;33(4):407–9.
94. Furuya M, Miyaoka T, Yasuda H, et al. Marked improvement in delirium with ramelteon: five case reports. Psychogeriatrics 2012;12(4):259–62.
95. Page VJ, Davis D, Zhao XB, et al. Statin use and risk of delirium in the critically ill. Am J Respir Crit Care Med 2014;189(6):666–73.
96. Morandi A, Hughes CG, Thompson JL, et al. Statins and delirium during critical illness: a multicenter, prospective cohort study. Crit Care Med 2014;42(8):1899–909.
97. Dautzenberg PL, Mulder LJ, Olde Rikkert MG, et al. Delirium in elderly hospitalised patients: protective effects of chronic rivastigmine usage. Int J Geriatr Psychiatry 2004;19(7):641–4.
98. van den Bliek BM, Maas HA. Successful treatment of three elderly patients suffering from prolonged delirium using the cholinesterase inhibitor rivastigmine. Ned Tijdschr Geneeskd 2004;148(43):2149 [author reply: 2149]; [in Dutch].
99. Moretti R, Torre P, Antonello RM, et al. Cholinesterase inhibition as a possible therapy for delirium in vascular dementia: a controlled, open 24-month study of 246 patients. Am J Alzheimers Dis Other Demen 2004;19(6):333–9.

100. Adams F, Fernandez F, Andersson B. Emergency pharmacotherapy of delirium in the critically ill cancer patient. Psychosomatics 1986;27(1 Suppl):33–8.
101. Fernandez F, Holmes VF, Adams F, et al. Treatment of severe, refractory agitation with a haloperidol drip. J Clin Psychiatry 1988;49(6):239–41.
102. Riker RR, Fraser GL, Cox PM. Continuous infusion of haloperidol controls agitation in critically ill patients. Crit Care Med 1994;22(3):433–40.
103. Sanders KM, Minnema MA, Murray GB. Low incidence of extrapyramidal symptoms in treatment of delirium with intravenous haloperidol and lorazepam in the intensive care unit. J Intensive Care Med 1989;4(5):201–4.
104. Ziehm SR. Intravenous haloperidol for tranquilization in critical care patients: a review and critique. AACN Clin Issues Crit Care Nurs 1991;2(4):765–77.
105. Breitbart W, Gibson C, Tremblay A. The delirium experience: delirium recall and delirium-related distress in hospitalized patients with cancer, their spouses/caregivers, and their nurses. Psychosomatics 2002;43(3):183–94.
106. Straker DA, Shapiro PA, Muskin PR. Aripiprazole in the treatment of delirium. Psychosomatics 2006;47(5):385–91.
107. Boettger S, Breitbart W. An open trial of aripiprazole for the treatment of delirium in hospitalized cancer patients. Palliat Support Care 2011;9(4):351–7.
108. Adams F. Neuropsychiatric evaluation and treatment of delirium in cancer patients. Adv Psychosom Med 1988;18:26–36.
109. Ayd FJ Jr. Haloperidol: twenty years' clinical experience. J Clin Psychiatry 1978; 39(11):807–14.
110. Sanders KM, Murray GB, Cassem NH. High-dose intravenous haloperidol for agitated delirium in a cardiac patient on intra-aortic balloon pump. J Clin Psychopharmacol 1991;11(2):146–7.
111. Stern TA. Continuous infusion of haloperidol in agitated, critically ill patients. Crit Care Med 1994;22(3):378–9.
112. Tesar GE, Murray GB, Cassem NH. Use of high-dose intravenous haloperidol in the treatment of agitated cardiac patients. J Clin Psychopharmacol 1985;5(6): 344–7.
113. Tune L. The role of antipsychotics in treating delirium. Curr Psychiatry Rep 2002; 4(3):209–12. Available at: http://www.ncbi.nlm.nih.gov/entrez/query.fcgi? cmd=Retrieve&db=PubMed&dopt=Citation&list_uids=12003684.
114. Naksuk N, Thongprayoon C, Park JY, et al. Clinical impact of delirium and antipsychotic therapy: 10-Year experience from a referral coronary care unit. Eur Heart J Acute Cardiovasc Care 2015. [Epub ahead of print].
115. Wilt JL, Minnema AM, Johnson RF, et al. Torsade de pointes associated with the use of intravenous haloperidol. Ann Intern Med 1993;119(5):391–4.
116. Lawrence KR, Nasraway SA. Conduction disturbances associated with administration of butyrophenone antipsychotics in the critically ill: a review of the literature. Pharmacotherapy 1997;17(3):531–7.
117. Shapiro BA, Warren J, Egol AB, et al. Practice parameters for intravenous analgesia and sedation for adult patients in the intensive care unit: an executive summary. Society of Critical Care Medicine. Crit Care Med 1995;23(9): 1596–600.
118. Khasati N, Thompson J, Dunning J. Is haloperidol or a benzodiazepine the safest treatment for acute psychosis in the critically ill patient? Interact Cardiovasc Thorac Surg 2004;3(2):233–6.
119. NICE, National Institute for Health and Care Excellence. Delirium: diagnosis, prevention and management (Clinical guideline; no. 103). National Guideline

Clearinghouse; 2010. Available at: http://www.nice.org.uk/nicemedia/live/13060/49909/49909.pdf. Accessed July 30, 2011.

120. Young J, Murthy L, Westby M, et al. Diagnosis, prevention, and management of delirium: summary of NICE guidance. BMJ 2010;341:c3704.

121. Jacobi J, Fraser GL, Coursin DB, et al. Clinical practice guidelines for the sustained use of sedatives and analgesics in the critically ill adult. Crit Care Med 2002;30(1):119–41.

122. American Psychiatric Association. Guideline watch: practice guideline for the treatment of patients with delirium. In: Cook IA, editor. American Psychiatric Association Practice guidelines. Washington, DC: American Psychiatric Association; 2004. p. 1–4.

123. Lonergan E, Britton AM, Luxenberg J, et al. Antipsychotics for delirium. Cochrane Database Syst Rev 2007;(2):CD005594.

124. Ozbolt LB, Paniagua MA, Kaiser RM. Atypical antipsychotics for the treatment of delirious elders. J Am Med Dir Assoc 2008;9(1):18–28.

125. Alao AO, Moskowitz L. Aripiprazole and delirium. Ann Clin Psychiatry 2006; 18(4):267–9.

126. Eremenko AA, Chernova EV. Treatment of delirium in the early postoperative period after cardiac surgery. Anesteziol Reanimatol 2014;(3):30–4 [in Russian].

127. Djaiani G, Silverton N, Fedorko L, et al. Dexmedetomidine versus propofol sedation reduces delirium after cardiac surgery: a randomized controlled trial. Anesthesiology 2016;124(2):362–8.

128. Pandharipande PP, Sanders RD, Girard TD, et al. Effect of dexmedetomidine versus lorazepam on outcome in patients with sepsis: an a priori-designed analysis of the MENDS randomized controlled trial. Crit Care 2010;14(2):R38.

129. Carrasco G, Baeza N, Cabré L, et al. Dexmedetomidine for the treatment of hyperactive delirium refractory to haloperidol in nonintubated ICU patients: a nonrandomized controlled trial. Crit Care Med 2016;44(7):1295–306.

130. Choi JY, Kim JM, Kwon CH, et al. Use of dexmedetomidine in liver transplant recipients with postoperative agitated delirium. Transplant Proc 2016;48(4):1063–6.

131. Liu X, Xie G, Zhang K, et al. Dexmedetomidine vs propofol sedation reduces delirium in patients after cardiac surgery: a meta-analysis with trial sequential analysis of randomized controlled trials. J Crit Care 2017;38:190–6.

132. Bourgeois JA, Koike AK, Simmons JE, et al. Adjunctive valproic acid for delirium and/or agitation on a consultation-liaison service: a report of six cases. J Neuropsychiatry Clin Neurosci 2005;17(2):232–8.

133. Sher Y, Miller AC, Lolak S, et al. Adjunctive valproic acid in management-refractory hyperactive delirium: a case series and rationale. J Neuropsychiatry Clin Neurosci 2015;27(4):365–70.

134. Burt T. Donepezil and related cholinesterase inhibitors as mood and behavioral controlling agents. Curr Psychiatry Rep 2000;2(6):473–8.

135. Bruera E, Strasser F, Shen L, et al. The effect of donepezil on sedation and other symptoms in patients receiving opioids for cancer pain: a pilot study. J Pain Symptom Manage 2003;26(5):1049–54.

136. Fisher RS, Bortz JJ, Blum DE, et al. A pilot study of donepezil for memory problems in epilepsy. Epilepsy Behav 2001;2(4):330–4.

137. Gleason OC. Donepezil for postoperative delirium. Psychosomatics 2003;44(5):437–8.

138. Haase U, Rundshagen I. Pharmacotherapy–physostigmine administered post-operatively. Anasthesiol Intensivmed Notfallmed Schmerzther 2007;42(3): 188–9 [in German].
139. Hori K, Tominaga I, Inada T, et al. Donepezil-responsive alcohol-related prolonged delirium. Psychiatry Clin Neurosci 2003;57(6):603–4.
140. Kaufer DI, Catt KE, Lopez OL, et al. Dementia with Lewy bodies: response of delirium-like features to donepezil. Neurology 1998;51(5):1512.
141. Kobayashi K, Higashima M, Mutou K, et al. Severe delirium due to basal forebrain vascular lesion and efficacy of donepezil. Prog Neuropsychopharmacol Biol Psychiatry 2004;28(7):1189–94.
142. Logan CJ, Stewart JT. Treatment of post-electroconvulsive therapy delirium and agitation with donepezil. J Ect 2007;23(1):28–9.
143. Palmer TR. Donepezil in advanced dementia, or delirium? J Am Med Dir Assoc 2004;5(1):67.
144. Rabinowitz T. Delirium: an important (but often unrecognized) clinical syndrome. Curr Psychiatry Rep 2002;4(3):202–8.
145. Weizberg M, Su M, Mazzola JL, et al. Altered mental status from olanzapine overdose treated with physostigmine. Clin Toxicol (Phila) 2006;44(3):319–25.
146. Wengel SP, Roccaforte WH, Burke WJ. Donepezil improves symptoms of delirium in dementia: implications for future research. J Geriatr Psychiatry Neurol 1998;11(3):159–61.
147. Gaudreau JD, Gagnon P, Roy MA, et al. Association between psychoactive medications and delirium in hospitalized patients: a critical review. Psychosomatics 2005;46(4):302–16.
148. Wengel SP, Burke WJ, Roccaforte WH. Donepezil for postoperative delirium associated with Alzheimer's disease. J Am Geriatr Soc 1999;47(3):379–80.
149. Brown DV, Heller F, Barkin R. Anticholinergic syndrome after anesthesia: a case report and review. Am J Ther 2004;11(2):144–53.
150. Funk W, Hollnberger H, Geroldinger J. Physostigmine and anaesthesia emergence delirium in preschool children: a randomized blinded trial. Eur J Anaesthesiol 2008;25(1):37–42.
151. Stern TA. Continuous infusion of physostigmine in anticholinergic delirium: case report. J Clin Psychiatry 1983;44(12):463–4.
152. Lipowski ZJ. Delirium, clouding of consciousness and confusion. J Nerv Ment Dis 1967;145(3):227–55.
153. Beaver KM, Gavin TJ. Treatment of acute anticholinergic poisoning with physostigmine. Am J Emerg Med 1998;16(5):505–7.
154. Richardson WH 3rd, Williams SR, Carstairs SD. A picturesque reversal of antimuscarinic delirium. J Emerg Med 2004;26(4):463.
155. Eyer F, Pfab R, Felgenhauer N, et al. Clinical and analytical features of severe suicidal quetiapine overdoses–a retrospective cohort study. Clin Toxicol (Phila) 2011;49(9):846–53.
156. Hail SL, Obafemi A, Kleinschmidt KC. Successful management of olanzapine-induced anticholinergic agitation and delirium with a continuous intravenous infusion of physostigmine in a pediatric patient. Clin Toxicol (Phila) 2013;51(3): 162–6.
157. Burns MJ, Linden CH, Graudins A, et al. A comparison of physostigmine and benzodiazepines for the treatment of anticholinergic poisoning. Ann Emerg Med 2000;35(4):374–81.

158. Bayindir O, Guden M, Akpinar B, et al. Ondansetron hydrochloride for the treatment of delirium after coronary artery surgery. J Thorac Cardiovasc Surg 2001; 121(1):176–7.
159. Giacino JT, Whyte J, Bagiella E, et al. Placebo-controlled trial of amantadine for severe traumatic brain injury. N Engl J Med 2012;366(9):819–26.
160. Hammond FM, Bickett AK, Norton JH, et al. Effectiveness of amantadine hydrochloride in the reduction of chronic traumatic brain injury irritability and aggression. J Head Trauma Rehabil 2014;29(5):391–9.
161. Sawyer E, Mauro LS, Ohlinger MJ. Amantadine enhancement of arousal and cognition after traumatic brain injury. Ann Pharmacother 2008;42(2):247–52.
162. Wheaton P, Mathias JL, Vink R. Impact of early pharmacological treatment on cognitive and behavioral outcome after traumatic brain injury in adults: a meta-analysis. J Clin Psychopharmacol 2009;29(5):468–77.
163. Van Reekum R, Bayley M, Garner S, et al. N of 1 study: amantadine for the amotivational syndrome in a patient with traumatic brain injury. Brain Inj 1995;9(1): 49–53.
164. Sullinger D, Gilmer A, Jurado L, et al. Development, implementation, and outcomes of a delirium protocol in the surgical trauma intensive care unit. Ann Pharmacother 2016. [Epub ahead of print].
165. Smith CD, Grami P. Feasibility and effectiveness of a delirium prevention bundle in critically ill patients. Am J Crit Care 2016;26(1):19–27.
166. Dale CR, Kannas DA, Fan VS, et al. Improved analgesia, sedation, and delirium protocol associated with decreased duration of delirium and mechanical ventilation. Ann Am Thorac Soc 2014;11(3):367–74.
167. Li J, Dong C, Zhang H, et al. Study of prevention and control of delirium in ventilated patients by simulating blockage of circadian rhythm with sedative in intensive care unit. Zhonghua Wei Zhong Bing Ji Jiu Yi Xue 2016;28(1):50–6 [in Chinese].
168. Reade MC, Eastwood GM, Bellomo R, et al. Effect of dexmedetomidine added to standard care on ventilator-free time in patients with agitated delirium: a randomized clinical trial. JAMA 2016;315(14):1460–8.
169. Su X, Meng ZT, Wu XH, et al. Dexmedetomidine for prevention of delirium in elderly patients after non-cardiac surgery: a randomised, double-blind, placebo-controlled trial. Lancet 2016;388(10054):1893–902.
170. Rosenzweig AB, Sittambalam CD. A new approach to the prevention and treatment of delirium in elderly patients in the intensive care unit. J Community Hosp Intern Med Perspect 2015;5(4):27950.
171. Palacios-Ceña D, Cachón-Pérez JM, Martínez-Piedrola R, et al. How do doctors and nurses manage delirium in intensive care units? A qualitative study using focus groups. BMJ Open 2016;6(1):e009678.
172. Michaud CJ, Bullard HM, Harris SA, et al. Impact of Quetiapine treatment on duration of hypoactive delirium in critically ill adults: a retrospective analysis. Pharmacotherapy 2015;35(8):731–9.
173. Wallace DJ, Angus DC, Seymour CW, et al. Critical care bed growth in the United States. A comparison of regional and national trends. Am J Respir Crit Care Med 2015;191(4):410–6.
174. Society of Critical Care Medicine. Critical care statistics in the United States. Society of Critical Care Medicine; 2012. Available at: http://www.sccm.org/Communications/Pages/CriticalCareStats.aspx.
175. Wunsch H, Guerra C, Barnato AE, et al. Three-year outcomes for Medicare beneficiaries who survive intensive care. JAMA 2010;303(9):849–56.

176. Siddiqi N, House AO, Holmes JD. Occurrence and outcome of delirium in medical in-patients: a systematic literature review. Age Ageing 2006;35(4):350–64.
177. Witlox J, Eurelings LS, de Jonghe JF, et al. Delirium in elderly patients and the risk of postdischarge mortality, institutionalization, and dementia: a meta-analysis. JAMA 2010;304(4):443–51.
178. Ely EW, Shintani A, Truman B, et al. Delirium as a predictor of mortality in mechanically ventilated patients in the intensive care unit. JAMA 2004;291(14): 1753–62.
179. Pisani MA, Kong SY, Kasl SV, et al. Days of delirium are associated with 1-year mortality in an older intensive care unit population. Am J Respir Crit Care Med 2009;180(11):1092–7.
180. van den Boogaard M, Peters SA, van der Hoeven JG, et al. The impact of delirium on the prediction of in-hospital mortality in intensive care patients. Crit Care 2010;14(4):R146.
181. Zhang Z, Pan L, Ni H. Impact of delirium on clinical outcome in critically ill patients: a meta-analysis. Gen Hosp Psychiatry 2013;35(2):105–11.
182. Salluh JI, Wang H, Schneider EB, et al. Outcome of delirium in critically ill patients: systematic review and meta-analysis. BMJ 2015;350:h2538.
183. Mekontso Dessap A, Roche-Campo F, Launay JM, et al. Delirium and circadian rhythm of melatonin during weaning from mechanical ventilation: an ancillary study of a weaning trial. Chest 2015;148(5):1231–41.
184. Dittrich T, Tschudin-Sutter S, Widmer AF, et al. Risk factors for new-onset delirium in patients with bloodstream infections: independent and quantitative effect of catheters and drainages-a four-year cohort study. Ann Intensive Care 2016;6(1):104.
185. Pompei P, Foreman M, Rudberg MA, et al. Delirium in hospitalized older persons: outcomes and predictors. J Am Geriatr Soc 1994;42(8):809–15.
186. Jackson JC, Gordon SM, Hart RP, et al. The association between delirium and cognitive decline: a review of the empirical literature. Neuropsychol Rev 2004; 14(2):87–98.
187. Murray AM, Levkoff SE, Wetle TT, et al. Acute delirium and functional decline in the hospitalized elderly patient. J Gerontol 1993;48(5):M181–6.
188. Newman MF, Grocott HP, Mathew JP, et al. Report of the substudy assessing the impact of neurocognitive function on quality of life 5 years after cardiac surgery. Stroke 2001;32(12):2874–81.
189. Pandharipande PP, Girard TD, Jackson JC, et al. Long-term cognitive impairment after critical illness. N Engl J Med 2013;369(14):1306–16.
190. van den Boogaard M, Schoonhoven L, Evers AW, et al. Delirium in critically ill patients: impact on long-term health-related quality of life and cognitive functioning. Crit Care Med 2012;40(1):112–8.
191. Brummel NE, Jackson JC, Pandharipande PP, et al. Delirium in the ICU and subsequent long-term disability among survivors of mechanical ventilation. Crit Care Med 2014;42(2):369–77.
192. Gross AL, Jones RN, Habtemariam DA, et al. Delirium and long-term cognitive trajectory among persons with dementia. Arch Intern Med 2012;172(17): 1324–31.
193. Davis DH, Muniz Terrera G, Keage H, et al. Delirium is a strong risk factor for dementia in the oldest-old: a population-based cohort study. Brain 2012; 135(Pt 9):2809–16.
194. Gunther ML, Morandi A, Krauskopf E, et al. The association between brain volumes, delirium duration, and cognitive outcomes in intensive care unit survivors:

the VISIONS cohort magnetic resonance imaging study*. Crit Care Med 2012; 40(7):2022–32.

195. Morandi A, Rogers BP, Gunther ML, et al. The relationship between delirium duration, white matter integrity, and cognitive impairment in intensive care unit survivors as determined by diffusion tensor imaging: the VISIONS prospective cohort magnetic resonance imaging study*. Crit Care Med 2012;40(7):2182–9.

196. Dew MA, Kormos RL, DiMartini AF, et al. Prevalence and risk of depression and anxiety-related disorders during the first three years after heart transplantation. Psychosomatics 2001;42(4):300–13.

197. DiMartini A, Dew MA, Kormos R, et al. Posttraumatic stress disorder caused by hallucinations and delusions experienced in delirium. Psychosomatics 2007; 48(5):436–9.

198. Jones C, Griffiths RD, Humphris G, et al. Memory, delusions, and the development of acute posttraumatic stress disorder-related symptoms after intensive care. Crit Care Med 2001;29(3):573–80.

199. Stukas AA Jr, Dew MA, Switzer GE, et al. PTSD in heart transplant recipients and their primary family caregivers. Psychosomatics 1999;40(3):212–21.

200. Wade D, Hardy R, Howell D, et al. Identifying clinical and acute psychological risk factors for PTSD after critical care: a systematic review. Minerva Anestesiol 2013;79(8):944–63.

201. Ritchie J, Steiner W, Abrahamowicz M. Incidence of and risk factors for delirium among psychiatric inpatients. Psychiatr Serv 1996;47(7):727–30.

202. González M, de Pablo J, Fuente E, et al. Instrument for detection of delirium in general hospitals: adaptation of the confusion assessment method. Psychosomatics 2004;45(5):426–31.

203. O'Keeffe S, Lavan J. The prognostic significance of delirium in older hospital patients. J Am Geriatr Soc 1997;45(2):174–8.

204. Leslie DL, Marcantonio ER, Zhang Y, et al. One-year health care costs associated with delirium in the elderly population. Arch Intern Med 2008;168(1):27–32.

205. Kean J, Trzepacz PT, Murray LL, et al. Initial validation of a brief provisional diagnostic scale for delirium. Brain Inj 2010;24(10):1222–30.

206. Schindler BA, Shook J, Schwartz GM. Beneficial effects of psychiatric intervention on recovery after coronary artery bypass graft surgery. Gen Hosp Psychiatry 1989;11(5):358–64.

207. Wanich CK, Sullivan-Marx EM, Gottlieb GL, et al. Functional status outcomes of a nursing intervention in hospitalized elderly. Image J Nurs Sch 1992;24(3): 201–7.

208. Milisen K, Foreman MD, Abraham IL, et al. A nurse-led interdisciplinary intervention program for delirium in elderly hip-fracture patients. J Am Geriatr Soc 2001; 49(5):523–32.

209. Marcantonio ER, Flacker JM, Wright RJ, et al. Reducing delirium after hip fracture: a randomized trial. J Am Geriatr Soc 2001;49(5):516–22.

210. Tabet N, Hudson S, Sweeney V, et al. An educational intervention can prevent delirium on acute medical wards. Age Ageing 2005;34(2):152–6.

211. Wong CP, Chiu PK, Chu LW. Zopiclone withdrawal: an unusual cause of delirium in the elderly. Age Ageing 2005;34(5):526–7.

212. Vidan M, Serra JA, Moreno C, et al. Efficacy of a comprehensive geriatric intervention in older patients hospitalized for hip fracture: a randomized, controlled trial. J Am Geriatr Soc 2005;53(9):1476–82.

213. Lundstrom M, Olofsson B, Stenvall M, et al. Postoperative delirium in old patients with femoral neck fracture: a randomized intervention study. Aging Clin Exp Res 2007;19(3):178–86.

214. Caplan GA, Harper EL. Recruitment of volunteers to improve vitality in the elderly: the REVIVE study. Intern Med J 2007;37(2):95–100.

215. Benedict L, Hazelett S, Fleming E, et al. Prevention, detection and intervention with delirium in an acute care hospital: a feasibility study. Int J Older People Nurs 2009;4(3):194–202.

216. Schweickert WD, Pohlman MC, Pohlman AS, et al. Early physical and occupational therapy in mechanically ventilated, critically ill patients: a randomised controlled trial. Lancet 2009;373:1874–82.

217. Holroyd-Leduc JM, Abelseth GA, Khandwala F, et al. A pragmatic study exploring the prevention of delirium among hospitalized older hip fracture patients: applying evidence to routine clinical practice using clinical decision support. Implement Sci 2010;5:81.

218. Bjorkelund KB, Hommel A, Thorngren KG, et al. Reducing delirium in elderly patients with hip fracture: a multi-factorial intervention study. Acta Anaesthesiol Scand 2010;54:678–88.

219. Colombo R, Corona A, Praga F, et al. A reorientation strategy for reducing delirium in the critically ill. Results of an interventional study. Minerva Anestesiol 2012;78:1026–33.

220. Gagnon P, Allard P, Gagnon B, et al. Delirium prevention in terminal cancer: assessment of a multicomponent intervention. Psychooncology 2012;21:187–94.

221. Martinez FT, Tobar C, Beddings CI, et al. Preventing delirium in an acute hospital using a non-pharmacological intervention. Age Ageing 2012;41:629–34.

222. Kaneko T, Jianhui C, Ishikura T, et al. Prophylactic consecutive administration of haloperidol can reduce the occurrence of postoperative delirium in gastrointestinal surgery. Yonago Acta Med 1999;179–84.

223. Kalisvaart K, de Jonghe J, Bogaards M, et al. Haloperidol prophylaxis for elderly hip-surgery patients at risk for delirium: a randomized placebo-controlled study. J Am Geriatr Soc 2005;53:1658–66.

224. Wang EH, Mabasa VH, Loh GW, et al. Haloperidol dosing strategies in the treatment of delirium in the critically ill. Neurocrit Care 2012;16:170–83.

225. Neufeld KJ, Yue J, Robinson TN, et al. Antipsychotic medication for prevention and treatment of delirium in hospitalized adults: a systematic review and meta-analysis. J Am Geriatr Soc 2016;64:705–14.

226. Berggren D, Gustafson Y, Eriksson B, et al. Postoperative confusion after anesthesia in elderly patients with femoral neck fractures. Anesth Analg 1987;66:497–504.

227. Williams-Russo P, Urquhart BL, Sharrock NE, et al. Post-operative delirium: predictors and prognosis in elderly orthopedic patients. J Am Geriatr Soc 1992;40:759–67.

228. Aizawa K, Kanai T, Saikawa Y, et al. A novel approach to the prevention of postoperative delirium in the elderly after gastrointestinal surgery. Surg Today 2002;32:310–4.

229. Maldonado JR, Wysong A, van der Starre PJ, et al. Dexmedetomidine and the reduction of postoperative delirium after cardiac surgery. Psychosomatics 2009;50:206–17.

230. Shehabi Y, Grant P, Wolfenden H, et al. Prevalence of delirium with dexmedetomidine compared with morphine based therapy after cardiac surgery: a

randomized controlled trial (DEXmedetomidine COmpared to Morphine-DEX-COM Study). Anesthesiology 2009;111:1075–84.

231. Rubino AS, Onorati F, Caroleo S, et al. Impact of clonidine administration on delirium and related respiratory weaning after surgical correction of acute type-A aortic dissection: results of a pilot study. Interact Cardiovasc Thorac Surg 2010;10:58–62.

232. Jakob SM, Ruokonen E, Grounds RM, et al. Dexmedetomidine vs midazolam or propofol for sedation during prolonged mechanical ventilation: two randomized controlled trials. JAMA 2012;307:1151–60.

233. de Jonghe A, Korevaar JC, van Munster BC, et al. Effectiveness of melatonin treatment on circadian rhythm disturbances in dementia. Are there implications for delirium? A systematic review. Int J Geriatr Psychiatry 2010;25:1201–8.

234. de Jonghe A, van Munster BC, van Oosten HE, et al. The effects of melatonin versus placebo on delirium in hip fracture patients: study protocol of a rando-mised, placebo-controlled, double blind trial. BMC Geriatr 2011;11:34.

235. Liptzin B, Laki A, Garb JL, et al. Donepezil in the prevention and treatment of post-surgical delirium. Am J Geriatr Psychiatry 2005;13:1100–6.

236. Sampson EL, Raven PR, Ndhlovu PN, et al. A randomized, double-blind, pla-cebo-controlled trial of donepezil hydrochloride (Aricept) for reducing the inci-dence of postoperative delirium after elective total hip replacement. Int J Geriatr Psychiatry 2007;22:343–9.

237. Oldenbeuving AW, de Kort PL, Jansen BP, et al. A pilot study of rivastigmine in the treatment of delirium after stroke: a safe alternative. BMC Neurol 2008;8:34.

238. Gamberini M, Bolliger D, Lurati Buse GA, et al. Rivastigmine for the prevention of postoperative delirium in elderly patients undergoing elective cardiac sur-gery–a randomized controlled trial. Crit Care Med 2009;37:1762–8.

239. van Eijk MM. Treatment of the delirious critically ill patient. Netherlands Journal of Critical Care 2012;16:200–10.

240. Breitbart W, Marotta R, Platt MM, et al. A double-blind trial of haloperidol, chlor-promazine, and lorazepam in the treatment of delirium in hospitalized AIDS pa-tients. Am J Psychiatry 1996;153:231–7.

241. Sipahimalani A, Masand PS. Olanzapine in the treatment of delirium. Psychoso-matics 1998;39:422–30.

242. Schwartz TL, Masand PS. Treatment of delirium with quetiapine. Prim Care Com-panion J Clin Psychiatry 2000;2:10–2.

243. Kim KS, Pae CU, Chae JH, et al. An open pilot trial of olanzapine for delirium in the Korean population. Psychiatry Clin Neurosci 2001;55:515–9.

244. Horikawa N, Yamazaki T, Miyamoto K, et al. Treatment for delirium with risperi-done: results of a prospective open trial with 10 patients. Gen Hosp Psychiatry 2003;25:289–92.

245. Sasaki Y, Matsuyama T, Inoue S, et al. A prospective, open-label, flexible-dose study of quetiapine in the treatment of delirium. J Clin Psychiatry 2003;64:1316–21.

246. Kim KY, Bader GM, Kotlyar V, et al. Treatment of delirium in older adults with quetiapine. J Geriatr Psychiatry Neurol 2003;16:29–31.

247. Liu CY, Juang YY, Liang HY, et al. Efficacy of risperidone in treating the hyper-active symptoms of delirium. Int Clin Psychopharmacol 2004;19:165–8.

248. Mittal D, Jimerson NA, Neely EP, et al. Risperidone in the treatment of delirium: results from a prospective open-label trial. J Clin Psychiatry 2004;65:662–7.

249. Parellada E, Baeza I, de Pablo J, et al. Risperidone in the treatment of patients with delirium. J Clin Psychiatry 2004;65:348–53.

250. Pae CU, Lee SJ, Lee CU, et al. A pilot trial of quetiapine for the treatment of patients with delirium. Hum Psychopharmacol 2004;19:125–7.
251. Han CS, Kim YK. A double-blind trial of risperidone and haloperidol for the treatment of delirium. Psychosomatics 2004;45:297–301.
252. Hu H, Deng W, Yang H. A prospective random control study comparison of olanzapine and haloperidol in senile delirium. Chongging Medical Journal 2004;1234–7.
253. Skrobik YK, Bergeron N, Dumont M, et al. Olanzapine vs haloperidol: treating delirium in a critical care setting. Intensive Care Med 2004;30:444–9.
254. Toda H, Kusumi I, Sasaki Y, et al. Relationship between plasma concentration levels of risperidone and clinical effects in the treatment of delirium. Int Clin Psychopharmacol 2005;20:331–3.
255. Lee KU, Won WY, Lee HK, et al. Amisulpride versus quetiapine for the treatment of delirium: a randomized, open prospective study. Int Clin Psychopharmacol 2005;20:311–4.
256. Takeuchi T, Furuta K, Hirasawa T, et al. Perospirone in the treatment of patients with delirium. Psychiatry Clin Neurosci 2007;61:67–70.
257. Maneeton B, Maneeton N, Srisurapanont M. An open-label study of quetiapine for delirium. J Med Assoc Thai 2007;90:2158–63.
258. Devlin JW, Roberts RJ, Fong JJ, et al. Efficacy and safety of quetiapine in critically ill patients with delirium: a prospective, multicenter, randomized, double-blind, placebo-controlled pilot study. Crit Care Med 2010;38:419–27.
259. Kim SW, Yoo JA, Lee SY, et al. Risperidone versus olanzapine for the treatment of delirium. Hum Psychopharmacol 2010;25:298–302.
260. Tahir TA, Eeles E, Karapareddy V, et al. A randomized controlled trial of quetiapine versus placebo in the treatment of delirium. J Psychosom Res 2010;69:485–90.
261. Grover S, Mattoo SK, Gupta N. Usefulness of atypical antipsychotics and choline esterase inhibitors in delirium: a review. Pharmacopsychiatry 2011;44:43–54.
262. Hakim SM, Othman AI, Naoum DO. Early treatment with risperidone for subsyndromal delirium after on-pump cardiac surgery in the elderly: a randomized trial. Anesthesiology 2012;116:987–97.
263. Kishi Y, Kato M, Okuyama T, et al. Delirium: patient characteristics that predict a missed diagnosis at psychiatric consultation. Gen Hosp Psychiatry 2007;29:442–5.
264. Tagarakis GI, Voucharas C, Tsolaki F, et al. Ondasetron versus haloperidol for the treatment of postcardiotomy delirium: a prospective, randomized, double-blinded study. J Cardiothorac Surg 2012;7:25.
265. Yoon HJ, Park KM, Choi WJ, et al. Efficacy and safety of haloperidol versus atypical antipsychotic medications in the treatment of delirium. BMC Psychiatry 2013;13:240.
266. Maneeton B, Maneeton N, Srisurapanont M, et al. Quetiapine versus haloperidol in the treatment of delirium: a double-blind, randomized, controlled trial. Drug Des Devel Ther 2013;7:657–67.

Assessment and Management of Toxidromes in the Critical Care Unit

J.J. Rasimas, MD, PhD, FAPM[a],*, Courtney M. Sinclair, BA[b]

KEYWORDS

- Toxidrome • Delirium • Antidote • Physostigmine • Flumazenil • Naloxone
- Psychosomatic

KEY POINTS

- In cases of suspected toxidrome exposure, whether it be purposeful, accidental, or iatrogenic, toxidromic presentation that is consistent with the history and physical examination should guide the judicious use of antidotes.
- Although surveys of available agents in the environment (e.g., home, hospital ward) can be useful aids to the diagnostic process, the patient's vital signs and physical examination are the best guides to medical intervention.
- The focus of treatment always should be the patient and the patient's symptoms, not the toxin or the assays that may or may not identify it.
- Good supportive care with prioritized attention to emergent physiologic needs is the cornerstone of management; detailed assessment and reassessment with synthesis of data over time is essential to this process.
- Pharmacologic interventions should be targeted to underlying toxic pathophysiology whenever possible with attention to not exacerbating delirium and minimizing its severity and duration.

INTRODUCTION

Psychiatrists must be concerned about toxic states, primarily because poisoned patients often have made choices that led to the exposure and its consequences, and those choices have mental health determinants and implications. But consulting psychiatrists may play a broader role in the critical care management of patients affected

Disclosures: None.
[a] Consultation - Liaison Psychiatry, Hennepin County Medical Center, University of Minnesota, 701 Park Avenue, R7.255, Minneapolis, MN 55415, USA; [b] Veterinary and Biomedical Sciences, University of Minnesota, 1988 Fitch Avenue, Saint Paul, MN 55108, USA
* Corresponding author.
E-mail address: joseph.rasimas@hcmed.org

Crit Care Clin 33 (2017) 521–541
http://dx.doi.org/10.1016/j.ccc.2017.03.002
0749-0704/17/© 2017 Elsevier Inc. All rights reserved.

by medications and other substances that goes far beyond psychiatric assessment and disposition planning after recovery from overdose. Toxic delirium abounds in the intensive care unit (ICU), where care interventions have as much or more to do with patients' neuropsychological functioning and experiences there as the critical illnesses they suffer.[1,2] Although psychiatric education offers some expertise in clinical pharmacology to inform differential diagnostic considerations of medication and substance toxicity, formal medical toxicology training for psychiatrists is rare.[3]

The most important diagnostic factor in uncovering a toxic etiology is the clinician's openness to the possibility of its existence. Therefore, a consulting psychiatrist, already prepared to perform the detail-oriented work of sorting out behavioral manifestations of disease, can be a vital asset at the bedside if also attuned to the role of purposeful, accidental, and iatrogenic exposures in the ICU. This article summarizes the presentation, evaluation, and treatment of toxidromes relevant to the work of acute psychosomatic medicine.

GENERAL APPROACH

Because the brain is the organ most commonly affected by acute poisoning, any patient whose behavior, level of consciousness, or established neuropsychiatric baseline are disturbed should prompt concerns about toxicity.[4] From the standpoint of central nervous system (CNS) function and diagnosis by the *Diagnostic and Statistical Manual of Mental Disorders*, the presence of delirium is therefore a major reason to suspect a toxic etiology. It is not only the symptomatic management of delirial states that defines much of consultation-liaison (C-L) psychiatry in the hospital setting, but also the medical detective work necessary to ascertain the possible causes of the syndrome.

Often, substance-related toxicity is not considered because of patients' purposeful deception or impairments in communication due to age, language barriers, underlying CNS ailment, or manifestations of the toxic exposure, itself. Physicians also are disinclined to look toward their own interventions as a primary cause for harm, thus further diminishing their attunement to toxic states induced by iatrogeny. Even in medical inpatients with many comorbid conditions that can affect brain function, adverse effects of the drugs used to treat those illnesses are likely to be the most common cause of delirium.[5] Toxicity from medications or other substances should be considered in patients who acutely develop seizures, coma, respiratory distress, shock, arrhythmias, metabolic acidosis, severe vomiting and diarrhea, or other puzzling multisystem disorders without known etiology.[6] The possibility even needs to be considered of substances being brought into the hospital and ingested by patients after an episode of care has commenced.

A detailed review of the history and medical record is essential to make sense of the time-course of evolution of a toxic or withdrawal state. Special attention should be paid to the first set of vital signs and physical examination documented, ideally before any medical interventions have been performed that would alter the phenomenology of the presenting problem. Data from emergency medical personnel can be particularly informative. The timing of significant changes in autonomic status, peripheral reflexes, behavior, and cognition also should be noted, with reference to medications given. Then, any subsequent shifts in patterns of autonomic indices and behavior during the hospital course should open the possibility of a new toxic process mediated by either the treatment process itself or withdrawal from discontinued substances.

Certain constellations of signs and symptoms, commonly called toxidromes, may suggest poisoning by a specific class of compounds (**Table 1**). The findings represent direct physiologic manifestations of the pharmacology of the agents in question, thus providing objective clinical data about the status of the patient and what has been

Table 1 Toxidromes	
Drug Class (Examples)	**Clinical Manifestations**
Anticholinergics (atropine, antihistamines, scopolamine, antispasmodics, tricyclic antidepressants, phenothiazines, antiparkinsonian agents, Jimson weed, psychedelic mushrooms)	Agitation, hallucinations, abnormal movements (eg, carphology), tachycardia, mydriasis, dry membranes, hyperthermia, decreased bowel sounds, urinary retention, flushed/dry skin
Cholinergics (organophosphates, carbamate insecticides, cholinesterase inhibitors)	Hypersalivation, lacrimation, urinary/fecal incontinence, gastrointestinal cramping, emesis (SLUDGE), bradycardia, diaphoresis, miosis, pulmonary edema, weakness, paralysis, muscle fasciculations
Opioids (oxycodone, hydrocodone, hydromorphone, fentanyl, morphine, propoxyphene, codeine, heroin)	Central nervous system (CNS) depression, respiratory compromise, miosis, bradycardia, hypotension, hypothermia, pulmonary edema, hyporeflexia, seizures
Sedative/Hypnotics (benzodiazepines, nonbenzodiazepine GABA agonists, barbiturates, ethanol, chloral hydrate, ethchlorvynol, meprobamate)	CNS depression, hyporeflexia, slow respirations, hypothermia, hypotension, and bradycardia (mild)
Sympathomimetics (psychostimulants, amphetamines, pseudoephedrine, phenylephrine, ephedrine, cocaine)	Hypertension, tachycardia, arrhythmias, agitation, paranoia, hallucinations, mydriasis, nausea, vomiting, abdominal pain, piloerection
Neuroleptics (chlorpromazine, promethazine, prochlorperazine, fluphenazine, perphenazine, haloperidol, olanzapine, quetiapine)	Hypotension, arrhythmias, oculogyric crisis, trismus, dystonia, ataxia, parkinsonism, neuroleptic malignant syndrome, anticholinergic manifestations (some)
Serotonergics (selective serotonin reuptake inhibitors, tricyclic antidepressants, monoamine oxidase inhibitors, buspirone, tramadol, fentanyl, synthetic stimulants, dextromethorphan)	Akathisia, tremor, agitation, hyperthermia, hypertension, diaphoresis, hyperreflexia, clonus, lower extremity muscular hypertonicity, diarrhea

ingested. Recognition of such patterns can be informative, but clinical pictures are not always so obvious. Polydrug overdoses may result in overlapping and confusing mixed syndromes. Pharmacokinetic drug compartmentalization also is a factor, with peripheral manifestations not always matching up with those reflecting toxicity in the CNS. Nevertheless, recognizing the dominant features of particular classes of pharmacologic toxicities can be a vital diagnostic and therapeutic starting point to psychosomatic consultation in the ICU.

TOXIDROMES

The toxic syndromes most frequently encountered in the emergency and ICU setting are detailed in the following sections. The causes vary, with anticholinergic toxicity, sedative toxicity, and serotonin syndrome being common after suicidal overdose, cholinergic and opioid toxicity often being accidental or secondary to a recreational drug misadventure, and almost any syndrome potentially resulting from iatrogenic interventions. The most commonly used antidotes for these conditions, and for other toxic states not discussed in detail, are provided as a reference for the ICU psychiatrist in **Table 2**. Their specific indications are discussed under each toxidrome subsection below.

Table 2
Emergency antidotes

Toxin	Antidote	Dosing
Acetaminophen	N-acetylcysteine (NAC)	IV or PO/NG: 140 mg/kg over 1 h, then 70 mg/kg over 1 h q4h × 5 doses; then reassess toxin clearance, PT/INR, and transaminases.[a]
Anesthetics (local) and some cardiotoxins	Lipid emulsion	IV: 1 mL/kg bolus of a 20% solution followed by 0.25 mL/kg per min infusion to maintain cardiovascular stability.[b]
Anticholinergics	Physostigmine	IV: 2 mg over 4 min in adolescents and adults, may repeat q1-2h prn; 20 µg/kg (1 mg maximum) in children, may repeat q1-2h prn.
Benzodiazepines and non-benzodiazepine hypnotics	Flumazenil	IV: 0.5 mg over 30 s in adults, Consider lower doses in children; may use 0.005–0.01 mg/kg at 0.2 mg/min rate in children; may repeat q30–60 min prn.
β-Adrenergic blockers	Glucagon[c]	IV: 50 µg/kg over 1–2 min up to 10 mg maximum followed by hourly infusion of half to full initial dose.
Calcium channel blockers	Calcium	IV: 1–2 g calcium (10% CaCl$_2$ solution) over 5 min in adults; 20–30 mg/kg per dose in children (may repeat).
	Insulin[c]	IV: 0.5–1 U/kg bolus followed by 0.5–1 U/kg per h continuous infusion.
	Glucose	IV: 25 g (as 50 mL of D$_{50}$W) in adults; 0.5 g/kg (as D$_{25}$W) in children (to maintain euglycemia in patients treated with insulin).
Cyanide, hydrogen sulfide	Sodium nitrite	IV: 300 mg over 2–5 min in adults; 0.2 mL/kg over 2–5 min in children.
	Sodium thiosulfate	IV: 12.5 g bolus in adults; 0.5 g/kg bolus (maximum 12.5 g) in children.
	Hydroxocobalamin (preferred)	IV: 70 mg/kg over 15 min.
Digitalis glycosides	Digoxin immune Fab	IV: 10–20 vials over 30 min for acute empiric dosing, otherwise based on serum digoxin concentration if known.
Ethylene glycol, methanol	Fomepizole (preferred)	IV: 15 mg/kg over 30 min, then 10 mg/kg q12h × 4 doses, then 15 mg/kg q12h as needed until nontoxic.
	Ethanol	IV: 10 mL/kg of 10% vol/vol solution, then 1.5 mL/kg per h continuous infusion until nontoxic; double rate during dialysis.
Iron	Deferoxamine	IV: start 5 mg/kg per h continuous infusion and titrate to 15 mg/kg per h as tolerated, total daily dose 6–8 g.
Isoniazid, hydrazine, and monomethylhydrazine	Pyridoxine	IV: 5 g in adults; 1 g in children.

Indication	Antidote	Dosing
Lead	Dimercaprol (BAL)	IM: 75 mg/m^2 q4h, first dose to precede edetate calcium disodium (CaNa$_2$ EDTA). Contraindicated if peanut allergic.
	CaNa$_2$ EDTA	IV: 1500 mg/m^2/d by continuous infusion.
	Succimer (DMSA)	PO: 10 mg/kg q8h for 5 d, then q12 h for 14 d in adults; 350 mg/m^2 in children (same course).
Methemoglobin-forming oxidants	Methylene blue	IV: 1–2 mg/kg over 5 min with 30 mL fluid flush, may repeat 1 mg/kg once.
Methotrexate	Folinic acid (leucovorin)	IV: 100 mg/m^2 over 15–30 min q3–6h for several days with absence/resolution of bone marrow toxicity.
Neuroleptics	Bromocriptine	PO: 5 mg q12h increasing to effect, as high as 10 mg q6h.
	Dantrolene	IV: 3–10 mg/kg over 15 min with oral doses of 25–600 mg/d to maintain response.
Opioids and centrally acting α2 agonists (eg, clonidine, guanfacine, tizanidine)	Naloxone	IV: Start 0.05 mg with repeat dosing every 15 s to reversal of respiratory depression and/or unconsciousness; once achieved, repeat the same total dose q1h prn. Higher doses (1–2 mg or more) may be useful in α2-adrenergic agonist toxicity.[7]
Organophosphates and carbamates	Atropine	IV: 1–2 mg doubled every 3–5 min until bronchorrhea resolves in adults; 0.03 mg/kg in children, similar titration.
	Pralidoxime (2-PAM)	IV: 1–2 g over 30 min, then up to 500 mg/h in adults; 25–50 mg/kg over 30–60 min, then 10–20 mg/kg per h in children.[d]
Snakebite (rattlesnake, copperhead, cottonmouth)	Crotalidae Polyvalent Immune Fab	IV: 4 vials typical minimum first dose in normal saline. Scheduled and prn regimens are effective going forward.
Sulfonylureas	Octreotide	SC: 50 μg q6-12h in adults, 1.25 μg/kg (max 50 μg) q6h in children.
Tricyclic antidepressants (and related compounds with sodium channel blocking properties)	Sodium bicarbonate	IV: 50 mEq per dose to address acidemia and/or ECG signs of sodium channel blockade. For an isotonic solution to continue alkaline fluid resuscitation, mix 150 mEq NaHCO$_3$ (typically 3 ampules) and 40 mEq KCl in 1 L D$_5$W. Goal serum pH 7.5–7.55.
Valproic acid	L-Carnitine	Clinically ill: IV: 100 mg/kg (max 6 g) over 30 min, then 15 mg/kg q4h. Clinically well: PO: 100 mg/kg per d (max 3 g) divided q6h.

Abbreviations: D$_5$W, a solution of 5% dextrose in water; D$_{25}$W, a solution of 25% dextrose in water; D$_{50}$W, a solution of 50% dextrose in water; ECG, electrocardiogram; IM, intramuscular; INR, international normalized ratio; IV, intravenous; PO, by mouth; NG, nasogastric; q, every; SC, subcutaneous; prn, as needed.

[a] This is one of many N-acetylcysteine regimens in use in the United States. The best regimen to use in different clinical situations remains under investigation.

[b] Intravenous lipid emulsion has been used in patients critically ill from a variety of different toxins using varying regimens.

[c] Glucagon is still used as a diagnostic aid in beta-blocker poisoning, but has largely been supplanted by other agents, including high-dose insulin, for ongoing treatment.

[d] Use of pralidoxime in carbamate poisoning is controversial, as there is some concern for worsening muscular weakness.

Anticholinergics

The anticholinergic syndrome occurs frequently because many common medications and other xenobiotics have anticholinergic properties. From sleep aids to muscle relaxants to antipsychotics, almost any medicinal compound whose generic moniker ends in "-pine," "-zine," or "-amine" has the potential to disrupt cholinergic function in the CNS with resulting delirium. Polypharmacy is a major concern, particularly in the elderly, as a number of commonly used drugs not typically classified as anticholinergics do have the potential to interfere with this critically important neurotransmitter.[8] Cholinergic activity is the primary mediator of attention, concentration, memory, reasoning, planning, and, to a large extent, communicating and understanding through language. Antimuscarinic toxicity in the CNS causes delirium, frequently accompanied by mumbling speech and carphology, aimless "picking" movements of the fingers. Psychomotor activity is generally of high frequency and low amplitude when patients are awake. Vivid visual hallucinosis of living creatures occurs. Deep tendon reflexes are often hyperdynamic, with a few beats of inducible clonus not uncommon. Other peripheral effects also are observed, but because most anticholinergics are lipophilic, the impact on brain function may be much more evident than effects on other organ systems. Inhibition of secretory functions of the integument can yield dry mouth, flushed skin, and impaired heat dissipation, so undressing behavior in a state of confused discomfort is common.[9] Suppression of cholinergic inhibition of heart rate may produce tachycardia. Unopposed sympathetic drive of the ciliary apparatus produces pupillary dilation. Cholinergic function also is required for normal peristalsis and bladder emptying, so this syndrome may be accompanied by fecal and urinary retention, as well. The duration of CNS effects typically exceeds that of peripheral symptoms[10] due to the chemical preference of the toxins for fatty tissues and their slow diffusion back out of the central compartment once they have accumulated there.

Most patients recover with removal of offending agents and supportive therapy, but delirium may last for days after an acute overdose of anticholinergics, and considerably longer if medications that contribute to the problem continue to be administered. Physostigmine may be a useful diagnostic tool and may serve as an efficacious antidote to rapidly target the cause of delirium. This tertiary amine readily crosses the blood-brain barrier and makes more acetylcholine available for neuronal function via reversible inhibition of cholinesterase within approximately 15 minutes of an intravenous (IV) dose. However, the antidote is relatively short-acting, with a plasma cholinesterase inhibition half-life of less than 90 minutes.[11] Therefore, even though its lipophilicity may prolong restorative effects in the CNS, repeat dosing of physostigmine is typically necessary in the setting of severe anticholinergic toxicity.

Physostigmine is indicated in patients with anticholinergic delirium caused by a variety of compounds from prescription medications to botanic hallucinogens (eg, Jimson Weed) (Box 1). Primarily on the basis of 2 case reports of asystole,[12] its use has been curtailed in the setting of a possible tricyclic antidepressant (TCA) overdose or possible polysubstance toxicity. However, more than 3 decades of extensive clinical experience since then have documented its safety and utility in anticholinergic states induced by medications that affect cardiac conduction.[13,14] The largest study to date (nearly 1200 patients, many with polydrug overdoses) found no induced arrhythmias and a low incidence of precipitated seizures with proper weight-based dosing: 0.05 mg/kg IV at a rate not to exceed 0.5 mg/min, with doses no more frequent than hourly.[15] Patients were confused and/or sedate, not profusely diaphoretic, and potentially exposed to an anticholinergic agent; no other contraindications were

Box 1
Antimuscarinic compounds for which physostigmine is antidotal

"Pure" anticholinergics
  Atropine
  Scopolamine
  Hyoscyamine

Cyclic antidepressants
  Doxepin
  Amitriptyline
  Nortriptyline
  Imipramine
  Clomipramine
  Desipramine
  Protriptyline
  Amoxapine
  Maprotiline

Antiparkinson agents
  Benztropine
  Trihexyphenidyl
  Biperiden

Antispasmodics
  Dicyclomine
  Oxybutynin
  Tolterodine
  Propantheline
  Clidinium

Muscle Relaxants
  Baclofen
  Carisoprodol
  Cyclobenzaprine
  Orphenadrine
  Glutethimide

Antihistamines
  Hydroxyzine
  Diphenhydramine
  Doxylamine
  Pyrilamine
  Chlorpheniramine
  Brompheniramine
  Clemastine

Antiemetics
  Promethazine
  Prochlorperazine
  Meclizine
  Dimenhydrinate

Antipsychotics
  Quetiapine
  Olanzapine
  Clozapine
  Asenapine
  Loxapine
  Chlorpromazine
  Fluphenazine
  Trifluoperazine
  Perphenazine
  Thioridazine

Mesoridazine
Thiothixene

Botanicals[a]
Jimson weed (*Datura stramonium*)
Angel's trumpet (*Brugmansia* spp)
Deadly nightshade (*Atropa belladonna*)
Mandrakes (*Bryonia alba* and *Mandragora* spp)
Henbane (*Hyoscyamus niger*)
Bittersweet (*Celastrus scandens*)
Lupins (*Lupinus* spp)
Fly agaric (*Amanita muscaria*)

[a] Potentially beneficial for central nervous system manifestations of exposure to all plants in the family Solanaceae.

imposed. In this study, more than 80% of patients had a positive response to antidotal treatment, and no serious adverse effects were observed. More than 300 patients were poisoned with TCAs, and roughly 95% of those individuals benefited from physostigmine. Side effects may include enuresis, stooling, nausea, and vomiting; they are transient, but keeping the head of a patient's bed elevated is advised. A baseline electrocardiogram (ECG) is recommended, and if terminal right axis deviation is present (indicated by elevation of the R-wave in lead aVR) or frank widening of the QRS complex is observed, then pretreatment with an IV dose of lorazepam is recommended right before a test dose of physostigmine to prevent seizures.[16] Bradyarrhythmias are rare, but cardiac monitoring is suggested by some toxicologists,[17] and required by many hospital pharmacy policies.

Cholinergics

The cholinergic syndrome is uncommon, but important to recognize because lifesaving treatment is available. Cholinergic toxicity produces a patient who presents "wet," as opposed to the anticholinergic syndrome, which often causes the patient to be "dry." The wetness is manifest by profuse sweating and excessive activity of the exocrine system, often accompanied by vomiting, diarrhea, and urinary incontinence. The mnemonic "SLUDGE" highlights specific elements of the syndrome: salivation, *l*acrimation, *u*rination, *d*efecation, *g*astrointestinal cramping, and emesis. The CNS (eg, confusion, seizures, coma) and skeletal muscles (eg, weakness, fasciculations, hyporeflexia) also can be involved, so the neuropsychiatric examination is important in diagnosis. Cholinergic excess is frequently caused by accidental organophosphate or carbamate pesticide exposure, which may occur through dermal contamination.[18] Such commercial/industrial agents and cholinesterase inhibitors used therapeutically for dementia can be used in suicide attempts, as well. Cholinergic effects also are the cause of toxicity from "nerve gases" like sarin and from mistaken ingestion of *Clitocybe* and *Inocybe* mushrooms. A not uncommon scenario of milder toxicity (but presenting with delirium) is accidental self-poisoning by a patient with dementia who takes repeat doses of a cognitive-enhancing drug due to forgetfulness about medication adherence.[19] It is also possible to develop toxic cholinergic "rebound" after abrupt cessation of excessive misuse of medications with anticholinergic properties (eg, diphenhydramine, quetiapine).[20] Mild forms of the toxidrome can be managed with discontinuation of offending agents and/or resumption of tapering doses of the overused anticholinergic drug, with supportive care. Recognition of critical illness should prompt the use of atropine (or perhaps glycopyrrolate if CNS manifestations are not significant) and, in some cases of severe toxicity, the cholines-terase regenerator pralidoxime.[21]

Sedative/Hypnotics

When administered in sufficient dosage, sedative/hypnotics cause general anesthesia with diminished reflex activity and a complete loss of awareness. Sedation can be profound, but it is rare that benzodiazepine toxicity, alone, results in significant respiratory depression. Barbiturates, however, are sufficiently potent to produce shock and respiratory failure. "Pure" GABA-ergic toxidromes can sometimes be distinguished on the basis of history, lethargy or coma, relatively preserved pulmonary function, and the absence of constricted pupils (see **Table 1**). Patients also can be confused and disinhibited by benzodiazepines such that they display intermittent agitation, despite the CNS depression typically produced by these agents. This phenomenon, along with prolongation of delirial and comatose states, is a major iatrogenic complication of care in the ICU setting. Continuous infusions of midazolam remain common practice,[22] even though interrupted regimens have been associated with decreased sedative use, lower rates of delirium, fewer complications, and shorter lengths of stay; and thus appear in the most current practice guidelines for critical care.[23] Even intermittent use of benzodiazepines can yield neuropsychiatric complications with the potential to contribute to long-term sequelae, so recognition of and definitive treatment for sedative toxicity is critical.

When offending toxins operate at the benzodiazepine-binding site of the GABA-A receptor complex, reversal of this syndrome can be accomplished with the administration of flumazenil. It should not, however, be used in the setting of active toxicity from agents that are highly proarrhythmic or proconvulsant, because adverse events can result.[24] With careful attention to neurologic status and autonomic indices, physical examination can identify patients (non-hyperreflexic, without tachycardia or significant hypertension) who can safely receive a potentially therapeutic test dose of flumazenil. If individual IV doses are kept low (0.2–0.5 mg) and delivered over 30 seconds, the incidence of arrhythmias and seizures, even in patients who take benzodiazepines chronically, is negligible.[25] A state of anxiety may emerge from the reversal of stupor,[26] but supportive psychological presence is all that is required to manage such a side effect from the antidote.[25] Withdrawal is possible, but because such an outcome cannot be predicted and the effects will be transient, a low dose of flumazenil can be used safely[27] as an initial alternative to the standard practice, relatively lacking in an evidence base, of scheduling a protracted taper of benzodiazepines for all patients who have been sedated for extended periods in the ICU.[23,28] Therapeutic effects include facilitation of extubation, restoration of wakefulness and cognition, and relief of disinhibition with the result that patients can advance to calm participation in their own care. Flumazenil is short-acting; multiple doses may be necessary to maintain the effect, so after initial benefit is achieved, repeating 0.5-mg doses every hour as needed is recommended.[25]

Although their mechanisms of action differ somewhat from benzodiazepines, the toxic effects of nonbenzodiazepine sedatives (eg, zolpidem, zaleplon, and zopiclone) will respond to flumazenil. Flumazenil will not reverse either the effects of barbiturates or those of other sedatives that work via distinct mechanisms like ion channel modulation. Although not a specific antidote, as it is in the setting of benzodiazepine toxicity, flumazenil has been used with benefit in some cases of muscle relaxant overdose.[29] See **Box 2** for a list of toxins for which flumazenil may be antidotal. The suggestion of increased central GABA activity in the pathophysiology of hepatic encephalopathy

> **Box 2**
> **Sedating compounds for which Flumazenil is antidotal**
>
> Benzodiazepines
>   Lorazepam
>   Oxazepam
>   Temazepam
>   Clorazepate
>   Alprazolam
>   Clonazepam
>   Diazepam
>   Triazolam
>   Estazolam
>   Midazolam
>   Chlordiazepoxide
>   Meprobamate
>   Flunitrazepam
>
> Muscle relaxants
>   Carisoprodol (Meprobamate)[a]
>   Metaxalone
>   Chlorzoxazone
>   Methocarbamol
>
> Nonbenzodiazepines
>   Imidazopyridines
>   Zolpidem
>   Pyrazolopyrimidines
>   Zaleplon
>   Cyclopyrrolones
>   Zopiclone
>   Eszopiclone
>
> Botanicals
>   Uncaria hook (*Uncaria macrophylla*)
>   Yokukansan (*Uncaria rhynchophylla*)
>
> [a] Meprobamate is a metabolite of carisoprodol with benzodiazepinelike GABA-ergic activity. The parent compound has anticholinergic activity and barbituratelike GABA-ergic activity.

and some limited clinical success indicate that flumazenil also may help to treat the neuropsychiatric complications of liver failure.[30]

Opioids

Toxicity from opioids progresses from analgesia to anesthetic CNS depression, coma, and death. Respiratory depression is particularly pronounced with opioid overdose, and the tidal volume or respiratory rate can be diminished before decreases in blood pressure or pulse occur. Sympatholysis is profound, and central to the toxidrome that leads to morbid and mortal outcomes with greater frequency than any other class of compounds.[31] Patients will have minimal respiratory drive and quickly develop manifestations of shock. Miosis also is characteristic and, in pure opioid toxicity, a fairly reliable finding.[32] A patient "found down" after several hours following opioid exposure will frequently have laboratory and imaging results consist with hypoxic and hypovolemic injury to multiple organ systems, including kidneys, liver, lungs, heart, skeletal muscle, and CNS. Damage to the latter is of greatest concern, as such injuries can leave patients who survive profoundly impaired and dependent on a high level of care indefinitely. In cases in which 4 or 5 days have passed since exposure, and patients continue to display neurologic impairments in the absence of other obvious causes, MRI of the brain typically reveals hyperintensities on diffusion-weighted imaging (DWI) in watershed areas in patients with anoxic injury.[33] Injury patterns may vary, but involvement of perirolandic areas or even more diffuse DWI and T2 fluid-attenuated inversion recovery abnormalities typically indicate more severe CNS damage.[34] Although some patients, particularly those who are younger, can make remarkable recoveries despite strikingly abnormal MRI findings, imaging still can be helpful for assessment and initial treatment planning after the acute phase of toxicity has been addressed.

Patients with opioid toxicity require high-level critical care with aggressive fluid resuscitation and vasopressor support, especially if there is any significant delay in coming to treatment. Noncardiogenic pulmonary edema with progression to acute respiratory distress syndrome is common. Rhabdomyolysis combined with hypotensive renal damage can result in a need for hemodialysis, sometimes for weeks. Compartment syndrome can produce massive elevations in serum creatine kinase levels; this laboratory test abnormality will lag the time of damage by 8 hours or more, so it is important to perform a detailed physical examination of all major muscle groups at time of presentation after any significant "down time" to identify areas of vascular compromise. Areas of skin reddening or blistering, sometimes called "barbiturate burns" can mark areas of prolonged pressure injury from time spent in deep coma.[35,36]

The diagnosis of opioid overdose is often confirmed using naloxone or nalmefene in adequate doses that reverse the toxidrome.[37] These mu receptor antagonists reliably reverse coma and respiratory depression if used shortly after an opioid overdose. Depending on the clinical scenario, lack of response is essentially diagnostic of another etiology for obtundation; in a patient with multisystem injury from opioid toxicity (see above), however, it is an ominous sign of prolonged CNS anoxia. Naloxone has an elimination half-life of approximately 1 hour, whereas that of nalmefene is more than 10 hours, thus making the latter antidote potentially useful in the case of opioid toxicity from a long-acting drug (eg, methadone).[38] In most patients, naloxone is the preferred agent, because a shorter-acting antidote allows for more careful titration of toxidrome reversal without precipitation of withdrawal. Medical toxicologists recommend assisted ventilation while preparing a low dose of 0.05 mg and then titrating upward every 15 seconds or so until an adequate response is achieved.[39] As soon as spontaneous respirations and calm wakefulness are restored, noting the total dose required is useful, because then the same naloxone dose can be repeated every 30 to 60 minutes as needed. Higher doses increase the likelihood of agitated withdrawal without added benefit to neurologic or respiratory status, especially in chronic users of opioids. Most opioids will require 0.4 mg or less of naloxone for adequate reversal. Exceptions include pentazocine[40] and buprenorphine,[41] partial agonists of mu receptors that have high binding affinity. The same may be true of some synthetic novel abusable opioids,[42] but an upward titration of antidote is still important to avoid dangerous withdrawal. Ongoing monitoring after antidote administration is vital, because cardiopulmonary symptoms are not reversed as durably as CNS depression, and life-threatening symptoms can recur.

Sympathomimetics

The sympathomimetic syndrome is usually seen after acute or chronic abuse of cocaine, amphetamines, or decongestants, the latter of which are often ingested in combination over-the-counter products. Pseudoephedrine and phenylephrine are the most common. Both are alpha-adrenergic agonists, with the former carrying some beta-stimulatory activity as well.[43] Ephedrine has nonspecific adrenergic effects, and is found in herbal preparations used recreationally to enhance energy, or as adjuncts to fitness regimens.[44,45] Cathinones and related designer drugs of abuse also produce this toxidrome.[46] Ketamine, with its potential to increase the presynaptic release of catecholamines,[47] also can exacerbate sympathomimesis.

Blood pressure is elevated, the pulse is rapid, pupils are typically dilated, and piloerection may be seen. Mild toxicity rarely leads to cardiac complications, but large overdoses of sympathomimetic agents can produce hypertensive crisis, intracranial hemorrhage, arrhythmias, cardiovascular compromise, and shock. Seizures occur, and the postictal state can contribute to alterations in mental status. Some compounds (eg, cocaine) cause seizures and arrhythmias due to their ability to interact with neuronal and cardiac sodium channels,[48] so sodium bicarbonate infusions are essential in the critical care of severely poisoned patients. Otherwise, no specific antidotes exist. Symptomatic management and supportive care are required. Benzodiazepines serve as the cornerstone of acute treatment because they attenuate catecholamine release, alleviate hypertension, prevent seizures, and provide helpful sedation.[49] Beta-blockers tend to be used with caution, because they can leave alpha-adrenergic stimulation unopposed. Vasodilators, such as hydralazine, nitroprusside, or phentolamine, are typically preferred for treatment of severe hypertension that does not respond quickly to benzodiazepines. There has been some recent consideration of the alpha-2 adrenergic agonist dexmedetomidine to manage these cases by targeting the underlying pathophysiology of the toxidrome[50]; if used, doses should be kept in the range of high alpha-2 specificity (≤ 0.5 µg/kg per hour) to avoid exacerbating hypertension via peripheral alpha-1 agonism.[51] Transition to clonidine or guanfacine may have a role after initial stability is achieved.

Patients may be agitated and even psychotic with manic symptoms and/or paranoid delusions.[52–54] The simple pharmacology and easy administration of haloperidol may make this agent preferable in the ICU management of these cases when an adjunct to benzodiazepines is needed. Psychiatric sequelae from some sympathomimetic toxins can linger long after physical symptoms have resolved, demanding attention to acute mental health care needs with subsequent abstinence and, sometimes, ongoing treatment with antipsychotic medications.[52] Atypical neuroleptics may be preferable once the critical illness period has passed, because they can have a more beneficial impact on mood, treat punding, and avoid movement side effects to which some patients may be more prone on account of their stimulant misuse.[55] As a general principle, it is important to appreciate that the clinical picture overlaps with serotonin syndrome, as these compounds have multiple mechanisms by which they enhance catecholamine activity.

Serotonergics

Serotonergic agents cause critical illness in various clinical scenarios, including suicidal overdoses, unintentional combined polypharmacy, and drug abuse misadventures involving cocaine, designer psychedelic stimulants, and dextromethorphan. The latter is a synthetic analog of codeine that is frequently abused by adolescents,[56] and is occasionally used alone or coingested with other compounds in suicide attempts. Its desirable and harmful effects are mediated by glutamatergic modulation and a collection of proserotonergic actions, including inhibition of serotonin reuptake mechanisms, direct serotonin receptor agonism, and even serotonin release.[57,58] Because most cases of serotonin syndrome can be traced to pharmacologic conditions in which more than 1 mechanism of serotonin enhancement is engaged,[59] it is not surprising that dextromethorphan alone can cause severe toxicity. As most recreational drugs capable of producing euphoria or hallucinosis operate via serotonin release or direct agonism, abusing such a drug in the context of treatment with antidepressants is a common etiologic combination.[60] Bupropion, although not often classified as a robustly serotonergic drug,[61] produces a toxic overdose picture in which patients invariably meet clinical criteria for serotonin syndrome[62] and can be exceptionally sick.[63]

The serotonin toxic picture is one characterized by neuromuscular excess, hyperthermia, and altered mental status. Hyperactive delirium with high-amplitude psychomotor unrest of variable frequency is observed. Classic signs of lower extremity muscle rigidity, hyperreflexia, and especially robust ankle clonus help to distinguish this toxidrome from anticholinergic poisoning (see **Table 1**). Muscle breakdown from hypertonicity, severe agitation, and/or seizure activity is a serious concern. Metabolic acidosis is a serious threat to integrity of organ function. In contrast to anticholinergic poisoning, the skin is typically not dry and the abdomen not quiet, but the 2 toxidromes with their manifestations of delirium, hyperthermia, reactive tachycardia, hyperreflexia, and intermittent agitation can be difficult to distinguish on clinical examination alone. Failure of lethargy, confusion, and/or agitation to resolve with physostigmine can help to distinguish serotonin syndrome from anticholinergic delirium.[15] It is helpful to consider serotonergic toxicity on a continuum of severity, recognizing that relatively mild anxiety, paresthesias, akathisia, and/or tremor can be the result of drug side effects,[59] although, they can be hard to distinguish from underlying psychiatric problems for which the drugs may have been prescribed. This may be especially true in the ICU setting in which other drug effects are also in play, and intubation of patients interferes with their ability to communicate their symptoms, emotions, and perceptions. As a result, the commonly used "analgosedative" fentanyl cannot be recommended for use in toxicology patients in the ICU, as it is proserotonergic and can fuel a toxic delirial state in conjunction with antidepressants and other agents.[64]

Because the clinical picture of serotonin syndrome can mimic neuroleptic malignant syndrome (NMS), antipsychotic medications should be used with extreme caution in the initial management of this delirium if the exposure history is at all unclear. In addition to differences in precipitating medications, NMS typically results in more generalized and severe muscle rigidity without hyperreflexia.[59,65] Benzodiazepines treat restlessness and agitation in both conditions and can provide neuromuscular relaxation that reduces fever and prevents rhabdomyolysis and renal injury, even though cognitive impairment may persist. Benzodiazepines are, indeed, the cornerstone of treatment for serotonin syndrome to calm autonomic unrest, prevent arrhythmias and seizures, and reduce agitation.[59] Hyperthermia must be addressed with aggressive cooling techniques. Restraints must be avoided, as ongoing agitation with restricted movement can result in more heat generation, rhabdomyolysis, and lethal acidosis. When benzodiazepines are ineffective, barbiturates or propofol are used, occasionally augmented with paralytics.[59] The serotonin antagonist cyproheptadine has been used, but it requires oral dosing and therefore displays limited efficacy in the critical care setting[66]; it is also anticholinergic at higher doses, with the potential to worsen delirium and hyperthermia. Augmentation of therapy with antipsychotic agents that antagonize serotonin receptors (eg, chlorpromazine, risperidone) has been attempted, but with limited efficacy data and concerns about their accompanying pharmacologic activities.[59] As in toxic states of sympathomimesis, centrally acting alpha-2 agonists (eg, dexmedetomidine) are under consideration, especially in light of their lower deliriogenic potential as compared with benzodiazepines.[67] It is important to be aware that serotonin toxicity can persist well beyond the time when pharmacokinetic profiles of the offending agents might predict their clearance, because the toxin in this syndrome is serotonin, and once a "storm" of neurotransmitter function has been incited, resolution depends not only on the exogenous substances but also on factors of physiology inherent to the patient.

Neuroleptics

Toxidromes involving antipsychotic medications can be variable and complex, reflecting the pharmacology of chemically diverse agents. Dopamine receptor antagonism is the central activity of all these drugs, but only high-potency, first-generation agents like haloperidol are likely to manifest a toxicity profile primarily reflective of that action. Many are anticholinergic, so in excessive doses, they may produce confusion and hallucinosis consistent with that toxidrome (see above), for which physostigmine is antidotal (see **Box 1**). It is also important to note, however, that although phenothiazines and newer, structurally unrelated antipsychotic medications have anticholinergic effects, they may not be sufficient to offset dopamine antagonism in the nigrostriatal pathway. As a result, movement disorder symptoms can accompany their use in therapeutic dose ranges. In these scenarios, anticholinergic agents, such as benztropine and diphenhydramine, are effective in reversing dystonias and acute parkinsonian effects. Noting this conundrum, we advise bearing in mind Paracelsus' foundational principle of medical toxicology, "*sola dosis facit venenum*,"[68] and approaching patients with suspected toxicity from neuroleptics differently based on the particular dosing and physiologic circumstances.

In the acute, purposeful overdose situation, patients are typically sedate with slowed motor activity from the effects of D2 antagonism, and also profoundly affected by anticholinergia if the agent in question has that activity. The latter will often be clinically dominant to the extent that use of physostigmine may help not only to clear confusion, but also to avoid intubation from concerns about obtundation.[15] Extrapyramidal effects (EPS) are rarely encountered in the setting of a suicidal ingestion of antipsychotic medication, whether it be a typical or atypical agent. The serotonin antagonism of atypical neuroleptics is not toxicologically relevant, apart from its potential to exacerbate sedation via mechanisms lacking a pharmacologic antidote; recovery comes only with tincture of time. Most neuroleptics have the capacity to antagonize alpha1-adrenergic receptors, so in conjunction with dopamine blockade (and in some cases, H1-histamine blockade), the result is hypotension. Fluid resuscitation is usually sufficient, although a brief period of vasopressor support may be necessary. Tachycardia may manifest from both alpha2-adrenergic blockade and anticholinergic effects. The greatest potential for lethality after a large ingestion of antipsychotic medication comes in the form of more serious arrhythmias.[69]

Although much attention has been paid to the differences between and among different compounds with respect to QT prolongation potential via potassium efflux antagonism,[70–72] the reality is that all antipsychotics come with a risk of *torsades de pointes* when taken in overdose.[73] The peak risk is observed, in most cases, approximately 6 hours after exposure; however, the greatest impact on myocardial rhythmicity can be delayed due to ongoing drug absorption after oral overdose. Management requires cardiac monitoring, supplementation with magnesium, and optimization of potassium and other electrolyte concentrations in serum. Sodium bicarbonate is not effective in preventing polymorphic ventricular arrhythmias; however, there are older antipsychotic medications capable of causing cardiac arrest via sodium channel blockade in similar fashion to TCAs. Thioridazine and mesoridazine overdoses will manifest with QRS widening on ECG, so treatment with sodium bicarbonate is central to prevention of ventricular arrhythmias in those cases,[74] along with

Box 3
Case study

A 27-year-old woman with schizoaffective disorder and addiction to alcohol and methamphetamine presented in near-coma to the intensive care unit (ICU) after suspected purposeful overdose of her psychiatric medications. Her prescriptions included olanzapine, fluoxetine, hydroxyzine, and gabapentin. Initially, she had a blood pressure of 136/73 mm Hg, heart rate of 111 beats per minute, a core temperature of 38°C, profound lethargy, purposeless movements of the arms with a tremor, and symmetric hyperreflexia with 1 beat of ankle clonus. Her electrocardiogram revealed no abnormalities apart from sinus tachycardia, and her laboratory studies were unremarkable. Without consideration of antidotal therapy, she was given benzodiazepines and then intubated with the procedure facilitated by succinylcholine and propofol. Infusions of propofol and fentanyl were maintained overnight, and then weaned down with a plan to extubate, because there was no discernible pulmonary pathology. Unfortunately, the patient exhibited agitated confusion. Instead of progressing to extubation under such circumstances, infusions were maintained at lower rates and she was given haloperidol in accordance with the ICU protocol for management of delirium. Records of the next physical examination document a blood pressure of 145/90 mm Hg, heart rate of 131 beats per minute, a core temperature of 38.1°C, and heightened reflexes with 4 beats of inducible ankle clonus. Critical care physicians recognized the potential problem of having given fentanyl to a patient with suspected recent exposures to fluoxetine and methamphetamine, and halted the opioid infusion. A few doses of 2 mg lorazepam were given on the second day in ICU. In the interest of minimizing the use of propofol, haloperidol doses were increased to 5 mg every 4 hours to manage agitation. Delirium persisted with no improvement on the third ICU day when the vital signs and neurologic examination were more in line with the initial presentation. Propofol was maintained in low-dose titration at the discretion of nursing staff, with a further increase in haloperidol to 10-mg doses as needed atop the previously scheduled regimen. On day 4 in the ICU, the patient's agitation was finally diminished, with breakthrough unrest only when her body was repositioned. Nursing staff noted her to be somewhat stiff when rolling for toileting, and paged medical staff about a fever of 39°C that afternoon. Acetaminophen was prescribed. A workup was undertaken for infectious causes of fever the next day; assays revealed a white blood count of 14/nL (increased over the 11/nL on admission) and broad-spectrum antibiotics were ordered. Vital signs were not severely abnormal, but varied over the course of the next day, while the body temperature remained above 39°C despite increase in fluid delivery and treatment with acetaminophen. The medication regimen was continued for another day until a psychiatric consultation was placed to "assist with management of prolonged delirium in the wake of a suicide attempt by a patient with drug abuse; no clear source of infection, not responding to haloperidol." A detailed interview, of course, could not be conducted, but the psychiatrist noted rigidity of all 4 limbs and normal deep tendon reflexes. A review of the medical record indicated that the patient had received a total of 125 mg haloperidol in the preceding 120 hours. A diagnosis of neuroleptic malignant syndrome (NMS) was proposed, with a recommendation to halt haloperidol, give sedative medications, institute aggressive cooling measures, and consider adding bromocriptine if rigidity were to persist. Abnormalities in vital signs, physical examination, and behavior became progressively less severe over the subsequent 6 days, and, despite developing a catheter-related urinary tract infection, the patient was finally able to leave the ICU nearly 3 weeks after her overdose.

The case highlights difficulties in managing the evolving course of a toxic patient in the ICU affected not only by a purposeful polysubstance ingestion, but also the medications used in critical care. There was a brief phase of serotonin toxicity due to the interaction between fentanyl and the compounds already present in the patient's tissues: fluoxetine and methamphetamine. Even though this toxidrome was quickly recognized, the less common problem of NMS eluded detection in the days following. Escalating doses of haloperidol created the problem, perhaps exacerbated by the olanzapine overdose. Attention to the vital signs and neuromuscular status would have provided guidance earlier in the clinical course and prevented the toxidrome from yielding a protracted ICU stay. Another point is that the patient's initial presentation was consistent with anticholinergic syndrome secondary to the effects of olanzapine, and physostigmine would have targeted the underlying cause of that confused agitation such that the subsequent iatrogenic toxic deliria could have been avoided.

attention to impaired repolarization. In general, older medications such as these are considerably more cardiotoxic in overdose than atypical agents.[69]

NMS is the potentially lethal complication that more commonly comes to mind in discussion of these medications. In the acute overdose scenario, however, NMS is extremely rare. NMS manifests under circumstances of ongoing treatment with anti-psychotic medications, with the risk being higher during phases of escalating doses. The risk is also greater with high-potency dopamine blockers. Thus, a patient who has been prescribed neuroleptics and presents to hospital in an altered state of health and behavior, or a patient whose clinical picture changes significantly in the ICU after having been treated with neuroleptics, must have NMS on the list of differential diagnostic considerations. It may aptly be viewed as the most severe manifestation of the contin-uum of EPS (akathisia, dystonia, parkinsonism) that overwhelms whole-body neural homeostasis.[75] The toxidrome reflects an idiopathic reaction resulting in severe mus-cle rigidity, hyperthermia, autonomic instability, and altered mental status; it requires discontinuation of antipsychotic medication and aggressive symptom-focused medi-cal interventions. Along with discontinuation of antipsychotics in favor of benzodiaze-pines, toxicologists recommend the use of dopamine receptor agonists (eg, bromocriptine) and turn to dantrolene sodium if severe muscle rigidity is fueling hyper-thermia and/or rhabdomyolysis that will not respond to sedatives and paralytics.[76]

Noting the overlap of the features of NMS with serotonin syndrome (see above), the complexity of medication regimens in patients who may have these toxidromes, and the preference to avoid benzodiazepines[5] in favor of antipsychotic medications in the treatment of most delirial states,[77] efforts have been made to guide the process of distinguishing NMS from serotonin syndrome.[78] Unfortunately, these guidelines that highlight differences in white blood counts, transaminases, and fever intensity focus on the most critical forms of 2 toxidromes that present with a continuum of severity. In the interest of patient safety, NMS must be identified as early in its progres-sion as possible, so that offending agents may be discontinued; and at these stages, laboratory indices and temperature readings are not helpful. On the other hand, a very inclusive set of criteria has been proposed that may deny many patients therapeu-tic benefit from neuroleptics if NMS is overdiagnosed.[79] Laboratory assays for urinary metabolites of dopamine and serotonin have been proposed to distinguish the syn-dromes,[80] but without validation or widespread availability of the technique, focus must turn to each individual patient's physical presentation. Two features of physical examination that must be assessed carefully and tracked repeatedly may be most helpful in defining cases of NMS: skeletal muscle tonicity and deep tendon reflex activ-ity. Patients with muscular rigidity confined to the lower extremities along with hyper-reflexia are very unlikely to have evolving NMS. This presentation is consistent with serotonin toxicity, especially if ankle clonus is present. Those individuals without hyper-reflexia who have rigidity in all 4 limbs (even if fairly subtle) may indeed have early signs of toxicity from antipsychotic medication that could become very severe if the offend-ing agents are not discontinued. In the ICU setting, making this distinction can be chal-lenging; the case scenario outlines some of the complexities involved (**Box 3**).

SUMMARY

The toxidromes in this survey were chosen for review based on the combined variables of high epidemiologic frequency of cases in the ICU and availability of the drugs that cause them. Of course, there are countless other agents that can cause life-threatening compli-cations. Inhalants and toxic alcohols are readily available substances involved in addic-tion that can produce critical illness from effects on cardiac, pulmonary, and neurologic systems with psychiatric sequelae.[81–83] Over-the-counter products containing acet-aminophen, nonsteroidal anti-inflammatory drugs, and aspirin frequently land purposeful overdose patients in the ICU.[84–86] Carbon monoxide exposure causes CNS injury that can lead to delayed neuropsychiatric impairment long after recovery from critical illness.[87–91] In addition to maintaining a basic familiarity with the principles of diagnosis and management and antidotes for these other poisons (see **Table 2**), it is worthwhile for the C-L psychiatrist to keep an updated medical toxicology handbook for reference.[92]

Although not qualified to deliver all the necessary treatments for toxicology patients in every setting, the psychosomatic medicine specialist can be well-equipped to iden-tify toxidromes and investigate the underlying causes for them, as well. A thorough history (often gathered from several sources in the manner of a C-L psychiatrist) and astute physical examination are key to toxicologic diagnosis. As Georg Groddeck, by some called the father of psychosomatic medicine, suggested: the crucial question is "why" not merely "how" a particular disease state arises.[93]

In cases of suspected exposure, whether it be purposeful, accidental, or iatrogenic, toxidromic presentation that is consistent with the history should guide the judicious use of antidotes. Although surveys of available agents in the environment (eg, home, hospital ward) can be useful aids to the diagnostic process, the patient's vital signs and physical examination are the best guides to medical intervention. The focus of treatment always should be the patient and the patient's symptoms, not the toxin or the assays that may or may not discover it.[94] Good supportive care with prioritized attention to emergent physiologic needs is the cornerstone of management; detailed assessment and reassessment with synthesis of data over time is essential to this pro-cess. Removal of ongoing exposures and institution of selected treatments help to promote recovery from the toxicity of an ICU stay, and potentially reduce long-term impact on mental health and functionality.

REFERENCES

1. Davydow DS, Gifford JM, Desai SV, et al. Posttraumatic stress disorder in general intensive care unit survivors: a systematic review. Gen Hosp Psychiatry 2008;30: 421–34.
2. van den Boogaard M, Schoonhoven L, Evers AW, et al. Delirium in critically ill pa-tients: impact on long-term health-related quality of life and cognitive functioning. Crit Care Med 2012;40:112–8.
3. Ingels M, Marks D, Clark RF. A survey of medical toxicology training in psychiatry residency programs. Acad Psychiatry 2003;27:50–3.
4. Flomenbaum NE, Goldfrank LR, Hoffman RS, et al. Principles of managing the poisoned or overdosed patient. In: Flomenbaum NE, Goldfrank LR, Hoffman RS, et al, editors. Goldfrank's toxicologic emergencies. 8th edition. New York: McGraw-Hill; 2006. p. 42–50.
5. Maldonado JR. Delirium in the acute care setting: characteristics, diagnosis and treatment. Crit Care Clin 2008;24:657–722.
6. Donovan JW, Burkhart KK, Brent J. General management of the critically poisoned patient. In: Brent J, Wallace KL, Burkhart KK, et al, editors. Critical care toxicology: diagnosis and management of the critically poisoned patient. Philadelphia: Elsevier Mosby; 2005. p. 1–11.
7. Kulig K, Duffy J, Rumack BH, et al. Naloxone for treatment of clonidine overdose. JAMA 1982;247:1697.
8. Tune LE. Serum anticholinergic activity levels and delirium in the elderly. Semin Clin Neuropsychiatry 2000;5:149–53.

9. Maytal G, Smith FA, Stern TA. Naked patients in the general hospital: differential diagnosis and management strategies. Psychosomatics 2006;47:486–90.

10. Tune LE. Anticholinergic effects of medication in elderly patients. J Clin Psychiatry 2001;62:11–4.

11. Knapp S, Wardlow ML, Albert K, et al. Correlation between plasma physostigmine concentrations and percentage of acetylcholinesterase inhibition over time after controlled release of physostigmine in volunteer subjects. Drug Metab Dispos 1991;19:400–4.

12. Pentel P, Peterson CD. Asystole complicating physostigmine treatment of tricyclic antidepressant overdose. Ann Emerg Med 1980;9:588–90.

13. Burns MJ, Linden CH, Graudins A, et al. A comparison of physostigmine and benzodiazepines for the treatment of anticholinergic poisoning. Ann Emerg Med 2000;35:374–81.

14. Schneir AB, Offerman SR, Ly BT, et al. Complications of diagnostic physostigmine administration to emergency department patients. Ann Emerg Med 2003; 42:14–9.

15. Rasimas JJ, Sachdeva KK, Donovan JW. Revival of an antidote: bedside experience with physostigmine. J Am Assoc Emerg Psychiatr 2014;12:5–24.

16. Boehnert MT, Lovejoy FH Jr. Value of the QRS duration versus the serum drug level in predicting seizures and ventricular arrhythmias after an acute overdose of tricyclic antidepressants. N Engl J Med 1985;313:474–9.

17. Martin TG, Morris WD. Physostigmine. In: Brent J, Wallace KL, Burkhart KK, et al, editors. Critical care toxicology: diagnosis and management of the critically poisoned patient. Philadelphia: Elsevier Mosby; 2005. p. 1565–74.

18. Hodgson MJ, Parkinson DK. Diagnosis of organophosphate intoxication. N Engl J Med 1985;313:329.

19. Greene YM, Noviasky J, Tariot PN. Donepezil overdose. J Clin Psychiatry 1999; 60:56–7.

20. Glickman L. Diphenhydramine abuse and withdrawal. JAMA 1986;256:1894.

21. Eddleston M, Szinicz L, Eyer P, et al. Oximes in acute organophosphorus pesticide poisoning: a systematic review of clinical trials. QJM 2002;95(5):275–83.

22. Anifantaki S, Prinianakis G, Vitsaksaki E, et al. Daily interruption of sedative infusions in an adult medical-surgical intensive care unit: randomized controlled trial. J Adv Nurs 2009;65:1054–60.

23. Barr J, Fraser GL, Puntillo K, et al. Clinical practice guidelines for the management of pain, agitation, and delirium in adult patients in the intensive care unit. Crit Care Med 2013;41:263–306.

24. Seger DL. Flumazenil–treatment or toxin. J Toxicol Clin Toxicol 2004;42:209–16.

25. Rasimas JJ, Kivovich V, Sachdeva K, et al. Antagonizing the errors of history: bedside experience with flumazenil. J Am Assoc Emerg Psychiatry 2015;13:17–34.

26. Ngo AS, Anthony CR, Samuel M, et al. Should a benzodiazepine antagonist be used in unconscious patients presenting to the emergency department? Resuscitation 2007;74:27–37.

27. Breheny FX. Reversal of midazolam sedation with flumazenil. Crit Care Med 1992; 20:736–9.

28. Cammarano WB, Pittet JF, Weitz S, et al. Acute withdrawal syndrome related to the administration of analgesic and sedative medications in adult intensive care unit patients. Crit Care Med 1998;26:676–84.

29. Kim S. Skeletal muscle relaxants. In: Olson KR, Anderson IB, Benowitz NL, et al, editors. Poisoning and drug overdose. 5th edition. New York: McGraw-Hill; 2007. p. 341–3.

30. Ahboucha S, Butterworth RF. Pathophysiology of hepatic encephalopathy: a new look at GABA from the molecular standpoint. Metab Brain Dis 2004;19:331–43.
31. Mowry JB, Spyker DA, Brooks DE, et al. 2015 annual report of the American Association of Poison Control Centers' National Poison Data System (NPDS): 33rd annual report. Clin Toxicol (Phila) 2016;54:924–1109.
32. Sporer KA. Acute heroin overdose. Ann Intern Med 1999;130:584–90.
33. White ML, Zhang Y, Helvey JT, et al. Anatomical patterns and correlated MRI findings of non-perinatal hypoxic-ischaemic encephalopathy. Br J Radiol 2013;86(1021):20120464.
34. Muttikkal TJ, Wintermark M. MRI patterns of global hypoxic-ischemic injury in adults. J Neuroradiol 2013;40(3):164–71.
35. Holten C. Cutaneous phenomena in acute barbiturate poisoning. Acta Derm Venereol Suppl (Stockh) 1952;32:162–8.
36. Proudfoot AT, Donovan JW. Diagnosis of poisonings. In: Brent J, Wallace KL, Burkhart KK, et al, editors. Critical care toxicology: diagnosis and management of the critically poisoned patient. Philadelphia: Elsevier Mosby; 2005. p. 13–28.
37. Hoffman RS, Goldfrank LR. The poisoned patient with altered consciousness. Controversies in the use of a 'coma cocktail'. JAMA 1995;274:562–9.
38. Glass PS, Jhaveri RM, Smith LR. Comparison of potency and duration of action of nalmefene and naloxone. Anesth Analg 1994;78(3):536–41.
39. Hahn I-H, Nelson LS. Opioid antagonists. In: Brent J, Wallace KL, Burkhart KK, et al, editors. Critical care toxicology: diagnosis and management of the critically poisoned patient. Philadelphia: Elsevier Mosby; 2005. p. 1489–91.
40. Moore RA, Rumack BH, Conner CS, et al. Naloxone: underdosage after narcotic poisoning. Am J Dis Child 1980;134:156–8.
41. van Dorp E, Yassen A, Sarton E, et al. Naloxone reversal of buprenorphine-induced respiratory depression. Anesthesiology 2006;105:51–7.
42. Lucyk SN, Nelson LS. Novel synthetic opioids: an opioid epidemic within an opioid epidemic. Ann Emerg Med 2017;69:91–3.
43. Johnson DA, Hricik JG. The pharmacology of alpha-adrenergic decongestants. Pharmacotherapy 1993;13(6 Pt 2):110S–5S.
44. Food and Drug Administration, HHS. Final rule declaring dietary supplements containing ephedrine alkaloids adulterated because they present an unreasonable risk. Final rule. Fed Regist 2004;69(28):6787–854.
45. Nelson L, Perrone J. Herbal and alternative medicine. Emerg Med Clin North Am 2000;18(4):709–22.
46. Valente MJ, Guedes de Pinho P, de Lourdes Bastos M, et al. Khat and synthetic cathinones: a review. Arch Toxicol 2014;88:15–45.
47. Sleigh J, Harvey M, Voss L, et al. Ketamine–more mechanisms of action than just NMDA blockade. Trends Anaesth Crit Care 2014;4:76–81.
48. Beckman KJ, Parker RB, Hariman RJ, et al. Hemodynamic and electrophysiological actions of cocaine. Effects of sodium bicarbonate as an antidote in dogs. Circulation 1991;83:1799–807.
49. Young CC, Prielipp RC. Benzodiazepines in the intensive care unit. Crit Care Clin 2001;17:843–62.
50. Seyit M, Erdur B, Kortunay S, et al. A comparison of dexmedetomidine, moxonidine and alpha-methyldopa effects on acute, lethal cocaine toxicity. Iran Red Crescent Med J 2015;17:e18780.
51. Weerink MA, Struys MM, Hannivoort LN, et al. Clinical pharmacokinetics and pharmacodynamics of dexmedetomidine. Clin Pharmacokinet 2017. [Epub ahead of print].

52. Berman SM, Kuczenski R, McCracken JT, et al. Potential adverse effects of amphetamine treatment on brain and behavior: a review. Mol Psychiatry 2009; 14:123–42.
53. Dalton R. Mixed bipolar disorder precipitated by pseudoephedrine hydrochloride. South Med J 1990;83:64–5.
54. Lake CR, Tenglin R, Chernow B, et al. Psychomotor stimulant-induced mania in a genetically predisposed patient: a review of the literature and report of a case. J Clin Psychopharmacol 1983;3:97–100.
55. Rusyniak DE. Neurologic manifestations of chronic methamphetamine abuse. Psychiatr Clin North Am 2013;36:261–75.
56. Baker SD, Borys DJ. A possible trend suggesting increased abuse from Coricidin exposures reported to the Texas Poison Network: comparing 1998 to 1999. Vet Hum Toxicol 2002;44(3):169–71.
57. Burns JM, Boyer EW. Antitussives and substance abuse. Subst Abuse Rehabil 2013;4:75–82.
58. Chyka PA, Erdman AR, Manoguerra AS, et al. Dextromethorphan poisoning: an evidence-based consensus guideline for out-of-hospital management. Clin Toxicol (Phila) 2007;45:662–77.
59. Boyer EW, Shannon M. The serotonin syndrome. N Engl J Med 2005;352: 1112–20.
60. Kirschner RI, Cimikoski WJ, Donovan JW. Drug combinations associated with serotonin syndrome in patients admitted to a toxicology treatment center. Clin Toxicol 2008;46:612.
61. Foley KF, DeSanty KP, Kast RE. Bupropion: pharmacology and therapeutic applications. Expert Rev Neurother 2006;6:1249–65.
62. Dunkley EJ, Isbister GK, Sibbritt D, et al. The Hunter Serotonin Toxicity Criteria: simple and accurate diagnostic decision rules for serotonin toxicity. QJM 2003; 96:635–42.
63. Shepherd G, Velez LI, Keyes DC. Intentional bupropion overdoses. J Emerg Med 2004;27:147–51.
64. Pedavally S, Fugate JE, Rabinstein AA. Serotonin syndrome in the intensive care unit: clinical presentations and precipitating medications. Neurocrit Care 2014; 21:108–13.
65. Caroff SN. Neuroleptic malignant syndrome. In: Mann SC, Caroff SN, Keck PE, et al, editors. Neuroleptic malignant syndrome and related conditions. 2nd edition. Washington, DC: American Psychiatric Publishing; 2003. p. 1–44.
66. Isbister GK, Buckley NA, Whyte IM. Serotonin toxicity: a practical approach to diagnosis and treatment. Med J Aust 2007;187:361–5.
67. Constantin JM, Momon A, Mantz J, et al. Efficacy and safety of sedation with dexmedetomidine in critical care patients: a meta-analysis of randomized controlled trials. Anaesth Crit Care Pain Med 2016;35:7–15.
68. Deichmann WB, Henschler D, Holmsted B, et al. What is there that is not poison? A study of the Third Defense by Paracelsus. Arch Toxicol 1986;58:207–13.
69. Tan HH, Hoppe J, Heard K. A systematic review of cardiovascular effects after atypical antipsychotic medication overdose. Am J Emerg Med 2009;27(5):607–16.
70. Beach SR, Celano CM, Noseworthy PA, et al. QTc prolongation, torsades de pointes, and psychotropic medications. Psychosomatics 2013;54:1–13.
71. Glassman AH, Bigger JT Jr. Antipsychotic drugs: prolonged QTc interval, torsade de pointes, and sudden death. Am J Psychiatry 2001;158:1774–82.
72. Stöllberger C, Huber JO, Finsterer J. Antipsychotic drugs and QT prolongation. Int Clin Psychopharmacol 2005;20:243–51.

73. Hasnain M, Vieweg WV. QTc interval prolongation and torsade de pointes associated with second-generation antipsychotics and antidepressants: a comprehensive review. CNS Drugs 2014;28:887–920.
74. Buckley NA, Whyte IM, Dawson AH. Cardiotoxicity more common in thioridazine
overdose than with other neuroleptics. J Toxicol Clin Toxicol 1995;33:199–204.
75. Strawn JR, Keck PE Jr, Caroff SN. Neuroleptic malignant syndrome. Am J Psychiatry 2007;164:870–6.
76. Burns MJ. Neuroleptic malignant syndrome. In: Brent J, Wallace KL, Burkhart KK,
et al, editors. Critical care toxicology: diagnosis and management of the critically
poisoned patient. Philadelphia: Elsevier Mosby; 2005. p. 305–13.
77. Trzepacz PT, Meagher DJ, Leonard M. Delirium. In: Levenson JL, editor. Textbook of
psychosomatic medicine. 2nd edition. Arlington: APA Publishing; 2011. p. 71–114.
78. Perry PJ, Wilborn CA. Serotonin syndrome vs neuroleptic malignant syndrome: a
contrast of causes, diagnoses, and management. Ann Clin Psychiatry 2012;24:
155–62.
79. Gurrera RJ, Caroff SN, Cohen A, et al. An international consensus study of neuroleptic malignant syndrome diagnostic criteria using the Delphi method. J Clin
Psychiatry 2011;72:1222–8.
80. Sokoro AA, Zivot J, Ariano RE. Neuroleptic malignant syndrome versus serotonin
syndrome: the search for a diagnostic tool. Ann Pharmacother 2011;45(9):e50.
81. McMartin K, Jacobsen D, Hovda KE. Antidotes for poisoning by alcohols that
form toxic metabolites. Br J Clin Pharmacol 2016;81:505–15.
82. Tormoehlen LM, Tekulve KJ, Nañagas KA. Hydrocarbon toxicity: a review. Clin
Toxicol (Phila) 2014;52:479–89.
83. Wu LT, Howard MO. Psychiatric disorders in inhalant users: results from the national epidemiologic survey on alcohol and related conditions. Drug Alcohol
Depend 2007;88:146–55.
84. Hodgman MJ, Garrard AR. A review of acetaminophen poisoning. Crit Care Clin
2012;28:499–516.
85. Hunter LJ, Wood DM, Dargan PI. The patterns of toxicity and management of
acute nonsteroidal anti-inflammatory drug (NSAID) overdose. Open Access
Emerg Med 2011;3:39–48.
86. O'Malley GF. Emergency department management of the salicylate-poisoned patient. Emerg Med Clin North Am 2007;25:333–46.
87. Myers RA, DeFazio A, Kelly MP. Chronic carbon monoxide exposure: a clinical
syndrome detected by neuropsychological tests. J Clin Psychol 1998;54:555–67.
88. Asian S, Karcioglu O, Bilge F, et al. Post-interval syndrome after carbon monoxide
poisoning. Vet Hum Toxicol 2004;46:183–5.
89. Ku BD, Shin HY, Kim EJ, et al. Secondary mania in a patient with delayed anoxic encephalopathy after carbon monoxide intoxication. J Clin Neurosci 2006;13:860–2.
90. Lam SP, Fong SY, Kwok A, et al. Delayed neuropsychiatric impairment after carbon
monoxide poisoning from burning charcoal. Hong Kong Med J 2004;10:428–31.
91. Weaver LK. Clinical practice. Carbon monoxide poisoning. N Engl J Med 2009;
360:1217–25.
92. Olson KR, Anderson IB, Benowitz NL, et al. Poisoning and drug overdose. 7th
edition. New York: McGraw-Hill; 2017.
93. Groddeck G. The meaning of illness. New York: International Universities Press;
1977.
94. Rainey PM. Laboratory principles. In: Flomenbaum NE, Goldfrank LR,
Hoffman RS, et al, editors. Goldfrank's toxicologic emergencies. 8th edition.
New York: McGraw-Hill; 2006. p. 88–108.

Substance Use, Intoxication, and Withdrawal in the Critical Care Setting

CrossMark

Joseph H. Donroe, MD, MPH[a],*, Jeanette M. Tetrault, MD[b]

KEYWORDS

- Critical care • Substance-related disorders • Opioid-related disorders
- Stimulant-related disorders • Synthetic cannabinoid • Synthetic cathinone
- Cocaine • MDMA

KEY POINTS

- Effects of substance use, including intoxication and withdrawal, are commonly encountered, although often difficult to detect in critically ill patients.
- Management is directed at the specific intoxication or withdrawal syndrome.
- Comprehensive management of patients with complications related to substance use includes engagement in longitudinal management of the underlying substance use disorder.

INTRODUCTION

Substance use disorders are common, although the prevalence in the inpatient setting is not well defined. In 2012, it was estimated that 11% of adult hospitalizations involved substance use disorders alone or in combination with mental health disorders, likely an underestimation given the frequency of underdiagnosis of substance use disorders.[1] The most common diagnoses were alcohol-related disorders, drug-induced mental disorders, opioid-related disorders, cocaine-related disorders, and hallucinogen-related disorders. The most common demographic was male Medicaid or Medicare recipients between the ages of 18 and 44 (drug-induced mental health, opioids, hallucinogens) or 45 and 64 (alcohol, cocaine). From a community sample,

Disclosure Statement: The authors have nothing to disclose.
This article is an update of an article previously published in *Critical Care Clinics*, Volume 24, Issue 4, October 2008.
[a] Department of Internal Medicine, Yale University School of Medicine, St. Raphael Campus, Office M330, 1450 Chapel Street, New Haven, CT 06511, USA; [b] Department of Internal Medicine, Yale University School of Medicine, 367 Cedar Street, Suite 305, New Haven, CT 06510, USA
* Corresponding author.
E-mail address: joseph.donroe@yale.edu

approximately 19% of hospitalized patients had evidence of unhealthy substance use, of whom most were admitted to academic teaching service.[2] Recent trends point to increasing numbers of hospitalizations from overdose in persons with opioid use disorder (OUD), and intoxication with designer drugs such as synthetic cannabinoids (SCB), synthetic cathinones (bath salts), and 3,4-methylenedioxymethamphetamine (MDMA, ecstasy).[3–6]

The epidemiology of substance use disorders in the critical care setting is largely unknown. Estimates from one community hospital noted 14% of intensive care unit (ICU) admissions were non–tobacco substance related.[7] Furthermore, substance use has been identified as a risk factor for hospitalization for diabetic ketoacidosis (DKA), with longer subsequent ICU stays compared with DKA unrelated to substance use.[8] In addition, substance use is associated with injury and trauma, including motor vehicle injuries, falls, drownings, thermal injury, homicide, and suicide.[9–12] In the United States, up to half of trauma beds are occupied by patients involved in alcohol-related traffic accidents.[10,13] Management of critically ill or injured patients who use illicit substances is complicated by both the intoxicating and the withdrawal effects of those substances. This review addresses the presenting features and management of non–alcohol-related intoxication and withdrawal syndromes of commonly used illicit substances likely to impact the care of a critically ill patient. Complications of alcohol intoxication and withdrawal are reviewed separately. Substances with mild intoxication and withdrawal syndromes unlikely to influence the care of critically ill patients, such as nicotine and natural cannabis, are not covered.

GENERAL CRITICAL CARE ISSUES RELATED TO SUBSTANCE USE
Overdose

Overdose may be suspected from history taken from patients or family, or the recognition of an overdose syndrome. Importantly, when caring for a person with altered mental status from suspected intoxication, HIPAA (Health Insurance Portability and Accountability Act) does not prevent providers from obtaining information from or giving information to close relations if such disclosure is thought to be important to the care of the patient.[14] General management principles include providing basic life support and airway management, obtaining intravenous (IV) access, vital sign monitoring, reviewing all potential medications the patient may have access to, a focused examination, including evaluation of pupils and a search for transdermal patches and signs of injection drug use, such as "track marks," electrocardiogram, and basic laboratory work to review renal and liver function and to exclude other causes such as infection or myocardial infarction, as well as urine and serum toxicologies.[9]

Agitation

Agitation may result from intoxication or withdrawal, and management can depend on the specific substance or substances used. Management begins with providing a low stimulation environment. In terms of pharmacotherapy to manage agitation, benzodiazepines are often used. Antipsychotic medications can be used as second-line agents. Restraints should generally be avoided if possible and may worsen agitation and risk of sudden death, particularly in the setting of stimulant drug use.[15,16]

Withdrawal
Withdrawal syndromes are the response to abrupt discontinuation, decreased dosing, or altered metabolism of a substance to which there is physiologic dependence and are common to many substances. These syndromes commonly complicate the care of critically ill patients.[9,17,18] It may be especially challenging to treat patients with

substance withdrawal syndromes because of an unknown history of substance use, altered mental status, or complex physiologic responses resulting from the presenting illness, which can be confused with withdrawal.[19] In addition, patients may be withdrawing from several substances upon presentation. General principles regarding the management of substance withdrawal syndromes include use of a symptom-triggered approach, substitution of a long-acting replacement for the misused drug in gradual tapering doses, and establishing a plan for long-term management of the underlying substance use disorder.[20] When assessing for superimposed substance withdrawal, the critical care team must consider potential polysubstance use.

Iatrogenic Dependence

It is important to consider development of iatrogenic physiologic dependence on medications in patients (with or without a history of substance use disorder) who have extended hospitalizations. Patients with critical illness often require prolonged stays in the ICU as well as large cumulative doses of opioids and sedatives to facilitate pain control, anxiety, and sedation. Acute withdrawal syndromes may present in these patients as a result of rapid weaning for transitions to lower levels of care. Continuous infusions of opioids or benzodiazepines may place patients at higher risk for the development of acute withdrawal than would administration of these medications by bolus injection.[9] It is up to the critical care team, therefore, to consider implementation of weaning protocols, consisting of a 5% to 10% reduction per day, early on in the course of a patient's ICU stay.[21]

CRITICAL CARE ISSUES RELATED TO SPECIFIC SUBSTANCES
Opioids

In 2015, an estimated 2.6 million Americans over the age of 12 met criteria for OUD.[22] Opioids include substances that are derived directly from the opium poppy (such as morphine and codeine), the semisynthetic opioids (such as heroin and hydromorphone), and the purely synthetic opioids (such as methadone and fentanyl). Opioid medications primarily act as agonists at the μ-opioid receptor and may be prescribed or obtained illegally. Common means of administration include ingestion, nasal insufflation, inhalation, and injection via IV, intramuscular, or subcutaneous routes. In the course of managing critically ill patients with OUD, clinicians should be vigilant for associated comorbid medical conditions that can complicate care, such as acute bacterial infections, HIV, and hepatitis C (HCV) –related problems.[23,24]

Intoxication and overdose

Opioid intoxication leads to impaired judgment, psychomotor agitation or depression, and pupillary constriction (**Table 1**).[25] Opioid overdose should be suspected in patients with any combination of depressed mental status, decreased respiratory rate or chest wall rise, and miotic pupils.[26] Patients who are not protecting their airway, are hypoxemic or hypercarbic, or have a respiratory rate less than 10 to 12 breaths per minute should receive bag-valve mask ventilation and have IV naloxone administered.[26] Naloxone can also be administered intramuscularly, intranasally, or via endotracheal tube depending on the clinical scenario. Because the effects of naloxone only last 20 to 90 minutes, suspected overdoses involving long-acting opioids may require repeat dosing or IV infusion. Orotracheal intubation is required if the airway is difficult to maintain or respiratory rate does not improve after escalating doses of naloxone. Importantly, symptoms of opioid withdrawal should be expected after administration of naloxone in patients with physiologic opioid dependence.[9]

Substance	Intoxication	Withdrawal	Associated Complications
Opiates • Morphine, codeine Semisynthetic opioids • Heroin, buprenorphine, hydromorphone Synthetic opioids • Fentanyl, methadone	Depressed mental status Impaired judgment Pupillary constriction Hypoventilation	Fever, tachycardia, hypotension Restlessness, irritability, insomnia Yawning, diaphoresis, piloerection Mydriasis, lacrimation, rhinorrhea Nausea, diarrhea, abdominal pain Myalgia, arthralgia	Overdose death Injection-related infection HIV HCV

Table 1
Opioids intoxication and withdrawal in critically ill patients

Withdrawal

The severity of opioid withdrawal varies with the dose, duration of substance use, and route of administration.[27] The time to onset and duration of opioid withdrawal symptoms depend on the half-life of the drug being used. For example, withdrawal from heroin may begin 4 to 6 hours after the last use, may peak within 36 to 72 hours, and may last for 7 to 14 days, whereas withdrawal from methadone may not occur until 36 hours after the last use.[28,29] Symptoms include diarrhea and vomiting, thermoregulation disturbances, insomnia, muscle and joint pain, anxiety, and dysphoria. The severity of opioid withdrawal can be graded using instruments such as the Clinical Opioid Withdrawal Scale and Objective Opioid Withdrawal Scale, although neither scale has been validated in an ICU setting.[28] Although opioid withdrawal includes no life-threatening complications (unlike alcohol or benzodiazepine withdrawal syndrome), the acute opioid withdrawal syndrome causes marked discomfort, frequently leads to a relapse to drug use, complicates other medical and surgical conditions, and can strain patient-doctor relations.[28,29]

Management of opioid withdrawal begins by reassuring patients that their symptoms will be taken seriously, providing general supportive measures, and initiating specific pharmacologic treatment. Pharmacologic options include opioid agonist therapy (OAT, methadone, and buprenorphine), alpha-adrenergic agents, and other non–opioid medications that can provide symptom relief.[28] Studies indicate buprenorphine and methadone have similar effectiveness for managing withdrawal, and alpha 2 adrenergic agonists are more effective than placebo at preventing severe withdrawal.[30,31] The choice of pharmacotherapy, therefore, may be influenced by the presence and severity of patients' underlying medical comorbidities, patient preference, and medication interactions.[28,32] Methadone and buprenorphine not only have the advantage of stabilizing withdrawal but also can be continued for long-term management of OUD, depending on patient preference and provider availability. Whenever possible, hospitalized patients with OUD should be engaged in conversations about long-term management of their OUD.[28]

Careful initiation and titration of various medications can treat opioid withdrawal. Methadone initiated at 10 to 30 mg daily and slowly titrated to a total daily dose of 20 to 40 mg is usually sufficient to treat withdrawal symptoms.[28,33,34] Alternatively, buprenorphine can be initiated once moderate opioid withdrawal is evident using standard protocols.[35] Buprenorphine initiated too early can precipitate withdrawal. Limitations to the use of buprenorphine in the treatment of OUD in the ICU are its sublingual administration and issues with regard to pain control and sedation. Typical doses of clonidine used to treat opioid withdrawal range between 0.1 and 0.2 mg every 6 hours with close monitoring of blood pressure. Side effects include sedation, dry mouth, orthostatic hypotension, and constipation.

Pain management in patients with opioid use disorder, including patients receiving opioid agonist therapy

Acute pain related to trauma and surgical procedures is common in critically ill patients. Issues unique to patients with OUD include provider misconceptions, opioid tolerance and decreased pain threshold, and concurrent OAT.[28,36] Provider misconceptions include the notions that the medication used for OUD should cover the acute painful condition, use of opioids for analgesia may result in relapse, addition of opioid analgesia to opioid maintenance is likely to result in central nervous system (CNS) and respiratory depression, and complaints of pain may constitute "drug-seeking" behavior. In general, patients should be maintained on medications to treat OUD (treatment programs should be contacted to verify dose and to ensure easy transition from inpatient hospital stay back to the community) and supplemented with short-acting opioids titrated to pain relief as well as use of non–opioid medications and techniques to treat pain. In ICU patients, physiologic responses such as heart rate and blood pressure may have to be used to monitor pain relief in patients maintained on sedation and mechanical ventilation. It should be recognized that patients with a history of OUD will likely exhibit tolerance to opioid medications and may require higher than usual doses to treat pain.[28,36]

Treatment of acute pain in patients maintained on buprenorphine for opioid dependence may be especially challenging because buprenorphine has a higher affinity for the μ-opioid receptor than do other opioids. Options for pain management in patients maintained on buprenorphine include discontinuation of buprenorphine treatment and transition to full agonist opioids for treatment of pain; transition to methadone for treatment of OUD with additional opioids to treat pain; division of daily dose of buprenorphine to 3 to 4 times daily to take advantage of analgesic properties of the medication; or continuation of buprenorphine with titration of short-acting opioids.[28,36]

Benzodiazepines

Benzodiazepines are one of the most widely prescribed psychotropic medications in the United States[37] (**Table 2**). Benzodiazepine medications act at the gamma-aminobutyric acid (GABA) receptor to amplify the effect of circulating GABA, thus leading to increased inhibitory tone and clinical sedation, muscle relaxation, and anxiolysis.[38] They are commonly prescribed for anxiety and sleep disorders, abortive therapy for seizure disorders, and management of alcohol withdrawal. Benzodiazepines

Table 2
Benzodiazepine intoxication and withdrawal in critically ill patients

Substance	Intoxication	Withdrawal	Associated Complications
Short acting • Alprazolam, midazolam Intermediate acting • Lorazepam, oxazepam Long acting • Diazepam, clonazepam	Depressed mental status Impaired judgment Decreased attention and memory Slurred speech Incoordination	Tachycardia, hypertension Agitation, hallucinations Tremor, seizure	Overdose death, especially with coingested opioids

are most commonly administered by oral ingestion, and more lipophilic (eg, diazepam) and short-acting (eg, alprazolam) formulations are most reinforcing.[38,39] It is important to note that illicit benzodiazepines are commonly coingested with other illicit substances, such as opioids, increasing the risk for overdose.[40]

Intoxication and overdose

Benzodiazepine intoxication is marked by impaired judgment and attention, depressed mental status, incoordination, slurred speech, and unsteady gait.[41] The risk of death resulting from benzodiazepines when used in isolation is relatively small; however, the risk of overdose and death increases substantially when benzodiazepines are coadministered with opioid medications, or other CNS-depressing agents.[42,43] Management of suspected benzodiazepine overdose is supportive. Flumazenil has a high-binding affinity for the GABA-A receptor but weak intrinsic action and thus can be used to reverse the intoxicating effects of other benzodiazepines. Its use, however, has fallen out of favor in the management of patients with depressed mental status who have known or suspected benzodiazepine ingestion due to the risk of precipitating seizures and arrhythmias.[43,44] In addition, intentional overdoses often involve coingestion of multiple medications, and benzodiazepines may actually have a stabilizing effect if the coingestants are prone to cause seizures, such as tricyclic antidepressants. Flumazenil may have a role, however, in reversing iatrogenic benzodiazepine overdose, for example, during procedural sedation, particularly when the chronicity of benzodiazepine use and other coadministered medications is known to the provider.[44]

Withdrawal

Benzodiazepine withdrawal is characterized by autonomic hyperactivity and can result in agitation, hallucinations, tremor, and seizures.[9,41] The severity and duration of withdrawal symptoms depend, in part, on the half-life of the medication being used. Inpatient management follows the same treatment protocol as for alcohol withdrawal. Treatment generally consists of use of a long-acting benzodiazepine in tapering doses over time. The symptom-triggered approach has been shown to be as effective as the fixed-dose approach for the acute treatment of benzodiazepine withdrawal.[45] For patients who have been taking benzodiazepines chronically for anxiety, either prescribed or illicitly, a prolonged tapering schedule with a long-acting benzodiazepine and appropriate management of the underlying anxiety disorder should be considered in order to reduce the chance of relapse to benzodiazepine use upon hospital discharge.[46,47] Careful coordination of care with outpatient providers is necessary to minimize relapse.

Stimulants: Cocaine and Methamphetamine

The stimulant effects of systemically administered cocaine, derived from the *Erythroxylum coca* plant, are due to the reuptake inhibition of catecholamines at the synaptic cleft (**Table 3**). In the United States in 2006, 1.7 million people reported cocaine abuse or dependence.[48] Illicit cocaine is either snorted or injected as cocaine hydrochloride, or smoked in its free base form.

Methamphetamine was the fourth most common illicit substance responsible for Emergency Department (ED) visits in 2011, and prevalence of use may be increasing.[49,50] Methamphetamine is a highly addictive synthetic stimulant that stimulates catecholamine release and partially blocks catecholamine reuptake at the synaptic cleft. It is distributed in either a powder, a pill, or a highly purified crystalline form, referred to as "crystal meth." Methamphetamine is commonly smoked, injected, ingested, or nasally insufflated.

Table 3
Stimulant intoxication and withdrawal in critically ill patients

Substance	Intoxication	Withdrawal	Associated Complications
Cocaine • Cocaine hydrochloride • Crack (freebase cocaine) Methamphetamine • Powder D-methamphetamine hydrochloride • Crystal D-methamphetamine hydrochloride	Euphoria Increased attention Paranoia, anxiety, agitation Disorientation Hallucination	Depressed mood Fatigue Vivid dreams Insomnia Increased appetite Psychomotor retardation Agitation	Injection-related infection Rhabdomyolysis Hyperthermia Seizure Cardiovascular • Myocardial infarction, aortic dissection, myocarditis, cardiomyopathy, chest pain Cerebrovascular • Hemorrhagic and ischemic stroke Pulmonary • Pneumothorax, "crack lung," bronchospasm, diffuse alveolar hemorrhage, pulmonary edema, pulmonary hypertension, bronchiolitis obliterans, pulmonary infarction

Intoxication and overdose

Stimulant intoxication leads to euphoria, increased alertness, mydriasis, tachycardia and hypertension, and reduced appetite, with increasing doses causing anxiety and paranoia, aggressiveness, disorientation, and hallucinations.[41,50,51] Stimulants can lower the seizure threshold and cause hyperthermia and rhabdomyolysis.[52] Apart from the infectious-related complications from IV administration, the most clinically significant effects of stimulant use are on the cardiovascular, cerebrovascular, and pulmonary systems.

Catecholamine excess leads to potent vasoconstriction, tachycardia, and propensity for arrhythmia. Stimulant-related chest pain is a common symptom and can be caused by a myriad of effects, including myocardial infarction, aortic dissection, cardiomyopathy, myocarditis, pneumothorax, and pneumomediastinum.[50,53–55] Myocardial infarction occurs from the vasoconstrictive effects, increased myocardial oxygen demand, increased platelet aggregation, and accelerated atherosclerotic changes in chronic users.[53,55] Management of cocaine-induced myocardial ischemia is focused on decreasing platelet aggregation (aspirin), decreasing vasoconstriction and hypertension (nitrates, calcium channel blockers), decreasing overall sympathetic tone (benzodiazepines), and in the appropriate setting, early reperfusion therapy with a preference for percutaneous coronary intervention over thrombolysis due to a cocaine-mediated increased risk of intracerebral hemorrhage. Beta-blockers should generally be avoided because they can theoretically increase vasoconstriction.[53] Treatment of methamphetamine-related cardiovascular complications is less well described, although management should proceed in a similar fashion to cocaine-related complications.

Current and prior stimulant use are risk factors for both hemorrhagic and ischemic strokes. Hemorrhagic strokes are likely sequelae of elevations in blood pressure and aneurysm formation, whereas ischemic strokes are due to accelerated atherosclerosis and vasoconstriction.[54,56–58] Stroke management in patients with current or prior stimulant use is similar to management in patients without stimulant use. As in patients with acute myocardial ischemia, beta-blockers should be avoided.[54]

The pulmonary effects of inhaled stimulant use are more widely described for cocaine and include bronchospasm, pneumothorax, diffuse alveolar hemorrhage, pulmonary edema, pulmonary hypertension, bronchiolitis obliterans, eosinophilic lung disease, pulmonary infarction, and exacerbation of underlying lung disease.[53,59] "Crack lung" is a syndrome of fever, shortness of breath, pleuritic chest pain, hemoptysis, and hypoxemic respiratory failure occurring within 48 hours of free base crack inhalation. Management is supportive, and improvement is expected within 24 hours of presentation.[60]

Withdrawal

Cocaine withdrawal is characterized by depressed mood and any 2 of the following: fatigue, vivid dreams, sleep disturbance, increased appetite, psychomotor retardation, or agitation.[61] Cocaine withdrawal is typically mild and treated supportively.

Frequent methamphetamine use results in significant psychiatric withdrawal symptoms and intense craving following abrupt cessation. Depressive symptoms are a prominent feature of withdrawal and can last for several weeks.[50]

3,4-Methylenedioxymethamphetamine

MDMA, or ecstasy, is a popular club drug with potentially life-threatening side effects[62] (Table 4). The prevalence of use is unknown, although available data highlight an increasing number of ED-related visits with 10,227 in 2004, 17,888 in 2008, and 22,498 in 2011.[49] Formulations contain varying and unknown quantities of MDMA and may contain other drugs, including amphetamines, ketamine, dextromethorphan, acetaminophen, and caffeine.[62,63] MDMA stimulates serotonin, dopamine, and norepinephrine synaptic release and may also inhibit the reuptake of serotonin in the synaptic cleft. The clinical effects of MDMA ingestion begin within 1 hour and can last up to 6 hours.[63]

Intoxication and overdose

MDMA has stimulant and hallucinogenic properties, and intoxication typically results in elevated mood, empathy, and increased energy. Minor effects may include trismus, bruxism, tachycardia, xerostomia, and ataxia. Acute toxicity can include sudden death presumably from arrhythmia, hyperthermia, rhabdomyolysis, renal failure, serotonin syndrome, liver failure, and hyponatremia.[62,63] The risk of significant toxicity likely relates to individual factors (eg, polymorphism influencing MDMA metabolism), environmental factors (eg, temperature at the event where MDMA was ingested), and chemical factors (eg, the amount of MDMA and other substances present in the ingested pill).[62,64]

Table 4
3,4-Methylenedioxymethamphetamine intoxication and withdrawal in critically ill patients

Street Names	Intoxication	Withdrawal	Associated Complications
Ecstasy	Euphoria	Depressed mood	Sudden death (arrhythmia)
Molly	Increased empathy	Fatigue	Hyperthermia
E, Vitamin E	Increased energy		Rhabdomyolysis
XTC	Trismus		Acute kidney injury
Skittles	Bruxism		Acute liver failure
Many more…	Xerostomia		Serotonin syndrome
	Tachycardia		Hyponatremia

The constellation of hyperthermia, rhabdomyolysis, and multiorgan failure is a well-described syndrome associated with acute MDMA intoxication. The cause may be secondary excessive exertion without adequate hydration to balance the associated hyperthermia. Prolonged extreme hyperthermia may predict subsequent morbidity and mortality.[62] Temperatures greater than 42°C have been reported, and rapid cooling is an essential component of care. Dantrolene has reported benefits for MDMA-induced hyperthermia, particularly when severe, although its use has not been subject to randomized study.[62,64] Rhabdomyolysis can be significant with creatinine kinase levels increasing to the tens to hundreds of thousands units per liter. Management includes addressing the hyperthermia and aggressive IV fluid resuscitation.[65]

MDMA can independently cause serotonin syndrome, although the risk is higher if multiple drugs associated with serotonin syndrome are ingested, including amphetamines, cocaine, antidepressants, and opioids. Serotonin syndrome is characterized by altered mental status, increased muscle tone, clonus, hyperreflexia, and hyperthermia. Management of severe cases may include sedation, mechanical ventilation, rapid cooling, and pharmacologic paralysis.[62,66]

Hyponatremia results from a combination of MDMA-induced antidiuretic hormone release, increased thirst resulting from xerostomia, and intentional overhydration by users attempting to minimize the known effects of hyperthermia and dehydration.[67] The degree of hyponatremia can be significant and lead to cerebral edema. The patient can present with confusion and seizures and can rapidly decompensate to coma and death. Management of severely symptomatic patients, marked by encephalopathy and seizure, includes careful administration of hypertonic saline.[67]

MDMA has also been associated with acute hepatitis and in one study was reported as second only to antituberculosis medications in causing drug-induced acute liver failure.[68] Patients may present with encephalopathy, jaundice, abdominal pain, and raised bilirubin and transaminases. Treatment is supportive.[68,69]

Withdrawal

Withdrawal syndrome from chronic MDMA use is related to serotonin depletion and does not play a major role in the management of critically ill patients. Symptoms, including depression and fatigue, typically occur the day following use and can last up to 5 days.

Synthetic Cannabinoids

SCB have become increasing popular because of perceived safety, ease of access, favorable cost and legal status, and lack of detectability on routine toxicology screening (**Table 5**). ED visits related to SCB increased from 11,406 in 2010 to 28,531 in 2011.[49] Preparation of SCB for consumption typically begins with taking

Table 5			
Synthetic cannabinoid intoxication and withdrawal in critically ill patients			
Street Names	**Intoxication**	**Withdrawal**	**Associated Complications**
Spice	Euphoria	Anxiety	Psychosis
K2	Relaxation	Tachycardia,	Catatonia
Bliss	Anxiety, agitation	hypertension	Self-mutilation
Black Mamba	Tachycardia, hypertension	Tremor, diaphoresis	Seizure
Genie	Hallucination, delusion	Nausea	Myocardial infarction
Bombay Blue	Nausea	Nightmares	Acute kidney injury
Many more...			Serotonin syndrome

plant material, which may or may not have inherent psychoactive properties, and saturating it with SCB dissolved in a solvent. As the plant dries, the SCB remains on the plant material.[70] Administration may be via ingestion, insufflation, or inhalation. Similar to delta-9-tetrahydrocannabinol (THC), SCB bind the cannabinoid (CB) 1 and 2 receptors.[71] Stimulation of the CB1 receptors are thought to mediate the psychotropic effects. SCB and metabolites have higher affinity than THC for CB receptors, and SCBs have higher potency when compared with THC.[72,73]

Intoxication and overdose

The amount of SCB remaining on plant material after the preparation process varies, which in part accounts for its unpredictable potency. They are ingested primarily for the euphoric effects. Toxicity from SCBs includes tachycardia, agitation, drowsiness, hallucinations, delusions, hypertension, nausea, confusion, dizziness, and chest pain.[70,72] Less commonly, SCB toxicity can lead to severe psychiatric, nervous system, cardiovascular, renal, and gastrointestinal toxicity. Case reports of catatonia, seizure, self-mutilation, psychosis, cerebral ischemia, myocardial infarction, hyperemesis, acute kidney injury from tubular injury, and serotonin syndrome resulting from SCB use are noted in the literature.[4,70–72,74,75] Management of acute SCB intoxication is supportive with IV fluids for volume depletion and benzodiazepines, and less commonly, antipsychotics, for agitation or psychotic symptoms.[71]

Withdrawal

Discontinuation of SCB after chronic use has been associated with a withdrawal syndrome, including craving, anxiety, tachycardia, hypertension, nausea, tremor, diaphoresis, and nightmares.[70,73] Symptoms seem to appear soon after cessation, and the intensity correlates with the amount of daily SCB use.[71] The withdrawal syndrome is unlikely to be clinically significant in critically ill patients.

Synthetic Cathinones

Synthetic cathinones, commonly referred to as "bath salts" in the United States, are becoming increasingly more popular (**Table 6**). Adverse effects from their use are encountered more and more frequently in US hospitals with 6670 exposures reported in 2011.[5] Naturally occurring cathinones are derived from the *Catha edulis* (khat) plant, native to East Africa. Synthetic cathinones are derivatives of naturally occurring cathinones.[76,77] Pharmacologically, cathinones are thought to stimulate the presynaptic release of dopamine, norepinephrine, and serotonin and inhibit their reuptake.[77,78] Typical means of administration include nasal insufflation, inhalation, and oral ingestion, although IV, intramuscular, and intraocular administration have also been

Table 6
Synthetic cathinone (bath salts) intoxication and withdrawal in critically ill patients

Street Names	Intoxication	Withdrawal	Associated Complications
Cloud 9	Euphoria	Depressed mood	Psychosis
Vanilla Sky	Increased attention	Anxiety	Seizure, coma
Gold Rush	Sexual arousal	Sleep disorder	Hyperthermia
White Lightening	Anxiety, agitation	Paranoia	Blurred vision
Pure Ivory	Tachycardia, hypertension		Rhabdomyolysis
Ivory Wave	Hallucination, delusion		Respiratory failure
Stardust			Acute kidney injury
Wicked X			Hyponatremia
Many more…			Serotonin syndrome

described.[76,78] Similar to SCB, synthetic cathinones are not detected on routine toxicology testing; however, they may produce a false positive for methamphetamine and phencyclidine.

Intoxication and overdose

Clinically, the effects of synthetic cathinones are similar to other stimulants with euphoria, increased attention, sexual arousal, tachycardia, and hypertension.[76,78] After nasal insufflation and oral ingestion, effects are felt within 10 to 20 minutes and 15 to 45 minutes, respectively, and last 1 to 4 hours.[78] There is a spectrum of associated toxicities reported from synthetic cathinone use. Psychiatric manifestations account for a large portion of individuals seeking medical care and include mild agitation to severe psychosis. Anxiety, paranoia, and suicidal ideation have also been reported. Additional effects include seizure, coma, tachycardia, hypertension, hyperthermia, shortness of breath, chest pain, acute kidney injury, blurred vision, rhabdomyolysis, hyponatremia, respiratory failure, and serotonin syndrome among others.[5,76,78] Management is supportive, including IV fluids for dehydration, aggressive cooling for hyperthermia, and benzodiazepines for synthetic cathinone–induced agitation. Vigilance for other coingestions is important, because polysubstance use with synthetic cathinones is particularly common.[78]

Withdrawal

Chronic use of synthetic cathinones may lead to a withdrawal syndrome, including depression, anxiety, sleep disorder, paranoia, and cravings, although it is unlikely to play a significant role when managing critically ill patients.[76]

TRANSITIONS OF CARE FOR PATIENTS WITH SUBSTANCE USE DISORDERS

It is important not to lose sight of the underlying substance use disorder when caring for critically ill patients suffering from the effects of substance-induced intoxication, overdose, or withdrawal. The hospitalization, in fact, can be an important "engageable" moment for patients with substance use disorders. For example, hospital-initiated OAT paired with referral to outpatient addiction services can reduce discharges against medical advice and increase follow-up in postdischarge addiction treatment centers.[28,32] Appropriate referral sources include detoxification facilities, addiction recovery clinics, counseling services, and area 12-step programs.[79]

In addition, it is important to note that patients with substance use often have underlying psychiatric comorbidities, including mood disorders. Screening for and treatment of psychiatric disorders are essential parts of treatment of the underlying substance use and substance use disorders.[20]

SUMMARY

Intoxication and withdrawal from substance use is common among patients presenting to the ICU with critical illness and may complicate the treatment course. It is important for the critical care team to consider underlying substance use disorders and withdrawal syndromes in patients presenting for care. It may be difficult to obtain a history of these disorders as a result of altered mental status, and a patient's family should also be asked. In addition, it is important to consider polysubstance use in any patient presenting with intoxication or withdrawal.

General principles regarding the treatment of substance withdrawal include application of general resuscitative measures, including airway, breathing, and circulatory management. For specific withdrawal syndromes, substitution of a long-acting agent (which acts on the same receptor pathway as the misused substance) in tapering doses is the general rule. In addition, use of a symptom-triggered approach to the treatment of substance withdrawal decreases length of stay and cumulative medication administered.

Of the utmost importance is long-term planning and referral for patients with underlying substance use disorders to allow for the best chance for successful treatment of these debilitating, chronic conditions. Consultation with an addiction specialist can be particularly helpful in this regard.

REFERENCES

1. Heslin KC, Elixhauser A, Steiner CA. Hospitalizations involving mental and substance use disorders among adults, 2012: statistical brief #191. Rockville (MD): Healthcare Cost and Utilization Project (HCUP) Statistical Briefs; 2015.
2. Holt SR, Ramos J, Harma MA, et al. Prevalence of unhealthy substance use on teaching and hospitalist medical services: implications for education. Am J Addict 2012;21(2):111–9.
3. National Institute on Drug Abuse. Emerging Trends and Alerts. 2016. Available at: https://www.drugabuse.gov/drugs-abuse/emerging-trends-alerts. Accessed January 14, 2017.
4. Springer YP, Gerona R, Scheunemann E, et al. Increase in adverse reactions associated with use of synthetic cannabinoids - Anchorage, Alaska, 2015-2016. MMWR Morb Mortal Wkly Rep 2016;65(40):1108–11.
5. Warrick BJ, Hill M, Hekman K, et al. A 9-state analysis of designer stimulant, "bath salt," hospital visits reported to poison control centers. Ann Emerg Med 2013; 62(3):244–51.
6. Centers for Disease Control and Prevention. Emergency department visits after use of a drug sold as "bath salts"–Michigan, November 13, 2010-March 31, 2011. MMWR Morb Mortal Wkly Rep 2011;60(19):624–7.
7. Baldwin WA, Rosenfeld BA, Breslow MJ, et al. Substance abuse-related admissions to adult intensive care. Chest 1993;103(1):21–5.
8. Isidro ML, Jorge S. Recreational drug abuse in patients hospitalized for diabetic ketosis or diabetic ketoacidosis. Acta Diabetol 2013;50(2):183–7.
9. Jenkins DH. Substance abuse and withdrawal in the intensive care unit. Contemporary issues. Surg Clin North Am 2000;80(3):1033–53.
10. McCabe S. Substance use and abuse in trauma: implications for care. Crit Care Nurs Clin North Am 2006;18(3):371–85.
11. Cherpitel CJ. Alcohol and injuries: a review of international emergency room studies since 1995. Drug Alcohol Rev 2007;26(2):201–14.
12. Hadfield RJ, Mercer M, Parr MJ. Alcohol and drug abuse in trauma. Resuscitation 2001;48(1):25–36.
13. Socie E, Duffy RE, Erskine T. Substance use and type and severity of injury among hospitalized trauma cases: Ohio, 2004-2007. J Stud Alcohol Drugs 2012;73(2):260–7.
14. Donroe JH, Tetrault JM. Recognizing and caring for the intoxicated patient in an outpatient clinic. Med Clin N Am. In press.
15. Stratton SJ, Rogers C, Brickett K, et al. Factors associated with sudden death of individuals requiring restraint for excited delirium. Am J Emerg Med 2001;19(3): 187–91.

16. Otahbachi M, Cevik C, Bagdure S, et al. Excited delirium, restraints, and unexpected death: a review of pathogenesis. Am J Forensic Med Pathol 2010; 31(2):107–12.

17. Al-Sanouri I, Dikin M, Soubani AO. Critical care aspects of alcohol abuse. South Med J 2005;98(3):372–81.

18. Zapantis A, Leung S. Tolerance and withdrawal issues with sedation. Crit Care Nurs Clin North Am 2005;17(3):211–23.

19. Spies CD, Dubisz N, Neumann T, et al. Therapy of alcohol withdrawal syndrome in intensive care unit patients following trauma: results of a prospective, randomized trial. Crit Care Med 1996;24(3):414–22.

20. Schottenfeld RS, Chawarski MC, Pakes JR, et al. Methadone versus buprenorphine with contingency management or performance feedback for cocaine and opioid dependence [see comment]. Am J Psychiatry 2005;162(2):340–9.

21. Cammarano WB, Pittet JF, Weitz S, et al. Acute withdrawal syndrome related to the administration of analgesic and sedative medications in adult intensive care unit patients.[see comment]. Crit Care Med 1998;26(4):676–84.

22. U.S. Department of Health and Human Services (HHS), Office of the Surgeon General. Facing addiction in America: the surgeon general's report on alcohol, drugs, and health. Washington, DC: HHS; 2016.

23. O'Connor PG, Selwyn PA, Schottenfeld RS. Medical care for injection-drug users with human immunodeficiency virus infection [see comment]. N Engl J Med 1994; 331(7):450–9.

24. Cherubin CE, Sapira JD. The medical complications of drug addiction and the medical assessment of the intravenous drug user: 25 years later [see comment]. Ann Intern Med 1993;119(10):1017–28.

25. Dole VP. Narcotic addiction, physical dependence and relapse. N Engl J Med 1972;286(18):988–92.

26. Boyer EW. Management of opioid analgesic overdose. N Engl J Med 2012; 367(2):146–55.

27. Smolka M, Schmidt LG. The influence of heroin dose and route of administration on the severity of the opiate withdrawal syndrome. Addiction 1999;94(8):1191–8.

28. Donroe JH, Holt SR, Tetrault JM. Caring for patients with opioid use disorder in the hospital. CMAJ 2016;188(17–18):1232–9.

29. Tetrault JM, O'Connor PG. Management of opioid intoxication and withdrawal. In: Ries RK, Fiellin DA, Miller SC, et al, editors. Principles of addiction medicine. 5th edition. Chevy Chase (MD): American Society of Addiction Medicine; 2014. p. 668–84.

30. Gowing L, Farrell M, Ali R, et al. Alpha(2)-adrenergic agonists for the management of opioid withdrawal. Cochrane Database Syst Rev 2016;(5):CD002024.

31. Meader N. A comparison of methadone, buprenorphine and alpha(2) adrenergic agonists for opioid detoxification: a mixed treatment comparison meta-analysis. Drug Alcohol Depend 2010;108(1–2):110–4.

32. O'Connor PG, Samet JH, Stein MD. Management of hospitalized intravenous drug users: role of the internist. Am J Med 1994;96(6):551–8.

33. Substance Abuse and Mental Health Services Administration. Detoxification and substance abuse treatment. Treatment Improvement Protocol (TIP) Series, No. 45. HHS Publication No. (SMA) 13-4131. Rockville (MD): Substance Abuse and Mental Health Services Administration; 2006.

34. Kampman K, Jarvis M. American Society of Addiction Medicine (ASAM) National Practice Guideline for the use of medications in the treatment of addiction involving opioid use. J Addict Med 2015;9(5):358–67.

35. Center for Substance Abuse Treatment. Clinical guidelines for the use of buprenorphine in the treatment of opioid addiction. Treatment Improvement Protocol (TIP) Series 40. DHHS Publication No. (SMA) 04-3939. Rockville (MD): Substance Abuse and Mental Health Services Administration; 2004.
36. Alford DP, Compton P, Samet JH. Acute pain management for patients receiving maintenance methadone or buprenorphine therapy. Ann Intern Med 2006;144(2): 127–34.
37. Olfson M, King M, Schoenbaum M. Benzodiazepine use in the United States. JAMA Psychiatry 2015;72(2):136–42.
38. Preskorn SH. A way of conceptualizing benzodiazepines to guide clinical use. J Psychiatr Pract 2015;21(6):436–41.
39. O'Brien CP. Benzodiazepine use, abuse, and dependence. J Clin Psychiatry 2005;66(Suppl 2):28–33.
40. Longo LP, Johnson B. Addiction: part I. Benzodiazepines–side effects, abuse risk and alternatives. Am Fam Physician 2000;61(7):2121–8.
41. American Psychiatric Association. Diagnostic and statistical manual of mental disorders. 5th edition. Arlington (VA): American Psychiatric Association; 2013.
42. Park TW, Saitz R, Ganoczy D, et al. Benzodiazepine prescribing patterns and deaths from drug overdose among US veterans receiving opioid analgesics: case-cohort study. BMJ 2015;350:h2698.
43. Penninga EI, Graudal N, Ladekarl MB, et al. Adverse events associated with flumazenil treatment for the management of suspected benzodiazepine intoxication–a systematic review with meta-analyses of randomised trials. Basic Clin Pharmacol Toxicol 2016;118(1):37–44.
44. Sivilotti ML. Flumazenil, naloxone and the 'coma cocktail'. Br J Clin Pharmacol 2016;81(3):428–36.
45. McGregor C, Machin A, White JM. In-patient benzodiazepine withdrawal: comparison of fixed and symptom-triggered taper methods. Drug Alcohol Rev 2003;22(2):175–80.
46. Lader M, Tylee A, Donoghue J. Withdrawing benzodiazepines in primary care. CNS Drugs 2009;23(1):19–34.
47. Onyett SR. The benzodiazepine withdrawal syndrome and its management. J R Coll Gen Pract 1989;39(321):160–3.
48. Substance Abuse and Mental Health Services Administration (SAMHSA). Results from the 2006 National Survey on Drug Use and Health: national findings. Rockville (MD): Office of Applied Studies, DHHS Publication No. SMA 07–4293; 2007.
49. Substance Abuse and Mental Health Services Administration. Drug abuse warning network, 2011: national estimates of drug-related emergency department visits. Rockville (MD): Substance Abuse and Mental Health Services Administration; 2013.
50. Courtney KE, Ray LA. Methamphetamine: an update on epidemiology, pharmacology, clinical phenomenology, and treatment literature. Drug Alcohol Depend 2014;143:11–21.
51. Goldstein RA, DesLauriers C, Burda AM. Cocaine: history, social implications, and toxicity–a review. Dis Mon 2009;55(1):6–38.
52. Hanson GR, Jensen M, Johnson M, et al. Distinct features of seizures induced by cocaine and amphetamine analogs. Eur J Pharmacol 1999;377(2–3):167–73.
53. Boghdadi MS, Henning RJ. Cocaine: pathophysiology and clinical toxicology. Heart Lung 1997;26(6):466–83.
54. Schwartz BG, Rezkalla S, Kloner RA. Cardiovascular effects of cocaine. Circulation 2010;122(24):2558–69.

55. Kaye S, McKetin R, Duflou J, et al. Methamphetamine and cardiovascular pathology: a review of the evidence. Addiction 2007;102(8):1204–11.
56. Sordo L, Indave BI, Barrio G, et al. Cocaine use and risk of stroke: a systematic review. Drug Alcohol Depend 2014;142:1–13.
57. Toossi S, Hess CP, Hills NK, et al. Neurovascular complications of cocaine use at a tertiary stroke center. J Stroke Cerebrovasc Dis 2010;19(4):273–8.
58. Ho EL, Josephson SA, Lee HS, et al. Cerebrovascular complications of methamphetamine abuse. Neurocrit Care 2009;10(3):295–305.
59. Restrepo CS, Carrillo JA, Martinez S, et al. Pulmonary complications from cocaine and cocaine-based substances: imaging manifestations. Radiographics 2007; 27(4):941–56.
60. Mégarbane B, Chevillard L. The large spectrum of pulmonary complications following illicit drug use: features and mechanisms. Chem Biol Interact 2013; 206(3):444–51.
61. Sofuoglu M, Poling J, Gonzalez G, et al. Cocaine withdrawal symptoms predict medication response in cocaine users. Am J Drug Alcohol Abuse 2006;32(4): 617–27.
62. Armenian P, Mamantov TM, Tsutaoka BT, et al. Multiple MDMA (Ecstasy) overdoses at a rave event: a case series. J Intensive Care Med 2013;28(4):252–8.
63. Hall AP, Henry JA. Acute toxic effects of 'Ecstasy' (MDMA) and related compounds: overview of pathophysiology and clinical management. Br J Anaesth 2006;96(6):678–85.
64. Parrott AC. MDMA and temperature: a review of the thermal effects of 'Ecstasy' in humans. Drug Alcohol Depend 2012;121(1–2):1–9.
65. Eede HV, Montenij LJ, Touw DJ, et al. Rhabdomyolysis in MDMA intoxication: a rapid and underestimated killer. "Clean" ecstasy, a safe party drug? J Emerg Med 2012;42(6):655–8.
66. Davies O, Batajoo-Shrestha B, Sosa-Popoteur J, et al. Full recovery after severe serotonin syndrome, severe rhabdomyolysis, multi-organ failure and disseminated intravascular coagulopathy from MDMA. Heart Lung 2014;43(2):117–9.
67. Campbell GA, Rosner MH. The agony of ecstasy: MDMA (3,4-methylenedioxymethamphetamine) and the kidney. Clin J Am Soc Nephrol 2008;3(6):1852–60.
68. Andreu V, Mas A, Bruguera M, et al. Ecstasy: a common cause of severe acute hepatotoxicity. J Hepatol 1998;29(3):394–7.
69. Brncic N, Kraus I, Viskovic I, et al. 3,4-Methylenedioxymethamphetamine (MDMA): an important cause of acute hepatitis. Med Sci Monit 2006;12(11): CS107–9.
70. Mills B, Yepes A, Nugent K. Synthetic cannabinoids. Am J Med Sci 2015;350(1): 59–62.
71. Cooper ZD. Adverse effects of synthetic cannabinoids: management of acute toxicity and withdrawal. Curr Psychiatry Rep 2016;18(5):52.
72. Orsini J, Blaak C, Tam E, et al. The wide and unpredictable scope of synthetic cannabinoids toxicity. Case Rep Crit Care 2015;2015:5.
73. Nacca N, Vatti D, Sullivan R, et al. The synthetic cannabinoid withdrawal syndrome. J Addict Med 2013;7(4):296–8.
74. Centers for Disease Control and Prevention. Acute kidney injury associated with synthetic cannabinoid use-multiple states, 2012. MMWR Morb Mortal Wkly Rep 2013;62(6):93–8.
75. Monte AA, Bronstein AC, Cao DJ, et al. An outbreak of exposure to a novel synthetic cannabinoid. N Engl J Med 2014;370(4):389–90.

76. Kersten BP, McLaughlin ME. Toxicology and management of novel psychoactive drugs. J Pharm Pract 2015;28(1):50–65.

77. German CL, Fleckenstein AE, Hanson GR. Bath salts and synthetic cathinones: an emerging designer drug phenomenon. Life Sci 2014;97(1):2–8.

78. Prosser JM, Nelson LS. The toxicology of bath salts: a review of synthetic cathinones. J Med Toxicol 2012;8(1):33–42.

79. D'Onofrio G, Becker B, Woolard RH. The impact of alcohol, tobacco, and other drug use and abuse in the emergency department. Emerg Med Clin North Am 2006;24(4):925–67.

Novel Algorithms for the Prophylaxis and Management of Alcohol Withdrawal Syndromes–Beyond Benzodiazepines

CrossMark

José R. Maldonado, MD

KEYWORDS

- Alcohol withdrawal • Withdrawal prophylaxis • Benzodiazepines
- Anticonvulsant agents • Alpha-2 agonists • Delirium tremens

KEY POINTS

- Ethanol affects multiple cellular targets and neural networks; and abrupt cessation results in generalized brain hyper excitability, due to unchecked excitation and impaired inhibition.
- In medically ill, hospitalized subjects, most AWS cases (80%) are relatively mild and uncomplicated, requiring only symptomatic management.
- The incidence of complicated AWS among patients admitted to medical or critical care units, severe enough to require pharmacologic treatment, is between 5% and 20%.
- Despite their proven usefulness in the management of complicated AWS, the use of BZDP is fraught with potential complications.
- A systematic literature review revealed that there are pharmacologic alternatives, which are safe and effective in the management of all phases of complicated AWS.

BACKGROUND

Alcohol use disorders (AUDs) are maladaptive patterns of alcohol consumption manifested by symptoms leading to clinically significant impairment or distress.[1] Ethanol is the second most commonly abused psychoactive substance (second to caffeine) and AUD is the most serious drug abuse problem in the United States[2] and worldwide.[3] The lifetime prevalences of *Diagnostic and Statistical Manual of Mental Disorders*, 4th edition, alcohol abuse and dependence were 17.8% and 12.5%, respectively; the total lifetime prevalence for any AUD was 30.3%.[4] Alcohol consumption-related problems are the

Psychosomatic Medicine Service, Emergency Psychiatry Service, Department of Psychiatry and Behavioral Sciences, Stanford University School of Medicine, 401 Quarry Road, Suite 2317, Stanford, CA 94305-5718, USA
E-mail address: jrm@stanford.edu

Crit Care Clin 33 (2017) 559–599
http://dx.doi.org/10.1016/j.ccc.2017.03.012
0749-0704/17/© 2017 Elsevier Inc. All rights reserved.

third leading cause of death in the United States.[5] An estimated 10% to 33% of patients admitted to the intensive care unit (ICU) have an AUD,[6–8] with a concomitant doubling of mortality.[9–11] AUD increases the need for mechanical ventilation by 49%, whereas a diagnosis of alcohol withdrawal syndrome (AWS) is associated with longer mechanical ventilation.[7] Morbidity and mortality rates are 2 to 4 times higher among chronic alcoholics, due to infections, cardiopulmonary insufficiency, or bleeding disorders[11–17]; and are associated with prolonged ICU stays ($P = .0001$).[15] The author found that up to 30% of ICU patients require pharmacologic management of complicated AWS.[18]

NEUROBIOLOGICAL EFFECTS OF ALCOHOL

Alcohol has varying effects in the central nervous system (CNS), depending on volume ingested and the chronicity of its use. Ethanol acts on many cellular targets of several neuromodulators within many neural networks in the brain.[19] The abrupt cessation of alcohol results in generalized brain hyperexcitability because receptors previously inhibited by alcohol are no longer inhibited and inhibitory systems are not functioning properly (**Fig. 1**). AWS is mediated by several neurochemical mechanisms: (1) the alcohol-enhanced effect of γ-aminobutyric acid (GABA) inhibitory effect; (2) alcohol-mediated inhibition of N-methyl-D-aspartate (NMDA)-receptors, leading to their upregulation and increased responsiveness to the stimulating effect of glutamate (GLU); and (3) excess availability of norepinephrine (NE) due to desensitization of alpha-2 receptors and conversion from dopamine (DA). The results are the classic clinical symptoms of AWS, including anxiety, irritability, agitation, tremors, and signs of adrenergic excess, as well as, in its extreme forms, withdrawal seizures, and delirium tremens (DT).[17,20–23]

OVERVIEW OF ALCOHOL WITHDRAWAL SYNDROMES

AWS occurs after a period of absolute or, in some cases, relative abstinence from alcohol (ie, as soon as the blood alcohol level decreases significantly in habituated individuals). Therefore, it is possible for patients to experience AWS even with elevated blood alcohol concentration (BAC). Approximately 50% of alcohol-dependent

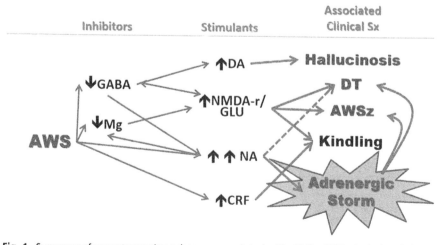

Fig. 1. Summary of neurotransmitter changes associated with AWSs. AWS, alcohol withdrawal syndrome; AWSz, alcohol withdrawal seizures; CRF, corticotropin-releasing factor; DA, dopamine; DT, delirium tremens; GABA, gamma-aminobutyric acid; GLU, glutamate; Mg, magnesium; NA, noradrenaline or norepinephrine; NMDA, N-methyl-D-aspartate receptor.

patients develop clinically relevant AWS.[24,25] Moreover, 10% to 30% of patients admitted to the hospital ICU experience AWS[7,8,26,27]; which is associated with increased morbidity and mortality.[28]

Typically, AWS begins within 6 to 24 hours after alcohol cessation or significant reduction of usual consumption, in habituated individuals (**Fig. 2, Table 1**).[29]

Uncomplicated withdrawal (so-called shakes) begins on the first day (as early as 12 hours after the last drink), peaking approximately 24 to 36 hours after relative or absolute abstinence. Approximately 80% of alcohol-dependent subjects will experience this and eventually recover without further complications.[30] Tremors, nervousness, irritability, nausea, and vomiting are the earliest and most common signs. In mild cases, withdrawal usually subsides in 5 to 7 days even without treatment. More severe symptoms lasting up to 10 to 14 days include coarse tremors (involving the upper extremities and tongue), anorexia, nausea, vomiting, psychological tension, general malaise, hypertension, autonomic hyperactivity, tachycardia, diaphoresis, orthostatic hypotension, irritability, vivid dreams, and insomnia.[23] Extrapyramidal symptoms may occur during AWS, even in patients not exposed to antipsychotic medications, after several weeks of continuous drinking or after an intensive brief binge episode.[31,32]

Alcohol withdrawal seizures (so-called rum fits) begin on the first day, peaking in approximately 12 to 48 hours (95% occurring in 7–38 hours) after a relative or absolute abstinence from alcohol. Grand mal seizures occur in up to 5% to 15% of patients experiencing AWS. Usually characterized by generalized motor seizures occurring during the course of AWS in the absence of an underlying seizure disorder.[30,33–35] The greater the amount of alcohol consumed, the greater the risk for seizures.[36–38] Approximately one-third of patients who develop AWS-seizures will only experience 1 seizure; whereas two-thirds will have multiple seizures, if untreated. Only a small minority (~3%) will develop status epilepticus; these patients often have an underlying seizure disorder.[30,35,39] Approximately one-third of patients who develop seizures go on to develop alcohol withdrawal delirium, or DTs.

Patients experiencing AWS may experience seizure activity that is not a direct consequence of the withdrawal itself. Alcohol-related seizures are defined as "adult onset seizures that occur in the setting of chronic alcohol dependence."[40] Yet alcohol withdrawal per se is the cause of seizures only in a subgroup of these patients.[40] In fact, approximately 50% of the seizures experienced by alcoholic subjects are a result of concurrent organic causes, such as cerebrovascular accidents, pre-existing epilepsy, toxic or metabolic conditions, structural brain lesions, nontraumatic intracranial lesions

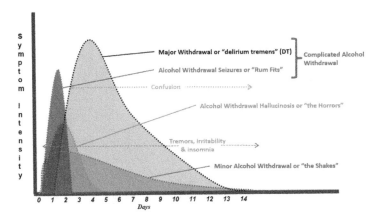

Fig. 2. Timing of alcohol withdrawal syndromes (AWS).

Table 1
Alcohol withdrawal syndromes

AWS	Time to Onset	Incidence	Manifestations
Uncomplicated Withdrawal (The Shakes)	Onset ~12 h, peak 24–36 h	80%	• Mild: tremors, nervousness, irritability, nausea, & vomiting are the earliest and most common signs • More severe symptoms lasting up to 10–14 d include coarse tremors (involving the upper extremities and tongue), anorexia, nausea, vomiting, psychological tension, general malaise, hypertension, autonomic hyperactivity, tachycardia, diaphoresis, orthostatic hypotension, irritability, vivid dreams, and insomnia
Alcohol Withdrawal Seizures (Rum Fits)	Onset ~12 h after cessation, peak 12–48 h	5%–15%	• Seizures are characterized by generalized motor seizures that occur during the course of alcohol withdrawal, usually in the absence of an underlying seizure disorder • The greater the amount of alcohol consumed the greater the risk for seizures • ~1/3 of subjects who develop alcohol withdrawal seizures will only experience 1 seizure, whereas 2/3 will have multiple seizures, often closely spaced, if untreated • Only 3% of cases will develop status epilepticus
Alcoholic Hallucinosis	Onset ~8 h after cessation, peak 24–96 h	As high as 30%	• Incidence seems related to length and amount of alcohol exposure • Usually consist of primarily visual misperceptions and tactile hallucinations • By definition, the sensorium is clear and vital signs are stable, differentiating it from alcohol withdrawal delirium (DTs), yet some signs of early withdrawal may be present
Alcohol Withdrawal Delirium (DTs)	Usually appear 1–3 d after cessation; peak intensity on 4–5th day	~5%	• In most cases (80%) the symptoms of DTs resolve within 72 h, in those that do not, the mortality rate in cases of DTs has been reported between 1% and 15% • When DTs are complicated by medical conditions the mortality rate may increase to 20% • DTs are differentiated from uncomplicated withdrawal by the presence of a profound confusional state (ie, delirium) • Symptoms commonly include confusion, disorientation, fluctuating or clouded consciousness, perceptual disturbances (eg, auditory or visual hallucinations or illusions), agitation, insomnia, fever, and autonomic hyperactivity terror, agitation, and primarily visual (sometimes tactile) hallucinations of insects, small animals, or other perceptual distortions can also occur

(eg, infections, tumors), illicit drug use, and traumatic brain injury (TBI).[41–43] In the case of other causes, the usual signs of AWS (eg, autonomic hyperactivity) may not be present and the patient's BAC is still elevated.[40,44] Focal brain lesions, such as TBI, stroke, and intracranial mass lesions, frequently cause partial rather than generalized seizures.[42,44,45]

Alcoholic hallucinosis begins on the first day (with onset as early as 8 hours after the last drink), peaking approximately 24 to 96 hours after a relative or absolute abstinence from alcohol. The incidence is as high as 30% but related to length and amount of alcohol exposure.[35,46,47] Alcoholic hallucinations usually consist of primarily visual misperceptions and tactile hallucinations (ie, formication).[23,48] Auditory hallucinations can occur but are usually mild, ranging from unformed sounds to accusatory voices, leading to fear and paranoia.[23,49] By definition, the sensorium is clear and vital signs (VS) are stable, differentiating it from DTs; yet some signs of uncomplicated withdrawal may be present. Symptoms resolve in hours to days and their presence have no predictive value regarding the possibility of developing DTs.[49] On rare occasions, hallucinations may persist after all other withdrawal symptoms have resolved.[50]

Alcohol withdrawal delirium usually appears 1 to 3 days after a relative or absolute abstinence, with a peak intensity on the fourth to fifth day. DTs occurs in approximately 5% of alcoholics.[51] In most cases (80%) the symptoms of DTs resolve within 72 hours.[30] Yet, in those that do not, the mortality rate may be as high as 15%[34,49,52–57]; or up to 20% when complicated by medical conditions. DTs is differentiated from uncomplicated withdrawal by the presence of a profound confusional state (ie, delirium). Symptoms commonly include confusion, disorientation, fluctuating or clouded consciousness, perceptual disturbances (eg, auditory or visual hallucinations or illusions), agitation, insomnia, fever, and autonomic hyperactivity. Terror, agitation, and primarily visual (but tactile hallucinations, formication), and other perceptual distortions can also occur. The confusion and mental status changes can last from a few days to several weeks, even after there has been resolution of the physical withdrawal symptoms. DTs-related deaths are usually the result of medical complications, including infections, cardiac arrhythmias, fluid and electrolyte abnormalities, pyrexia, poor hydration, hypertension, or suicide in response to hallucinations or delusions.

CLINICAL DILEMMA

Studies have shown that in medically ill, hospitalized subjects, most AWS cases are relatively mild and uncomplicated, requiring only symptomatic management (eg, anxiety, tremulousness, insomnia). Usually, the symptoms of uncomplicated AWS do not require medical intervention and disappear within 2 to 7 days. The unnecessary prophylaxis or treatment of patients feared to be at risk or experiencing AWS may lead to several unintended consequences, including sedation, falls, respiratory depression, and delirium.

The incidence of complicated AWS among patients admitted to medical or critical care units, severe enough to require pharmacologic treatment, is between 5% and 20%. When complicated AWS does occur, it is associated with an increased incidence of acute medical and surgical complications; increased ventilator, ICU, and hospital days; increased in-hospital morbidity and mortality; prolonged hospital stay; inflated health care costs; increased burden on nursing and medical staff; and further worsens cognitive functioning among withdrawing subjects.[58]

There is a positive correlation between the severity and duration of DTs symptoms and the occurrence of pneumonia, coronary heart disease, alcohol liver disease, and anemia.[59] The mortality of untreated, complicated AWS is approximately 15% to 20%, compared with 2%, when appropriately treated.

ALCOHOL WITHDRAWAL TREATMENT

The effective management of AWS includes a combination of supportive and pharmacologic measures. Supportive measures include the stabilization and management of comorbid medical problems, assessment and management of concurrent substance intoxication or withdrawal syndrome, and nutritional supplementation.

A recently published Cochrane Review, including 64 studies (n = 4309), evaluated benzodiazepine (BZDP) against placebos, BZDPs against other medications (including other anticonvulsants), and one BZDP against a different BZDP.[60] The data revealed that studies were small, had large heterogeneity, had variable assessment outcomes, and most did not reach statistical significance. Ultimately, the only statistically significant finding was that BZDPs were more effective than placebo for preventing withdrawal seizures; however, they were not shown to be superior to anticonvulsants or other agents. Some studies have suggested that BZDP use itself may be associated with the development of delirium.[61] In fact, others have found that BZDP use (and its amount) was an independent risk factor for the development of delirium.[62–70]

BENZODIAZEPINE-SPARING ALTERNATIVE FOR THE TREATMENT OF ALCOHOL WITHDRAWAL

The effectiveness of BZDP in managing AWS has been covered elsewhere and will not be repeated here.[71] Despite their proven usefulness in the management of complicated AWS, the use of BZDP is fraught with potential complications (**Box 1**). In an

---

Box 1
Potential problems with the use of benzodiazepines for alcohol withdrawal

- BZDPs represent the standard of care for the treatment of alcohol withdrawal and have been shown to prevent alcohol withdrawal seizures and DTs.[71]

- Yet there are potential problems with their use in the management of AWS.
  1. BZDPs have abuse liability (eg, iatrogenic BZDP dependence); concurrent alcohol or BZDP use 29% to 76%. (Ciraulo and colleagues, 1988)[224] This is problematic in an outpatient setting or when trying to discharge home a patient on moderate or high doses.
  2. BZDPs blunt cognition might hamper early attempts at rehabilitation and counseling.[75]
  3. BZDPs have significant interactions with alcohol, opioids, and other CNS depressants. If taken together, there can be additive respiratory depression and cognitive impairment.
  4. There are preclinical and clinical studies suggesting that BZDP use may increase craving, early relapse to alcohol use, and increased alcohol consumption.[91] (Poulos and Zack, 2004)
  5. The risk of developing BZDP-induced delirium is increased.[75]
  6. There is risk of psychomotor retardation, cognitive blunting, ataxia, and poor balance, and decreased mobility.
  7. Anxiolytic and hypnotic drugs, such as BZDPs and Z drugs (zaleplon, zolpidem, and zopiclone) were associated with significantly increased risk of mortality over a 7-year period, after adjusting for a range of potential confounders. (Weich and colleagues BMJ 2014)[232]
  8. There is increased compensatory up-regulation of NMDA and kainite-Rs and Ca^{2+} channels.
  9. Thalamic gating function is disrupted.
  10. There is increased risk of developing BZDP-induced delirium.[69]
  11. It can interfere with central cholinergic function muscarinic transmission at the level of the basal forebrain and hippocampus (ie, cause a centrally mediated acetylcholine deficient state).
  12. New evidence suggests that BZDP use may be associated with an increased risk of dementia. (de Gage and colleagues BMJ 2012)[222] and (de Gage and colleagues BMJ 2014)[223]
  13. It can interfere with physiologic sleep patterns (eg, decreased slow wave sleep and REM periods duration, REM latency, and REM deprivation).

attempt to avoid the extremes of undersedation or oversedation, and some of their side effects, the author decided to search for pharmacologic agents effective in the management of AWS beyond conventional BZDP-based protocols.

The author found that the available data support the use, safety, and efficacy of various alternatives to BZDP agents that, rather than substituting for ethanol, actually addressed the underlying pathophysiological derangements that underlie alcohol dependence and withdrawal syndromes. A systematic review of the literature revealed that pharmacologic alternatives to BZDPs were classified into one of 3 groups: non–BZDP-GABA-ergic agents; anticonvulsant agents, usually with glutamatergic or Calcium^{2+} (Ca^{2+}) channel modulator activity; and alpha-2 adrenergic (AAG) agonists.

Other γ-Aminobutyric Acid-ergic Agents

Propofol is a short-acting, lipophilic intravenous general anesthetic.[72] Although structurally distinct from other agents, its clinical action and effects on cerebral activity and intracranial dynamics are similar to short-acting barbiturates.[73] Propofol causes global CNS depression, presumably through direct activation of the GABA$_A$ receptor-chloride ionophore complex (increasing chloride conductance)[74] and by inhibiting the NMDA subtype of GLU receptor, possibly through an allosteric modulation of channel gating,[75] which may explain its effectiveness in treating status epilepticus and DTs.[76–78] There are 6 case reports on propofol's effectiveness in treating AWS in cases of nonresponsive to conventional therapy.[79–81] Its rapid onset and short half-life make it easy to titrate but may also create problems, especially when abruptly discontinued (ie, withdrawal). Common side effects include hypotension, bradycardia, and respiratory depression. Other significant side effects include decreased cerebral metabolism, propofol-induced hypertriglyceridemia (which has been causally associated with pancreatitis) and tachyphylaxis, and propofol infusion syndrome.[82–85] Of note, propofol has no US Food and Drug Administration (FDA) approval for the prophylaxis or treatment of AWS.

Antiepileptic Drugs

Antiepileptic drugs (AEDs) with GABA-ergic and GLU-Ca^{2+} channel modulator activity may be used. The routine use of AEDs, such as phenytoin, in cases of AWS is not recommended. A meta-analysis of randomized, placebo-controlled trials for the secondary prevention of AWS-seizures showed phenytoin was ineffective.[42]

Yet new promising data on the use of other anticonvulsants for the prophylaxis and treatment of ASW is emerging, including evidence for carbamazepine (CBZ), valproic acid (VPA), gabapentin (GAB), pregabalin, tiagabine, and vigabatrin. The mechanism by which these other agents exert their positive effects on the prevention and management of AWS is likely associated with their effects on GLU and Ca channels (**Table 2**). Of note, none of the anticonvulsant agents discussed here have FDA approval for the prophylaxis or treatment of AWS.

Carbamazepine

CBZ has effects on various types of channel receptors, including sodium (Na), Ca, and potassium (K), as well as neurotransmitter receptor systems, including adenosine, serotonin (5HT), DA, GLU, cyclic adenosine monophosphate (cAMP), and peripheral BZDP receptors.[86] Mechanisms of action include (1) its ability to stabilize the Na channels, reducing firing frequency[87–89]; (2) its potentiation of GABA receptors[90]; and (3) its inhibition of GLU release, likely contributing to its anticonvulsant properties.[86] CBZ has been in use in Europe for the treatment of AWS for more than 25 years.[91]

Table 2
Glutamate and calcium channel modulators

Drug	T ½	Product Availability	Bioavailability	Metabolism	Protein Binding	Mechanism Action
CBZ	25 h	po	~100%	Hepatic	55%	• Stabilizes neuronal membranes • Inhibits voltage-sensitive Na+ channels and/or Ca+ channels → ↓ cortical GLU release • Ca channel blockers • Excitatory amino acid antagonists
VPA	9–16 h	po or intravenous (IV)	90%	Hepatic conjugation	90%	• GABA transaminase inhibitor → ↑ GABA • Inhibits voltage-sensitive Na+ channels → ↓ cortical GLU release • ↓ Release of the epileptogenic amino acid, γ-hydroxybutyrate (GHB)
GAB	5–7 h	po	60%	None Renal excretion	<3%	• Voltage-gated Ca+ channel blockade → ↓ cortical GLU release • NMDA antagonism • Activation of spinal alpha-2 adrenergic receptors • Attenuation of Na+-dependent action potential
Vigabatrin	5–8 h	po	50%	None Significant renal excretion	~0%	• Block the reuptake of GABA & inhibits the catabolism of GABA → ↑GABA concentrations, no receptor agonist • Inhibition of voltage-sensitive Na+ channels
Tiagabine	7–9 h	po	90%	Hepatic, various Cytochromes P450 (CYP): CYP3A, CYP1A2, CYP2D6, or CYP2C19	96%	• Block the reuptake of GABA → ↑GABA concentrations, no receptor agonist • Inhibition of voltage-sensitive Na+ channels

Abbreviation: T ½, half-life.

CBZ is superior to placebo[92] and non-BZDP hypnotic agents, such as clomethaizole[93] and barbiturates,[94] in suppressing all aspects of AWS. Nine randomized, controlled studies (n = 800) have demonstrated the effectiveness of CBZ in alcohol detoxification, compared with BZDP **(Table 3)**.[91,93–105]

CBZ-treated subjects had an overall better response to treatment (ie, were calmer, less irritable, and less dysphoric)[92,96]; experienced superior and faster relief of symptoms, including anxiety, fear, and hallucinations[96,106]; had shortened duration of DTs[94,99,107]; and decreased incidence of AWS-seizures.[99,101,106,107] CBZ was found particularly useful in outpatient detoxification because it enabled the alcoholic to return to work more quickly[92,108] and had greater efficacy than BZDP in preventing post-treatment relapses to drinking.[91] Data suggest CBZ may be useful in the treatment of alcohol dependence and the reduction of cravings and recidivism.[91,109–111] Furthermore, it has a strong antikindling effect and lacks any misuse potential.[108]

CBZ is well-tolerated, rapidly absorbed after oral administration, and its metabolism is largely unaffected by liver damage.[112,113] There were no significant cardiovascular or hepatotoxic effects noted, and no adverse interactions when used with ethanol.[114] Reports suggest that CBZ improves sleep without rapid eye movement (REM)-suppression.[106]

Potential side effects include pruritus without rash (18.9%),[91] followed by dizziness, ataxia, headache, somnolence, dry mouth, orthostatic hypotension, vertigo, nausea, and vomiting (in up to 10% of patients).[115] A major concern is the risk of agranulocytosis or aplastic anemia, both potentially lethal conditions, occurring in less than 0.01%.[116] This was not reported in any of the studies cited.

Oxcarbazepine

An analogue of CBZ, oxcarbazepine (OXC) reduces high-voltage–dependent Ca channels of striatal and cortical neurons, thus reducing NMDA glutamatergic transmission associated with alcohol withdrawal states.[117] Unlike CBZ, oxazepam (OXA) is not associated with significant neurologic side effects or blood dyscrasias and is only a weak inducer of the P450 system.[118] Studies have shown OXC has comparable effects to CBZ in the treatment of AWS,[119–122] reducing both AWS symptoms and alcohol craving score, suggesting a role in relapse prevention.[123–126]

Valproic acid

VPA has effects at various types of channel receptors (eg, Na+, Ca+, K+) and neurotransmitter receptor systems (eg, GABA, GLU, 5HT, DA).[127] Mechanisms of action include increase in the turnover of GABA, inhibition of the NMDA subtype of GLU receptors, and the reduction of γ-hydroxybutyrate (GHB).[127]

Six randomized, controlled studies (n = 900 subjects) have demonstrated the effectiveness of VPA in alcohol detoxification when compared with BZDPs **(Table 4)**.[98,128–137] Compared with placebo, VPA-treated subjects experienced faster symptom resolution, required less adjunct medication, and experienced fewer seizures (5 in placebo vs none in VPA).[98,128,131] Compared with BZDP, VPA-treated subjects experienced better resolution of AWS symptoms ($P \leq .01$) and required less rescue medication.[130,132] Compared with CBZ, VPA-treated subjects reported faster symptom resolution, shorter course of AWS, fewer ICU transfers, a more favorable side-effect profile, and fewer withdrawal seizures.[133]

VPA's tolerability and safety are similar to that of CBZ.[127] The most significant adverse effects include teratogenic potential, thrombocytopenia, and idiosyncratic liver toxicity.[127] Compared with other AEDs, VPA causes fewer neurologic adverse effects and fewer skin rashes.[127]

Table 3
Glutamate and calcium channel modulators: carbamazepine

Study	Population	Intervention	AWS Definition	Outcome
Bjorkqvist et al,[95] 1976; DBPCRCT	O/P ETOH Rehabilitation settings-multicenter trial, N = 105	Placebo (PBO) vs CBZ: 800 mg d 1–2, 600 mg d 3–4, 400 mg d 5–6, 200 mg d 7	Clinical Institute Withdrawal Assessment for Alcohol, revised (CIWA-Ar)	• CBZ proved superior to PBO o Greater change in the total symptom score in the CBZ group than in the PBO o Subjects' ability to return to work improved significantly faster on CBZ
Ritola et al,[93] 1981 DB-BD	Male inpatients, N = 68	Chlormethiazole (CMT) vs CBZ: 400 mg d 0, 800 mg d 1–2, 600 mg d 3–4, 400 mg d 5–6	—	• 70% good to excellent results, both groups • CBZ improvement all areas, except depression • Fewer dropouts in CBZ group
Agricola et al,[96] 1982; DBRCT	University Med Center Substance Abuse I/P Unit, N = 60	CBZ 600 mg vs tiapride 600 mg	CIWA-Ar	• Both drugs were effective in the treatment of AWS o No significant difference was found with respect to total symptoms, score, and visual analog scale assessment • CBZ gave faster relief of symptoms and a superior response on anxiety, fear, & hallucinations • No progression to DTs
Flyngering et al,[94] 1984; DBRCT	Male inpatients, N = 72	Barbital vs CBZ: 400–1200 mg d 1, 200–600 mg d 2–6	—	• No overall difference between groups • AWS duration shorter (~9 h) in CBZ group • No difference in dropout rate
Malcolm et al,[97] 1989; DBRCT	VAMC, I/P unit, N = 66	Oxazepam (OXA) 120 mg/d vs CBZ 800 mg/d, tapering over 5 d	CIWA-Ar	• No differences between the 2 groups (both groups achieved maximum reduction of symptoms (CIWA-Ar) between days 4 and 5)

Study	Setting	Intervention	Scale	Results
Hillbom et al,[98] 1989; DBRCT	I/P Adults; N = 138	CBZ (max 1200/d) vs VPA (max 1200/d), vs PBO	Episodes of seizure (SZ) or DTs	• SZ episodes: CBZ (n = 2), VPA (n = 1), PBO (n = 3) • DTs: CBZ (n = 0), VPA (n = 2), PBO (n = 1)
Stuppaeck et al,[159] 1992; DBRCT	University Med Center Substance Abuse I/P Unit, N = 60	OXA 120 mg (÷) vs CBZ 800 mg (÷) tapering over 7 d	CIWA-Ar	• No clinical differences between the 2 groups • Greater progression to DTs & SZ in OXA group (OXA 7% & 3%, CLO 0% & 0%, respectively)
Malcolm et al,[91] 2002; DBRCT	University Medical Center Substance Abuse O/P clinic, N = 136	LOR 6–8 mg (÷) on day 1, tapering to 2 mg vs CBZ 600–800 mg on day 1, tapering to 200 mg	CIWA-Ar	• Both drugs were equally efficacious at treating AWS • CBZ had greater efficacy than LOR in preventing post-treatment relapses to drinking over the 12 d of follow-up • There was a greater reduction in anxiety symptoms, as measured by the Zung Anxiety Scale, in CBZ group
Lucht et al,[100] 2003; OL	I/P Adults; N = 127	Sx-triggered: Tiapride (≤1800 mg/d) + CBZ (≤1200 mg/d) vs CLOM (≤1200 mg/d) vs DIA (≤80 mg/d)	AWS	• No significant differences in AWS scores between the Tx groups throughout the study • No significant differences in SZs or DTs
Schik et al,[119] 2005	Single-blinded and randomized pilot study, N = 29 subjects	Oxcarbazepine (OXC) vs CBZ	—	• OXC group showed a significant decrease of AWS and reported significantly less craving for alcohol compared with the CBZ group • Subjectively experienced side effects, normalization of vegetative parameters, and improvement in cognitive processing speed was no different between groups

(continued on next page)

Table 3
(continued)

Study	Population	Intervention	AWS Definition	Outcome
Polycarpou et al,[101] 2005	Various, Cochrane Review, 48 studies, N = 3610 subjects	Anticonvulsant vs PBO comparison	CIWA-Ar	• For the ACA vs PBO comparison, therapeutic success tended to be more common among the ACA-treated subjects (relative risk [RR] 1.32, 95% CI 0.92–1.91) • ACA tended to show a protective benefit against SZs (RR 0.57; 95% CI 0.27–1.19) • For the subgroup analysis of CBZ vs BZDP; • A statistically significant protective effect was found for the anticonvulsant ($P = .02$) • Side-effects was less common in the ACA-group (RR 0.56; 95% CI 0.31–1.02)
Minozzi et al,[102] 2010	Various, Cochrane Review, 56 studies, N = 4076 subjects	Anticonvulsant vs PBO vs BZDPs	CIWA-Ar, AWSz, DTs	• CBZ was associated with a significant reduction in alcohol withdrawal symptoms (CIWA-Ar mean difference = −1.04, 95% CI −1.89 to −0.20) when compared with the BZDPs lorazepam and OXA
Barrons & Roberts,[103] 2010	Systematic review	Anticonvulsant vs PBO vs BZDPs	CIWA-Ar, AWSz, DTs	• CBZ was found safe and tolerable when administered at daily doses of 800 mg (fixed or tapered over 5–9 d) • CBZ was associated with a significant reduction in alcohol withdrawal symptoms as measured by CIWA-Ar

Abbreviations: (÷), in divided daily doses; ACA, anticonvulsant agents; CBZ, carbamazepine; CLOM, clomethiazole; DB-BD, double-blind; DBPCRCT, double blind, placebo controlled, randomized clinical trial; DBRCT, double blind randomized clinical trial; DIA, diazepam; *I/P*, in-patient; *O/P ETOH*, out-patient alcohol detoxification; Sx, symptom; Tx, treatment.

Gabapentin

GAB acts by inhibition of the neuronal Ca^{2+} channel and amplification of GABA synthesis.[138] Mechanisms of action include increased GABA-ergic tone and reduced glutamatergic tone through inhibition of GLU synthesis, modulation of Ca current, inhibition of Na channels, and reduction of NE and DA release, leading to a reversal of the low GABA–high GLU state found during AWS.[139–145]

An advantage to GAB use is its extrahepatic metabolism or elimination, particularly in alcoholic subjects with hepatic dysfunction.[146] Early animal data suggested the usefulness of GAB in the treatment of AWS.[145,147] GAB has performed as well as barbiturates[148] and BZDP, with subjects experiencing less craving, anxiety, and sedation.[149] Clinical data supporting the use of GAB in the management of AWS are summarized in **Table 5**.[139,150–152]

Other antiepileptic agents

Both lamotrigine and topiramate significantly reduced observer-rated and self-rated withdrawal severity, dysphoric mood, and supplementary diazepam administration when compared with placebo, and were as effective as diazepam.[153] Other drugs for which there is positive evidence for the treatment of AWS include pregabalin,[154–156] topiramate,[153,157] tiagabine,[158] and vigabatrin.[159] In addition, topiramate has shown promise in the treatment of alcohol dependence.[160–165]

In summary, "anticonvulsants appear to be more effective against a larger range of withdrawal symptoms than benzodiazepines, especially among alcoholics with moderate to severe withdrawal symptoms".[166] These agents "might have a further advantage to benzodiazepines in that they appear useful both for treating the acute withdrawal symptoms and, once abstinence has been achieved, for preventing relapse by modulating post-cessation craving and affective disturbance."[166]

Alpha-2 Adrenergic Receptor Agonist

AWS are characterized by a reduction in the inhibitory effects of GABA (disinhibition) and activation of the sympathetic nervous system (stimulation). The severity of AWS correlates positively with the amount of released NE.[167,168] Clinical data have shown significant elevations of cerebral spinal fluid 3-methoxy-4-hydroxyphenylglycol (a major NE metabolite) concentrations in subjects with active AWS, suggesting that enhanced NE turnover is causally associated with the severity of AWS.[167] Excess NE activity may indeed drive the excess GLU activity even further, contributing to agitation, psychosis, and even seizure activity.

AAG induces activation of inward rectifying G-protein-coupled K^+ channels and block voltage-gated Ca channels.[169] Activated alpha 2-adrenergic receptors will hyperpolarize neurons and inhibit the presynaptic release of GLU, aspartate, and NE.[170] This potentially contributes to its neuroprotective qualities against various sources of cerebral ischemic injury and explain the role of AAG in the management of AWS.[171] In addition, AAG decreased cerebellar cyclic guanosine 3',5'-monophosphate (cGMP), which correlates with their anesthetic and anticonvulsant effects.[172] Given the current understanding of the effects of chronic alcohol use in the CNS and the effects of AWS in the catecholamine system, it makes sense to consider the potential use of alpha-2 agonists in the management of AWS.[29,173] Data on the clinical effectiveness of AAG are summarized in **Table 6**.

The variability in clinical and side-effect profiles observed between the various alpha-2 agonists is related to differences in affinities for the 3 identified alpha-2 noradrenergic receptor subtypes: A, B, and C.[174–176] Alpha-2A receptor agonism promotes sedation, hypnosis, analgesia, sympatholysis, neuroprotection, and inhibition of

Table 4
Glutamate and calcium channel modulators: valproic acid

Study, N = 7	Population	Intervention	AWS Definition	Outcome
Lambie et al,[128] 1980; randomized, single-blind trial	I/P (Detoxification) Detox Unit, N = 49	VPA 400 mg tid × 7 d vs PBO	Severity of Sxs scale; occurrence of AWS	• There were 5 cases of SZ activity, all in the control group (none in VPA) • Physical symptoms disappeared slightly more quickly in the VPA-treated group than in the control group despite that 22 subjects in the control group were on CMT compared with only 5 subjects in the VPA group
Hillbom et al,[98] 1989; DBRCT	I/P Adults; N = 138	CBZ (maximum [max] 1200/d) vs VPA (max 1200/d) vs PBO	Episodes of SZ or DTs	• SZ episodes: CBZ (n = 2), VPA (n = 1), PBO (n = 3) • DTs: CBZ (n = 0), VPA (n = 2), PBO (n = 1)

Rosenthal et al,[129] 1998; open, randomized trial	I/P Detox Unit N = 42	VPA vs PHB
		Day 1–500 mg po stat loading dose, followed by 500 mg po 6 h later
		Day 2–500 mg po bid
		Day 3–500 mg po bid
		Day 4–250 mg po bid
		Day 5–250 mg po × 1
			ASQ	• This study offers confirmation that VPA is as effective as PHB in the management of AWS
				  ○ Subjective and objective ratings of abstinence symptoms and subjective mood disturbance decreased significantly in intensity in both groups over 5 d
				  ○ There were no withdrawal-related SZs or other acute sequelae

Myrick et al,[130] 2000; prospective, randomized, single-blind trial	I/P Detox Unit N = 11	LOR 2 mg for CIWA-Ar scores >6 vs VPA 500 mg tid for 4 d plus LOR 2 mg for CIWA-Ar >6	CIWA-Ar	• The group-by-CIWA-Ar score interaction was determined to favor VPA significantly ($P \le .01$) • Subjects in the VPA group seemed to use less LOR than those in the control group over the study period

Study	Setting	Intervention	Scale	Results
Reoux et al,[131] 2001; DBPCRCT	I/P Detox Unit, N = 36	VPA 500 mg tid × 7 d vs PBO in a double-blind manner OXA PRN in both as rescue	CIWA-Ar	• Use of VPA resulted in less use of OXA ($P<.033$) • The progression in severity of withdrawal symptoms (based on CIWA-Ar) was also significantly greater in the PBO group ($P<.05$)
Longo et al,[132] 2002; randomized, open-label study	I/P Detox Unit, N = 16	BZDP vs VPA (5 d detox) vs VPA (+6 wk maintenance) Loading dose of 20 mg/kg/d in 2 divided doses 6–8 h apart on day 1, then bid thereafter	CIWA-Ar	• AWS reduction occurred more rapidly and consistently in the VPA-treatment group than the BZDP-control group at 12 and 24 h intervals (based on CIWA-Ar scores), not statistically significant • Although the protocol allowed for the availability of a BZDP rescue in the event of VPA nonresponse, none of the VPA-treated subjects required prn BZDP
Eyer et al,[133] 2011; retrospective chart review	I/P Detox Unit, N = 827	CBZ (200 mg tid) vs VPA 300 mg tid)	CIWA-Ar	• VPA may offer some benefits compared with CBZ in the adjunct treatment of moderate-to-severe AWS ○ Shorter need for pharmacologic treatment ○ Fewer ICU transfers ○ A more favorable side-effect profile • Trend that VPA may be more effective than CBZ in reducing complications during AWS, especially WSz

Table 5
Glutamate and calcium channel modulators: Other anticonvulsant agents

Study, N = 11	Population	Intervention	AWS Definition	Outcome
Stuppaeck et al,[159] 1996; ROLCT	I/P Detox unit, N = 10	Vigabatrin 1 mg bid × 3 d Individuals were studied for a total of 7 d, OXA PRN	CIWA-Ar	• Overall, AWS suppression, as measured by CIWA-Ar seemed efficacious • 1 subject had a SZ on d 3 (even after having received OXA 250 mg over 2 previous days)
Myrick et al,[158] 2005; retrospective chart review	O/P Detox unit; N = 13	Tiagabine 2–4 mg bid vs OXA initiated at 30 mg bid to qid	CIWA-Ar	• Both TGB and BZDP-treated subjects were detoxified without serious side-effects • No subjects experienced DTs, SZs, or other complications
Mariani et al,[148] 2006; ROLCT	University Med Center Substance Abuse I/P Unit, N = 27	PHE vs GAB Day 1 GAB 1200 mg po loading dose, followed in 6 h with 600 mg po, followed in 6 h with 600 mg po (total of 2400 mg in the first 24 h) Day 2 600 mg po tid Day 3 600 mg po bid Day 4 600 mg po qd	CIWA-Ar	• There were no significant differences in the proportion of subjects in each group requiring rescue medication for breakthrough signs and symptoms of AWS • No group differences on alcohol withdrawal, craving, mood, irritability, anxiety, or sleep were observed • There were no serious adverse events on GAB group
Ponce et al,[122] 2005	I/P Detox unit; N = 84	BZDP vs OXC	CIWA-Ar side effects	• Both OXC and BZDP were equally efficient in preventing the appearance of epileptic complications and in reducing withdrawal symptoms • Overall, OXC produced fewer adverse events (P<.001) and offered fewer problems when it came to ending administration (P<.001)

Study	Sample	Intervention	Scale	Findings
Krupitsky et al,[153] 2007; PBO-controlled randomized single-blinded trial	I/P Detox Unit, N = 127	Assigned × 7 d to • PBO • Diazepam (DZP) 10 mg tid • Lamotrigine 25 mg qid • Memantine 10 mg tid • Topiramate 25 mg qid • Additional DZP rescue	CIWA-Ar	• All active medications significantly reduced withdrawal severity, dysphoric mood, and supplementary DZP administration vs PBO • The active medications did not differ from DZP • First systematic clinical evidence supporting the efficacy of several antiglutamatergic approaches for treating alcohol withdrawal symptoms
Myrick et al,[149] 2009; DBRCT	I/P Detox Unit, n = 100	Randomized to low-dose GAB (300 mg tid × 3 d, then 400 mg bid on d 4); high-dose GAB (400 mg tid × 3 d, then 400 mg bid on d 4); vs LOR (2 mg tid × 3 d, then 2 mg bid on d 4); follow-up up to 12 d	CIWA-Ar	• High-dose GAB was statistically superior but clinically similar to LOR ($P = .009$) • During treatment, LOR-treated participants had higher probabilities of drinking compared with GAB-treated ($P = .0002$) • Post-treatment, GAB-treated participants had less probability of drinking during the follow-up post-treatment period ($P = .2$ for 900 mg) compared with LOR-treated ($P = .55$) • The GAB groups also had less craving, anxiety, and sedation compared with LOR
Di Nicola et al,[155] 2010; OLP	N = 40	Pregabalin flexible dosing 200–450 mg/d for O/P treatment of mild-to-moderate AWS	CIWA-Ar	• Pregabalin was safe and tolerable and associated with a significant reduction in CIWA-Ar scores and alcohol craving
Muller et al,[229] 2010; OLOS	O/P Detox Program, N = 131	Levetiracetam, mean initial dose was 850 mg/d	AWSS score	• 93.1% completed the program successfully • The AWSS score decreased clearly over 5 d • The medication was well-tolerated • There was no treatment discontinuations due to side effects of levetiracetam • No serious medical complications, especially SZs or deliria, were observed during the detox • At the 6-mo follow-up, 57 subjects (43.5%) were still abstinent

(continued on next page)

Table 5
(continued)

Study, N = 11	Population	Intervention	AWS Definition	Outcome
Martinotti et al,[156] 2010; MCRSBCT	O/P Detox program, N = 111	Pregabalin vs tiapride vs lorazepam; multicenter; single-blind trial	CIWA-Ar	• All medications significantly reduced AWS, with pregabalin demonstrating significantly better treatment for headache and orientation withdrawal symptoms
Forg et al,[225] 2012; RPCT	I/P Detoxification, N = 42	For 6 d, participants either received pregabalin vs PBO according to a fixed dose schedule starting with 300 mg/d; with rescue DZP based on AWSS score	AWSS, CIWA-Ar and neuropsychological scales	• Pregabalin and PBO were equally safe and well-tolerated • No statistically significant difference was found comparing the total amount of additional DZP medication required in the 2 study groups • Pregabalin and PBO also showed similar efficacy according to alterations of scores of the AWSS, CIWA-Ar, and neuropsychological scales • The frequency of adverse events and dropouts did not differ between the both treatment groups
Stock et al,[231] 2013; DBRPCT	O/P VA Clinic, N = 26	GAB (1200 mg/d starting dose) vs chlordiazepoxide (100 mg/d starting dose) were administered according to a fixed-dose taper schedule over 6 d	Sleepiness, alcohol craving, and ataxia in addition to CIWA-Ar scores	• There were no significant differences in AWS symptoms by medication • GAB group reported decreased daytime sleepiness compared with those who received chlordiazepoxide

Abbreviations: DBRPCT, double; DZP, diazepam; PHE, phenobarbital; PRN, pro re nata, or as needed; qd, daily; ROLCT, randomized, open label, clinical trial; VA, Veterans Administration.

Table 6
Centrally acting alpha-2 adrenergic receptors agonists

Drug	Alpha-2 or alpha-1 Selectivity	dT ½	eT ½	Product Availability	Bioavailability	Protein Binding
Guanfacine	2640	2.5 h	17 h	po	~100%	70%
Dexmedetomidine	1600	6 min	2 h	IV	70%–80%	94%
Medetomidine	1200	—	—	—	—	—
Clonidine	220	11 min	13 h	po TDS IV	100% po 60% TDS	40%
Methyldopa	—	12 min	105 min	po/IV	50%	<20%
Guanabenz	—	60 min	6 h	Po	75%	90%

Abbreviations: dT ½, drug plasma half-life; eT ½, elimination half-life; TDS, transdermal system (or patch).

insulin secretion.[177,178] Alpha-2B receptor agonism suppresses shivering centrally, promotes analgesia at spinal cord sites, and induces vasoconstriction in peripheral arteries.[179] Alpha-2C receptor is associated with modulation of cognition, sensory processing, mood-induced and stimulant-induced locomotor activity, and regulation of epinephrine outflow from the adrenal medulla.[180,181] Although inhibition of NE release seems equally affected by all 3 alpha-2 receptor subtypes.[181] The hypotensive effects of alpha-2 agonists are attributable to their actions at alpha-2A and alpha-2C in the nucleus tractus solitaries.[182,183] Alpha-2A is densest in the PFC[184] and is primarily responsible for the cognitive enhancing effects of alpha-2 agonists. Meanwhile the alpha-2B subtype is found predominantly in the thalamus[183] and predominantly mediates alpha-2 agonists' sedative actions.[185]

There are data on 3 AAGs for the treatment of AWS: lofexidine, clonidine, and dexmedetomidine (DEX). Lofexidine has animal[186] and human[187,188] data supporting its effectiveness in the treatment of AWS but because it is not available in the United States, it is not discussed further.

Clonidine

Case reports confirmed the usefulness of adding clonidine (CLO) to help resolve AWS not responding to conventional sedative therapy.[189] Seven double-blind, placebo-controlled trials demonstrate CLO's utility in managing AWS (**Table 7**). When compared with BZDP, subjects on CLO experienced significantly lower mean withdrawal scores ($P<.02$), significantly lower mean systolic blood pressure ($P<.01$), and significantly lower mean heart rate ($P<.001$).[92,190–193] However, subjects in the CLO group experienced less anxiety and better cognitive recovery.[191] In addition, CLO provided better management of psychological symptoms (eg, anxiety, irritability, agitation) and CNS excitation (ie, seizures, DTs) associated with alcohol withdrawal.[92,189,191–196] No subject developed seizures or progressed to DTs.

Dexmedetomidine

DEX is a selective AAG with sedative, analgesic, anxiolytic, and sympatholytic properties, generally devoid of significant respiratory depression.[197] Its specificity for the alpha-2 receptor is 8 times that of CLO.[198,199] The FDA recently approved the use of DEX for sedation without intubation, which provides clinicians with an additional medication to treat patients with alcohol withdrawal who require ICU placement, while

Table 7
Centrally acting alpha-2 adrenergic receptors agonists in alcohol withdrawal syndrome

Study, N = 11	Population	Intervention	AWS Definition	Outcome
Bjorkqvist,[92] 1975; DBRPCT	I/P Detox Unit, N = 60	Fixed titration of po CLO (over 4 d) vs PBO	• Nurses evaluation • Self-report	• Self-rated and nurse observer–rated symptoms of alcohol withdrawal were significantly reduced with CLO as compared with PBO on day 2 of treatment ($P<.025$ and $P<.01$, respectively), with no hypotension • Subjects in the CLO group did better in every index measured: the movements and tremor improved faster; systolic blood pressure (BP), need for additional medication
Walinder et al,[195] 1981; ROL	I/P Detox Unit, N = 19	Fixed titration of po CLO vs fixed CBZ dose (200 mg tid) × 4 d	Comprehensive Psychopathological Rating Scale	• CLO treatment seems at least as effective as CBZ in suppression and management of the AWS
Wilkins et al,[196] 1983; randomized, crossover double-blind fashion	I/P Detox Unit, N = 11	Randomized, crossover double-blind fashion CLO vs PBO	Autonomic reactivity	• CLO significantly suppressed heart rate (HR; $P = .002$), arterial BP ($P = .006$), and an accumulated score of withdrawal symptoms and signs ($P = .004$)
Manhem et al,[193] 1985; DBRCT	I/P Detox Unit, N = 20	Fixed titration of po clonidine (0.15–0.3 mg qid) vs CMT (500–1000 mg qid) × 4 d	Alcohol withdrawal assessment scales (various) Autonomic reactivity	• During treatment, BP & HR were significantly lower following CLO compared with CMT ($P<.05$ for both) • CLO treatment reduced physical AWAS symptoms more effectively than CMT • Plasma NE and epinephrine levels were significantly lower in subjects treated with clonidine starting on day 1 of treatment ($P<.01$) • No specific adverse effects with clonidine, including SZs, were reported, although 1 subject in each group developed alcohol withdrawal delirium
Baumgartner & Rowen,[190] 1987; DBRPCT	I/P Detox Unit, N = 61	Fixed titration of chlordiazepoxide (50–150 mg/d, over 4 d) vs transdermal CLO (0.2–0.6 mg/d)	AWSS	• CLO mean AWAS score was significantly lower than CDP group ($P<.02$) • Mean systolic BP was significantly lower in CLO group ($P<.01$) • Mean HR was significantly lower in CLO group ($P<.001$) • No subject in either group developed SZs or progressed to DTs

Study	Setting	Intervention	Measures	Results
Baumgartner & Rowen,[191] 1991; DBRPCT	I/P Detox Unit, N = 50	Fixed titration of chlordiazepoxide (over 4 d) vs transdermal CLO (0.2-mg oral loading dose + 0.2 mg/24 h transdermal patches × 2 on day 1)	AWAS	• There was no significant difference in subject-reported subjective symptoms of alcohol withdrawal • Mean systolic and diastolic BP and pulse were significantly lower for subjects in the CLO group ($P<.001$ for all) • CLO group had a better response to therapy as assessed by the AWAS, less anxiety as assessed by the Ham-A Rating Scale ($P<.02$), better control of HR and BP; better cognitive recovery • No SZ or DTs in either group
Adinoff,[221] 1994; DBRPCT	I/P Detox Unit, N = 25	DZP (10 mg) vs APZ (1 mg) vs CLO (0.1 mg) vs PBO, all given q 1 h until AWS ratings dropped to <5	CIWA-Ar Autonomic reactivity	• APZ was significantly more efficacious than both clonidine and PBO in decreasing withdrawal symptoms but did not significantly decrease BP compared with DZP or PBO • DZP was more effective than clonidine and PBO on some measures of withdrawal • CLO decreased systolic BP significantly more than the other 2 active drugs and PBO but was no more effective than PBO in decreasing other symptoms of withdrawal

Dobrydnjov et al,[192] 2004; DBRCT	Surgical subjects, n = 45	DZP vs clonidine given preoperative to subjects undergoing transurethral resection of the prostate under spinal anesthesia	CIWA-Ar
			Autonomic reactivity
				• Median CIWA-Ar score: 12 vs 1 ($P<.001$)
				• Development of AWS: 80% vs 10% ($P<.002$)
				  o Anxiety: 67% vs 0% ($P<.001$)
				  o Agitation: 40% vs 0% ($P<.05$)
				  o Progression to DTs: 27% vs 7%
				• VS: hyperdynamic circulatory reaction observed in D group; slightly decreased mean arterial BP in CLO

(continued on next page)

Table 7
(continued)

Study, N = 11	Population	Intervention	AWS Definition	Outcome
Khan et al,[227] 2008; case control study	N = 35	CLO	—	• Predictors associated with increased mortality by univariate analysis: hyperthermia in the first 24 h of DTs diagnosis, persistent tachycardia, and use of restraints • Predictors associated with decreased mortality: an emergency department diagnosis of DTs, and use of clonidine
Lizotte et al,[228] 2014; retrospective chart review	ICU-AWS, N = 41	AWS who received adjunctive DEX or propofol	BZDP & haloperidol use; 2ry measures included AWSS and sedation scoring, analgesic use, IUC-LOS, rates of intubation, and adverse events	• Among the DEX and propofol groups, significant reductions in BZDP (P≤0001 and P = .043, respectively) and haloperidol (P≤0001 and P = .026, respectively) requirements were observed • Shorter LOS in the DEX group (123.6 h vs 156.5 h; P = .125) • Rates of intubation (14.7% vs 100%) and time of intubation (19.9 h vs 97.6 h; P = .002) were less in the DEX group • Incidence of hypotension was 17.6% in the DEX group vs 28.5% in the propofol group
Wong et al,[233] 2015; review	13 studies, ICU treatment of AWS using DEX	DEX as an adjunctive agent for the treatment of alcohol withdrawal in adult subjects	CIWA-Ar	• DEX seems well-tolerated, with an expected decrease in BP and HR SZs have occurred in subjects with alcohol withdrawal despite the use of DEX, with and without BZDPs

Abbreviations: AWAS, alcohol withdrawal assessment scales (various); D group, diazepam group; ICU-LOS, intensive care unit-length of stay; ROL, randomized, open label (trial).

avoiding the potential problems associated with the use of BZDPs, barbiturates, and propofol (ie, respiratory depression, need for endotracheal intubation, sepsis, and increased morbidity and mortality).[26]

Animal data demonstrated its efficacy in managing all phases of AWS.[200–203] Several clinical reports suggest DEX has been efficacious in cases in which BZDP has failed to effectively manage AWS.[197,204–211]

Guanfacine

Guanfacine (GUA), an even more selective alpha-2 or alpha-1 agent, causes less hypotension and is a better anxiolytic with less sedative side effects than CLO[212]; yet it is 25 times more potent than CLO at enhancing spatial working memory performance.[213] Its effectiveness in the management of AWS has been demonstrated in animal models[214,215] but no human data are available. Yet the author has effectively and safely used GUA in the management of complicated AWS and hyperactive delirium. This agent is particularly useful when transitioning patients off prolonged use of DEX. Given its relatively long half-life, this agent may have a lower incidence of noradrenergic rebound on discontinuation.[216]

DEVELOPMENT OF A NOVEL ALGORITHM FOR THE PROPHYLAXIS AND TREATMENT OF ALCOHOL WITHDRAWAL

The author's institution created a multidisciplinary taskforce, including members from all clinical departments, tasked with reviewing the available literature regarding AWS assessment methods and treatment algorithms. Concerns regarding potential problems with oversedation, negative neurologic sequelae, development of medication-induced delirium, and codependence issues between alcohol and BZDP sparked interest in developing a BZDP-sparing protocol. Based on the taskforce findings, we developed an alternative BZDP-sparing protocol for the prophylaxis and treatment of AWS; with BZDP allowed as rescue to breakthrough AWS (**Box 2, Fig. 3**). The ultimate goal was to decrease excessive BZDPs use and its related side effects.

Using the Prediction of Alcohol Withdrawal Severity Scale (PAWSS)[217] (**Fig. 4**), a tool validated in medically ill patients as reliable at identifying patients at high risk for complicated AWS, we could better tailor interventions and minimize excessive medication use and side effects.[58,217,218] Thus, patients at low risk for complicated AWS (ie, PAWSS <4) are only monitored, and antihistaminic agents offered for the management of insomnia and sleep but not given active treatment.

Patients scoring at high risk for complicated AWS (ie, PAWSS 4), undergo examination with a severity scale, such as the Clinical Institute Withdrawal Assessment for Alcohol, revised (CIWA-Ar)[219] or the Alcohol-Withdrawal Syndrome Scale AWSS).[220] If patient are currently not experiencing active AWS (ie, CIWA-Ar <15; AWSS <6)[220] they are placed on the prophylaxis protocol. The prophylaxis protocol is recommended for patients who (1) are at risk for complicated AWS but (2) who are not yet experiencing active AWS. By definition, a patient on active AWS should demonstrate signs of an adrenergic storm. The protocol calls for initiation of an alpha-2 agonist (either CLO or GUA; see **Box 2**). A patient experiencing severe hypotension, due to blood loss or sepsis, may not be able to tolerate the alpha-2 effect, in which case an antiglutamatergic-calcium-channel ($Ca^{2+}Ch$) modulator is indicated (either GAB or VPA). All patients are under ongoing surveillance for symptoms of clinical response or signs of AWS progression using a severity scale every 4 hours. Any patient whose withdrawal severity score rises despite adequate prophylactic management should be considered in active withdrawal and converted to the treatment protocol.

Box 2
Benzodiazepine-sparing: general management protocol

Assessment

Determine the patient's risk for AWS based on PAWSS score
  PAWSS less than 4: low risk, suggest continued monitoring and only symptomatic
  management
  PAWSS 4 or higher: high risk; prophylaxis management or active treatment is indicated,
  based on CIWA or AWSS[220] score (next)

Determine whether the patient is actively withdrawing; conduct CIWA or AWSS
  CIWA less than 15 (AWSS <6): not actively withdrawing; proceed with prophylaxis, if
  indicated
  CIWA 15 or higher (AWSS ≥6): patient already experiencing active AWS, proceed to
  treatment (not prophylaxis)

Decision algorithm

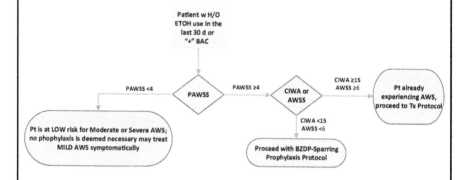

Monitoring

Monitor patient's progress with an AWS severity scale

AWS Severity	CIWA-Ar (Sullivan et al,[219] 1989; Shaw et al,[230] 1981; Holbrook,[226] 1999)	AWSS[220] (Wetterling et al, 1997[220]; 2006[234])
Mild	≤15	≤5
Moderate	16–20	6–9
Severe	≥20	≥10

Nonpharmacological management

1. Implement early mobilization techniques
   a. Aggressive physical therapy and occupational therapy as soon as it is medically safe to do so
      i. In bedridden patients, daily passive range of motion
      ii. The patient should out of bed as much as possible
         1. Get the patient up and moving as early as possible
   b. Patients out of bed as much as possible
   c. Provide patients with any required sensory aids (ie, eyeglasses, hearing aids)
   d. Promote as normal a circadian light rhythm as possible
      i. Environmental manipulations
         1. Light control (ie, lights on and curtains drawn during the day, off at night)
         2. Noise control (ie, provide ear plugs, turn off televisions, minimize night staff chatter)
      ii. Provide as much natural light as possible during the daytime

   e. If possible, provide the patient with at least a 6-hour period of protected nighttime sleep (ie, no blood draws, tests, and medication administrations unless absolutely necessary)

2. Provide adequate intellectual and environmental stimulation
   a. Encourage visitation by family and friends
   b. Minimize television use

3. Monitor for seizures

4. Fall precautions

5. Basic laboratory tests: creatinine clearance (CrCl), LFTs, electrocardiogram, volatile screen order, toxicology screening test (if not already done)

Fluid and nutritional replacement

1. Correct and monitor fluid balances and electrolytes
   a. Magnesium (Mg) [1.7–2.2 mg/dL]
   b. Na [135–145 mEq/L]
   c. K [3.7–5.2 mEq/L]

2. Vitamin supplementation
   a. Thiamine 500 mg IV, intramuscular (IM), or by mouth 3 times a day × 5 days
      • Followed by thiamine 100 mg IV, IM, or by mouth for rest of hospital stay (or up to 14 d)
   b. Folate 1 mg by mouth daily
   c. Multivitamin, 1 tab by mouth daily
   d. B complex vitamin 2 tabs by mouth daily
   e. Vitamin K 5 to 10 mg subcutaneously × 1 (if international normalized ratio is >1.3)

BZDP-sparing AWS pharmacological prophylaxis

• Prophylaxis is suggested in patients who (1) are at risk for complicated AWS but (2) who are not experiencing active AWS yet

• If CIWA15 or higher, the patient is actively experiencing AWS, switch to treatment order set
   a. Alpha-2 agents
      i. Clonidine transdermal 0.1 mg (2 patches)
      ii. Plus, administer clonidine 0.1 mg by mouth or IV every 8 hours (×3 doses)
      iii. Alternatively, may use GUA 0.5, 1 mg by mouth twice a day; GUA has better anxiolytic effect and is less hypotensive than clonidine
   b. If patient's VS unable to tolerate alpha-2 effect may instead use GAB
      i. Day 0: 1200 mg loading dose + 800 mg 3 times a day
      ii. Day 1 to 3: 800 mg by mouth 3 times a day
      iii. Day 4 to 5: 600 mg by mouth 3 times a day
      iv. Day 5 to 7: 300 mg by mouth 3 times a day
      v. Day 8: D/C
      vi. Do not use GAB in patients with severe renal dysfunction who are unable to clear GAB (ie, CrCl is <60)
   c. In patient at extremely high risk for severe AWS (ie, PAWSS ≥7 or BAC ≥300 on admission) use both clonidine and GAB, as above; GAB may also be used as an alternative to BZDPs in patients experiencing extreme levels of anxiety, even in the absence of objective signs of AWS
   d. For adjunct management of insomnia, may use (choose from the following)
      i. Melatonin 6 mg by mouth every HS, plus one PRN
      ii. Doxylamine 25 to 50 mg every HS, PRN
      iii. Hydroxyzine 50 mg by mouth every HS, PRN
      iv. Doxepin 10 mg by mouth every HS, PRN
      v. Zolpidem 10 mg by mouth every HS, PRN
   e. For adjunct management of anxiety, may use (choose of the following)
      i. Doxylamine 25 to 50 mg every HS, PRN
      ii. Hydroxyzine 50 mg by mouth every HS, PRN
   f. BZDPs should be used only in the case of a patient who experiences breakthrough symptoms of AWS, despite of implementation of the BZDP-sparing protocol, as signaled by a CIWA score 15 or higher (AWSS ≥6)[220] over 8 hours; in that case, switch to a BZDP-sparing treatment protocol; for breakthrough AWS:

     i. If CIWA-Ar greater than 15 (AWSS $\geq$6), lorazepam 1 mg q 4 hours
    ii. If CIWA-Ar greater than 20 (AWSS $\geq$10),[220] lorazepam 2 mg q 4 hours

BZDP-Sparing AWS: pharmacological treatment

- If CIWA less than 15, the patient is not actively experiencing AWS; switch to the prophylaxis order set
  a. Alpha-2 agents
     i. Transdermal clonidine 0.2 mg × 2 (total 0.4 mg)
     ii. Plus, administer clonidine 0.1 mg by mouth or IV every 8 hours (×3 doses)
     iii. Alternatively, may use guanfacine 1 mg, by mouth, twice a day 1 mg, by mouth, 3 times a day; GUA has better anxiolytic effect and is less hypotensive than clonidine
     iv. Closely monitor CIWA or AWSS every 4 hours; if AWS continues (eg, CIWA $\geq$15, AWSS $\geq$6), add VPA
  b. Plus, Ca^{2+}Ch modulator (GLU), either:
     i. GAB schedule (GAB can be used only if CrCl is greater than 60, must be renally dosed if CrCl <60)
        1. Day 0: 1200 mg loading dose plus 800 mg 3 times a day
        2. Day 1 to 3: 800 mg by mouth 3 times a day
        3. Day 4 to 5: 600 mg by mouth 3 times a day
        4. Day 5 to 7: 300 mg by mouth 3 times a day
        5. Day 8: D/C
     ii. VPA by mouth or IV
        1. Start VPA 250 mg by mouth or IV bid plus 500 mg every HS
        2. Cases of late severe AWS may require up to 1.5 gm in first 24 hours
        3. If Sx's escalate after 12 hours, increase total dose to 2 gm in divided doses
        4. If Sx's of AWS continue or worsen, add GAB
        Note: In the treatment protocol, clinicians are to use both an alpha-2 agonist plus an antiglutamatergic-Ca^{2+}Ch agent; GAB can be used if CrCl is less than 60; alternatively may use VPA
  c. For adjunct management of insomnia
     i. Melatonin 6 mg by mouth every 1800
     ii. Doxylamine 25 to 50 mg every HS, PRN
     iii. Hydroxyzine 50 mg by mouth every HS, PRN
     iv. Doxepin 10 mg every HS, PRN
     v. Zolpidem 10 mg by mouth every HS, PRN
  d. For breakthrough AWS (consider progression to rescue protocol, if the patient experiences a sustained elevation of the severity scale scores)
     i. If CIWA-Ar greater than 15 (AWSS >6), lorazepam 1 mg every 4 hours
     ii. If CIWA-Ar greater than 20 (AWSS $\geq$10),[220] lorazepam 2 mg every 4 hours
  e. Nonresponsive AWS, consider transfer to ICU; then add DEX drip, 0.4 µg/kg/h; titrate every 20 minutes to effect

BZDP-Sparing AWS: rescue treatment protocol

1. Alpha-2 agents
   a. Initiate DEX at 0.4 µg/kg/h (no loading)
   b. Titrate dose by 0.1 µg/kg/h every 20 minutes to effect or in response to an elevated assessment score (AWAS >10)
   c. There is no maximum dose, yet clinical experience suggests the maximum required DEX dose for alcohol withdrawal management is approximately 2.4 µg/kg/h

2. Valproic acid by mouth, or valproate sodium by IV
   a. Add VPA 250 mg by mouth or IV twice a day plus 500 mg every HS (if the patient is not already on it)
   b. It may be necessary to increase the dose to 500 mg twice a day plus 1000 mg every HS if the patient continues to be symptomatic after 12 to 24 hours
   c. If Sx's of AWS continue or worsen, add GAB

3. GAB schedule
   a. Day 0: 1200 mg loading dose plus 800 mg 3 times a day
   b. Day 1 to 3: 800 mg by mouth 3 times a day
   c. Day 4 to 5: 600 mg by mouth 3 times a day

   d. Day 5 to 7: 300 mg by mouth 3 times a day
   e. Day 8: D/C
4. The idea is to avoid BZDP, if possible, to minimize risk for delirium and prolonging BZDP or alcohol dependence
   a. Yet in some cases, lorazepam 2 mg by mouth or IV, every 1 hour PRN, may be used based on assessment scales or clinical picture, after the patient has been initiated on DEX and VPA (as above)
   b. If symptoms are severe (ie, AWSS $\geq$10), may use lorazepam 2 to 4 mg by mouth every 2 hours until the scores have dropped to the moderate range

Abbreviations: BAC, blood alcohol concentration; D/C, discontinue; HS, hora somni (or at bedtime); LFTs, Liver function tests; PRN, pro re nata, or as needed; Sx's, symptoms.

Patients scoring at high risk for complicated AWSS[220] (ie, PAWSS $\geq$4) and scoring on the active withdrawal range on a severity scale (ie, CIWA-Ar $\geq$15, AWSS $\geq$6) should be immediately transferred to the treatment protocol. An AAG (ie, CLO or GUA) at twice the dose of the prophylactic protocol, plus an antiglutamatergic-Ca^{2+}Ch modulator (choice of agent is made based on clinical circumstances and patient's characteristics) are initiated, as per protocol (see **Box 2**, **Fig. 3**).

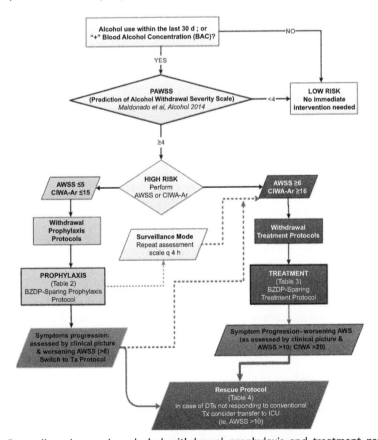

Fig. 3. Benzodiazepine-sparing alcohol withdrawal prophylaxis and treatment protocol. AWSS, Alcohol Withdrawal Syndrome Scale; BAC, blood alcohol concentration; BZDP, benzodiazepine; CIWA-Ar, Clinical Institute Withdrawal Assessment for Alcohol; PAWSS, Prediction of Alcohol Withdrawal Severity Scale.

Prediction of Alcohol Withdrawal Severity Scale (PAWSS)

Maldonado et al., 2014

Part A: Threshold Criteria:

("+" or "-", no point)

Have you consumed any amount of alcohol (i.e., been drinking) within the last 30 d? OR did the patient have a "+" BAL upon admission?   _____

IF the answer to either is YES, proceed with test:

Part B: Based on patient interview:

(1 point each)

1. Have you <u>ever</u> experienced previous episodes of alcohol withdrawal?   _____

2. Have you <u>ever</u> experienced alcohol withdrawal seizures?   _____

3. Have you <u>ever</u> experienced delirium tremens or DT's?   _____

4. Have you <u>ever</u> undergone alcohol rehabilitation treatment?

   (i.e., in-patient or out-patient treatment programs or AA attendance)   _____

5. Have you <u>ever</u> experienced blackouts?   _____

6. Have you combined alcohol with other "downers" like benzodiazepines or

   barbiturates during the last 90 d?   _____

7. Have you combined alcohol with any other substance of abuse

   during the last 90 d?   _____

8. Have you been recently intoxicated/drunk within the last 30 d?   _____

Part C: Based on clinical evidence:

(1 point each)

9. Was the patient's blood alcohol level (BAL) on presentation >200?   _____

10. Is there evidence of increased autonomic activity?

   (e.g., HR >120 bpm, tremor, sweating, agitation, nausea)   _____

Total Score: _____

Notes: Maximum score = 10. This instrument is intended as a <u>SCREENING TOOL</u>. The greater the number of positive findings, the higher the risk for the development of alcohol withdrawal syndromes. A score of ≥4 suggests HIGH RISK for moderate to severe AWS; prophylaxis and/or treatment may be indicated.

Fig. 4. PAWSS. (*From* Maldonado JR, Sher Y, Ashouri JF. The "Prediction of Alcohol Withdrawal Severity Scale" (PAWSS): systematic literature review and pilot study of a new scale for the prediction of complicated alcohol withdrawal syndrome. Alcohol 2014;48(4):375–90; with permission.)

VPA may be used as an alternative to GAB in cases of patients with severe renal dysfunction unable to clear GAB (creatinine clearance [CrCl] is <60). Once a patient has been stable for 2 days (48 hours), the clinician may begin a slow VPA titration by 250 mg per day until off. Do not use or discontinue its use if alanine aminotransferase (ALT) is greater than 150, aspartate aminotransferase (AST) is greater than 80, or if platelets decrease by 30% (from baseline) or are below 150, at baseline.

GAB and/or VPA may also be used as an alternative for patients unable to tolerate the hypotensive effect of an AAG agent.

Any patient whose withdrawal severity score rises despite of prophylactic management should be considered as deteriorating and thus requires more aggressive treatment. That usually includes first optimization of BZDP-sparing protocol by switching to the treatment protocol, minimal use of BZDP agents for breakthrough until stabilization, or implementation of the rescue protocol with the use of DEX.

SUMMARY

Current guidelines for the prophylaxis and management of AWS are based on the use of BZDPs. The rationale has always been that BZDPs effectively cover all phases of alcohol withdrawal. Yet clinical experience with the use of BZDPs suggests difficulties in implementing prophylaxis and treatment protocols adequately. The problem seems related to the way BZDPs are administered, whether objective physiologic or psychological methods are used to time dosing, and the type of BZDP agent used.

The author's clinical experience demonstrates that current BZDP-based, severity scale-triggered protocols can be fraught with complexities, breakthrough AWS, and significant side effects, particularly the development of BZDP-induced delirium. Available data suggest that non-BZDP agents may offer a safe and effective alternative for the prophylaxis and treatment of AWS.

The data for the use of non-BZDP agents are growing but larger, randomized, head-to-head studies comparing them with BZDP are necessary to assess efficacy and safety. In the author's experience, the use of a predictive tool to help identify patients at risk for complicated-AWS, in combination with monitoring by the use of severity scales, and coupled with the BZDP-sparing prophylaxis and treatment algorithms has been the best way to manage AWS while minimizing the side effects associated with BZDP use. In 4 years of experience, the use of the BZDP-sparing protocol has proven effective and safe. To date, there have been no significant adverse side effects requiring discontinuation of the protocol, no fatalities, no progression to alcohol withdrawal seizures, and no breakthrough DTs. Despite this positive experience, the author acknowledges that large, randomized studies are needed to confirm these findings.

REFERENCES

1. American Psychiatric Association. Diagnostic and statistical manual of mental disorders. 5th edition. Washington, DC: American Psychiatric Association; 2013.
2. Williams GD, Stinson FS, Lane JD, et al. Apparent per capita alcohol consumption: national, state and regional trends, 1977–1994. Washington, DC: NIAAA; 1996.
3. Lieber CS. Medical disorders of alcoholism. N Engl J Med 1995;333(16): 1058–65.
4. Hasin DS, Stinson FS, Ogburn E, et al. Prevalence, correlates, disability, and co-morbidity of DSM-IV alcohol abuse and dependence in the United States: results from the National Epidemiologic Survey on Alcohol and Related Conditions. Arch Gen Psychiatry 2007;64(7):830–42.
5. Mokdad AH, Marks JS, Stroup DF, et al. Actual causes of death in the United States, 2000 [see comment]. JAMA 2004;291(10):1238–45 [erratum appears in JAMA 2005;293(3):293–4].
6. Baldwin WA, Rosenfeld BA, Breslow MJ, et al. Substance abuse-related admissions to adult intensive care. Chest 1993;103(1):21–5.

7. de Wit M, Wan SY, Gill S, et al. Prevalence and impact of alcohol and other drug use disorders on sedation and mechanical ventilation: a retrospective study. BMC Anesthesiol 2007;7:3.

8. Gacouin A, Legay F, Camus C, et al. At-risk drinkers are at higher risk to acquire a bacterial infection during an intensive care unit stay than abstinent or moderate drinkers. Crit Care Med 2008;36(6):1735–41.

9. Moss M, Burnham EL. Alcohol abuse in the critically ill patient. Lancet 2006; 368(9554):2231–42.

10. Stanley KM, Amabile CM, Simpson KN, et al. Impact of an alcohol withdrawal syndrome practice guideline on surgical patient outcomes. Pharmacotherapy 2003;23(7):843–54.

11. Herve C, Gaillard M, Roujas F, et al. Alcoholism in polytrauma. J Trauma 1986; 26(12):1123–6.

12. Jensen NH, Dragsted L, Christensen JK, et al. Severity of illness and outcome of treatment in alcoholic patients in the intensive care unit. Intensive Care Med 1988;15(1):19–22.

13. Jurkovich GJ, Dragsted L, Christensen JK, et al. The effect of acute alcohol intoxication and chronic alcohol abuse on outcome from trauma. JAMA 1993; 270(1):51–6.

14. Moller AM, Tonnesen H. Smoking and alcohol intake in surgical patients: identification and information in Danish surgical departments. Eur J Surg 2001; 167(9):650–1.

15. Spies CD, Neuner B, Neumann T, et al. Intercurrent complications in chronic alcoholic men admitted to the intensive care unit following trauma. Intensive Care Med 1996;22(4):286–93.

16. Spies CD, Nordmann A, Brummer G, et al. Intensive care unit stay is prolonged in chronic alcoholic men following tumor resection of the upper digestive tract. Acta Anaesthesiol Scand 1996;40(6):649–56.

17. Spies CD, Rommelspacher H. Alcohol withdrawal in the surgical patient: prevention and treatment. Anesth Analg 1999;88(4):946–54.

18. Maldonado JR, Wise L. Clinical and financial implications of the timely recognition and management of delirium in the acute medical wards. J Psychosom Res 2003;55:151.

19. Krystal JH, Tabakoff B. Ethanol abuse, dependence, and withdrawal: neurobiology and clinical implications. In: Davis KL, Charney DS, Coyle JT, et al, editors. Neuropsychopharmacology: the fifth generation of progress. Philadelphia: Lippincott Williams and Wilkins.; 2002. p. 1425–43.

20. Hall W, Zador D. The alcohol withdrawal syndrome. Lancet 1997;349(9069): 1897–900.

21. Bayard M, McIntyre J, Hill KR, et al. Alcohol withdrawal syndrome. Am Fam Physician 2004;69(6):1443–50.

22. Littleton J. Neurochemical mechanisms underlying alcohol withdrawal. Alcohol Health Res World 1998;22(1):13–24.

23. Turner RC, Lichstein PR, Peden JG Jr, et al. Alcohol withdrawal syndromes: a review of pathophysiology, clinical presentation, and treatment. J Gen Intern Med 1989;4(5):432–44.

24. Lau K, Freyer-Adam J, Coder B, et al. Dose-response relation between volume of drinking and alcohol-related diseases in male general hospital inpatients. Alcohol Alcohol 2008;43(1):34–8.

25. Sannibale C, Fucito L, O'Connor D, et al. Process evaluation of an out-patient detoxification service. Drug Alcohol Rev 2005;24(6):475–81.

26. O'Brien JM Jr, Lu B, Ali NA, et al. Alcohol dependence is independently associated with sepsis, septic shock, and hospital mortality among adult intensive care unit patients. Crit Care Med 2007;35(2):345–50.
27. Suchyta MR, Beck CJ, Key CW, et al. Substance dependence and psychiatric disorders are related to outcomes in a mixed ICU population. Intensive Care Med 2008;34(12):2264–7.
28. Palmstierna T. A model for predicting alcohol withdrawal delirium. Psychiatr Serv 2001;52(6):820–3.
29. Maldonado J. An approach to the patient with substance use and abuse. Med Clin North Am 2010;94(6):1169–205, x–i.
30. Victor M, Adams RD. The effect of alcohol on the nervous system. Res Publ Assoc Res Nerv Ment Dis 1953;32:526–73.
31. Shen RY, Chiodo LA. Acute withdrawal after repeated ethanol treatment reduces the number of spontaneously active dopaminergic neurons in the ventral tegmental area. Brain Res 1993;622(1–2):289–93.
32. Shen WW. Extrapyramidal symptoms associated with alcohol withdrawal. Biol Psychiatry 1984;19(7):1037–43.
33. Mennecier D, Thomas M, Arvers P, et al. Factors predictive of complicated or severe alcohol withdrawal in alcohol dependent inpatients. Gastroenterol Clin Biol 2008;32(8–9):792–7.
34. Schuckit MA, Tipp JE, Reich T, et al. The histories of withdrawal convulsions and delirium tremens in 1648 alcohol dependent subjects. Addiction 1995;90(10):1335–47.
35. Victor M, Brausch C. The role of abstinence in the genesis of alcoholic epilepsy. Epilepsia 1967;8(1):1–20.
36. Isbell H, Fraser HF, Wikler A, et al. An experimental study of the etiology of rum fits and delirium tremens. Q J Stud Alcohol 1955;16(1):1–33.
37. Leone M, Bottacchi E, Beghi E, et al. Alcohol use is a risk factor for a first generalized tonic-clonic seizure. The ALC.E. (Alcohol and Epilepsy) Study Group. Neurology 1997;48(3):614–20.
38. Ng SK, Hauser WA, Brust JC, et al. Alcohol consumption and withdrawal in new-onset seizures. N Engl J Med 1988;319(11):666–73.
39. Aminoff MJ, Simon RP. Status epilepticus. Causes, clinical features and consequences in 98 patients. Am J Med 1980;69(5):657–66.
40. Rathlev NK, Ulrich AS, Delanty N, et al. Alcohol-related seizures. J Emerg Med 2006;31(2):157–63.
41. Gill JS, Shipley MJ, Tsementzis SA, et al. Alcohol consumption–a risk factor for hemorrhagic and non-hemorrhagic stroke. Am J Med 1991;90(4):489–97.
42. Rathlev NK, Medzon R, Lowery D, et al. Intracranial pathology in elders with blunt head trauma. Acad Emerg Med 2006;13(3):302–7.
43. Sonne NM, Tonnesen H. The influence of alcoholism on outcome after evacuation of subdural haematoma. Br J Neurosurg 1992;6(2):125–30.
44. Rathlev NK, Ulrich A, Fish SS, et al. Clinical characteristics as predictors of recurrent alcohol-related seizures. Acad Emerg Med 2000;7(8):886–91.
45. Rathlev NK, Ulrich A, Shieh TC, et al. Etiology and weekly occurrence of alcohol-related seizures. Acad Emerg Med 2002;9(8):824–8.
46. Brathen G. Alcohol and epilepsy. Tidsskr Nor Laegeforen 2003;123(11):1536–8 [in Norwegian].
47. Elton M. Alcohol withdrawal: clinical symptoms and management of the syndrome. Acta Psychiatr Scand Suppl 1986;327:80–90.

48. Sarff M, Gold JA. Alcohol withdrawal syndromes in the intensive care unit. Crit Care Med 2010;38(9 Suppl):S494–501.
49. Holloway HC, Hales RE, Watanabe HK. Recognition and treatment of acute alcohol withdrawal syndromes. Psychiatr Clin North Am 1984;7(4):729–43.
50. Lishman W. Organic psychiatry. The psychological consequences of cerebral disorder. Oxford (United Kingdom): Blackwell Scientific Publications; 1998.
51. Yost DA. Alcohol withdrawal syndrome. Am Fam Physician 1996;54(2):657–64, 669.
52. Campos J, Roca L, Gude F, et al. Long-term mortality of patients admitted to the hospital with alcohol withdrawal syndrome. Alcohol Clin Exp Res 2011;35(6): 1180–6.
53. Cushman P Jr. Delirium tremens. Update on an old disorder. Postgrad Med 1987;82(5):117–22.
54. Erwin WE, Williams DB, Speir WA. Delirium tremens. South Med J 1998;91(5): 425–32.
55. Hemmingsen R, Kramp P, Rafaelsen OJ. Delirium tremens and related clinical states. Aetiology, pathophysiology and treatment. Acta Psychiatr Scand 1979; 59(4):337–69.
56. Horstmann E, Conrad E, Daweke H. Severe course of delirium tremens. Results of treatment and late prognosis. Med Klin (Munich) 1989;84(12):569–73 [in German].
57. Monte R, Rabuñal R, Casariego E, et al. Analysis of the factors determining survival of alcoholic withdrawal syndrome patients in a general hospital. Alcohol Alcohol 2010;45(2):151–8.
58. Maldonado JR, Sher Y, Ashouri JF, et al. The "Prediction of Alcohol Withdrawal Severity Scale" (PAWSS): systematic literature review and pilot study of a new scale for the prediction of complicated alcohol withdrawal syndrome. Alcohol 2014;48(4):375–90.
59. Ungur LA, Neuner B, John S, et al. Prevention and therapy of alcohol withdrawal on intensive care units: systematic review of controlled trials. Alcohol Clin Exp Res 2013;37(4):675–86.
60. Schaefer TJ, Hafner JW. Are benzodiazepines effective for alcohol withdrawal? Ann Emerg Med 2013;62(1):34–5.
61. Marcantonio ER, Juarez G, Goldman L, et al. The relationship of postoperative delirium with psychoactive medications. JAMA 1994;272(19):1518–22.
62. Ely EW, Gautam S, Margolin R, et al. The impact of delirium in the intensive care unit on hospital length of stay. Intensive Care Med 2001;27(12):1892–900.
63. Gaudreau JD, Gagnon P, Roy MA, et al. Association between psychoactive medications and delirium in hospitalized patients: a critical review. Psychosomatics 2005;46(4):302–16.
64. Girard TD, Pandharipande PP, Ely EW. Delirium in the intensive care unit. Crit Care 2008;12(Suppl 3):S3.
65. Kudoh A, Takase H, Takahira Y, et al. Postoperative confusion increases in elderly long-term benzodiazepine users. Anesth Analg 2004;99(6):1674–8 [Table of contents].
66. Maldonado JR. Delirium in the acute care setting: characteristics, diagnosis and treatment. Crit Care Clin 2008;24(4):657–722.
67. Maldonado JR. Pathoetiological model of delirium: a comprehensive understanding of the neurobiology of delirium and an evidence-based approach to prevention and treatment. Crit Care Clin 2008;24(4):789–856.

68. Pain L, Jeltsch H, Lehmann O, et al. Central cholinergic depletion induced by 192 IgG-saporin alleviates the sedative effects of propofol in rats. Br J Anaesth 2000;85(6):869–73.
69. Pandharipande P, Shintani A, Peterson J, et al. Lorazepam is an independent risk factor for transitioning to delirium in intensive care unit patients. Anesthesiology 2006;104(1):21–6.
70. Tune LE, Bylsma FW. Benzodiazepine-induced and anticholinergic-induced delirium in the elderly. Int Psychogeriatr 1991;3(2):397–408.
71. Mayo-Smith MF. Pharmacological management of alcohol withdrawal. A meta-analysis and evidence-based practice guideline. American Society of Addiction Medicine working group on pharmacological management of alcohol withdrawal. JAMA 1997;278(2):144–51.
72. Smith I, White PF, Nathanson M, et al. Propofol. An update on its clinical use. Anesthesiology 1994;81(4):1005–43.
73. Mirski MA, Muffelman B, Ulatowski JA, et al. Sedation for the critically ill neurologic patient. Crit Care Med 1995;23(12):2038–53.
74. Hara M, Kai Y, Ikemoto Y. Propofol activates GABAA receptor-chloride ionophore complex in dissociated hippocampal pyramidal neurons of the rat. Anesthesiology 1993;79(4):781–8.
75. Orser BA, Bertlik M, Wang LY, et al. Inhibition by propofol (2,6 di-isopropylphenol) of the N-methyl-D-aspartate subtype of glutamate receptor in cultured hippocampal neurones. Br J Pharmacol 1995;116(2):1761–8.
76. Kuisma M, Roine RO. Propofol in prehospital treatment of convulsive status epilepticus. Epilepsia 1995;36(12):1241–3.
77. Merigian KS, Browning RG, Leeper KV. Successful treatment of amoxapine-induced refractory status epilepticus with propofol (diprivan). Acad Emerg Med 1995;2(2):128–33.
78. Stecker MM, Kramer TH, Raps EC, et al. Treatment of refractory status epilepticus with propofol: clinical and pharmacokinetic findings. Epilepsia 1998;39(1):18–26.
79. Coomes TR, Smith SW. Successful use of propofol in refractory delirium tremens. Ann Emerg Med 1997;30(6):825–8.
80. McCowan C, Marik P. Refractory delirium tremens treated with propofol: a case series. Crit Care Med 2000;28(6):1781–4.
81. Takeshita J. Use of propofol for alcohol withdrawal delirium: a case report. J Clin Psychiatry 2004;65(1):134–5.
82. Currier DS, Bevacqua BK. Acute tachyphylaxis to propofol sedation during ethanol withdrawal. J Clin Anesth 1997;9(5):420–3.
83. Devlin JW, Lau AK, Tanios MA. Propofol-associated hypertriglyceridemia and pancreatitis in the intensive care unit: an analysis of frequency and risk factors. Pharmacotherapy 2005;25(10):1348–52.
84. Diedrich DA, Brown DR. Analytic reviews: propofol infusion syndrome in the ICU. J Intensive Care Med 2011;26(2):59–72.
85. Leisure GS, O'Flaherty J, Green L, et al. Propofol and postoperative pancreatitis. Anesthesiology 1996;84(1):224–7.
86. Ambrosio AF, Soares-Da-Silva P, Carvalho CM, et al. Mechanisms of action of carbamazepine and its derivatives, oxcarbazepine, BIA 2-093, and BIA 2-024. Neurochem Res 2002;27(1–2):121–30.
87. Macdonald RL, Kelly KM. Antiepileptic drug mechanisms of action. Epilepsia 1993;34(Suppl 5):S1–8.

88. Marjerrison G, Jedlicki SM, Keogh RP, et al. Carbamazepine: behavioral, anticonvulsant and EEG effects in chronically-hospitalized epileptics. Dis Nerv Syst 1968;29(2):133–6.

89. Willow M, Gonoi T, Catterall WA. Voltage clamp analysis of the inhibitory actions of diphenylhydantoin and carbamazepine on voltage-sensitive sodium channels in neuroblastoma cells. Mol Pharmacol 1985;27(5):549–58.

90. Granger P, Biton B, Faure C, et al. Modulation of the gamma-aminobutyric acid type A receptor by the antiepileptic drugs carbamazepine and phenytoin. Mol Pharmacol 1995;47(6):1189–96.

91. Malcolm R, Myrick H, Roberts J, et al. The effects of carbamazepine and lorazepam on single versus multiple previous alcohol withdrawals in an outpatient randomized trial. J Gen Intern Med 2002;17(5):349–55.

92. Bjorkqvist SE. Clonidine in alcohol withdrawal. Acta Psychiatr Scand 1975;52(4):256–63.

93. Ritola E, Malinen L. A double-blind comparison of carbamazepine and clomethiazole in the treatment of alcohol withdrawal syndrome. Acta Psychiatr Scand 1981;64(3):254–9.

94. Flygenring J, Hansen J, Holst B, et al. Treatment of alcohol withdrawal symptoms in hospitalized patients. A randomized, double-blind comparison of carbamazepine (Tegretol) and barbital (Diemal). Acta Psychiatr Scand 1984;69(5):398–408.

95. Bjorkqvist SE, Isohanni M, Mäkelä R, et al. Ambulant treatment of alcohol withdrawal symptoms with carbamazepine: a formal multicentre double-blind comparison with placebo. Acta Psychiatr Scand 1976;53(5):333–42.

96. Agricola R, Mazzarino M, Urani R, et al. Treatment of acute alcohol withdrawal syndrome with carbamazepine: a double-blind comparison with tiapride. J Int Med Res 1982;10(3):160–5.

97. Malcolm R, Ballenger JC, Sturgis ET, et al. Double-blind controlled trial comparing carbamazepine to oxazepam treatment of alcohol withdrawal. Am J Psychiatry 1989;146(5):617–21.

98. Hillbom M, Tokola R, Kuusela V, et al. Prevention of alcohol withdrawal seizures with carbamazepine and valproic acid. Alcohol 1989;6(3):223–6.

99. Stuppaeck CH, Pycha R, Miller C, et al. Carbamazepine versus oxazepam in the treatment of alcohol withdrawal: a double-blind study. Alcohol Alcohol 1992;27(2):153–8.

100. Lucht M, Kuehn KU, Armbruster J, et al. Alcohol withdrawal treatment in intoxicated vs non-intoxicated patients: a controlled open-label study with tiapride/carbamazepine, clomethiazole and diazepam. Alcohol Alcohol 2003;38(2):168–75.

101. Polycarpou A, Papanikolaou P, Ioannidis JP, et al. Anticonvulsants for alcohol withdrawal. Cochrane Database Syst Rev 2005;(3):CD005064.

102. Minozzi S, Amato L, Vecchi S, et al. Anticonvulsants for alcohol withdrawal. Cochrane Database Syst Rev 2010;(3):CD005064.

103. Barrons R, Roberts N. The role of carbamazepine and oxcarbazepine in alcohol withdrawal syndrome. J Clin Pharm Ther 2010;35(2):153–67.

104. Franz M, Dlabal H, Kunz S, et al. Treatment of alcohol withdrawal: tiapride and carbamazepine versus clomethiazole. A pilot study. Eur Arch Psychiatry Clin Neurosci 2001;251(4):185–92.

105. Garcia-Borreguero D, Bronisch T, Apelt S, et al. Treatment of benzodiazepine withdrawal symptoms with carbamazepine. Eur Arch Psychiatry Clin Neurosci 1991;241(3):145–50.

106. Poutanen P. Experience with carbamazepine in the treatment of withdrawal symptoms in alcohol abusers. Br J Addict Alcohol Other Drugs 1979;74(2): 201–4.
107. Brune F, Busch H. Anticonvulsive-sedative treatment of delirium alcoholicum. Q J Stud Alcohol 1971;32(2):334–42.
108. Sillanpaa M, Sonck T. Finnish experiences with carbamazepine (Tegretol) in the treatment of acute withdrawal symptoms in alcoholics. J Int Med Res 1979;7(3): 168–73.
109. Ulrichsen J, Clemmesen L, Flachs H, et al. The effect of phenobarbital and carbamazepine on the ethanol withdrawal reaction in the rat. Psychopharmacology (Berl) 1986;89(2):162–6.
110. Messiha FS, Butler D, Adams MK. Carbamazepine and ethanol elicited responses in rodents. Alcohol 1986;3(2):131–3.
111. Strzelec JS, Czarnecka E. Influence of clonazepam and carbamazepine on alcohol withdrawal syndrome, preference and development of tolerance to ethanol in rats. Pol J Pharmacol 2001;53(2):117–24.
112. Pynnonen S, Bjorkqvist SE, Pekkarinen A. The pharmacokinetics of carbamazepine in alcoholics. In: Meinardi H, Rowan AJ, editors. Advances in epileptology. Amsterdam (The Netherlands): Swets and Zeitlinger; 1978. p. 285–9.
113. Pynnonen S, Mantyla R, Iisalo E. Bioavailability of four different pharmaceutical preparations of carbamazepine. Acta Pharmacol Toxicol (Copenh) 1978;43(4): 306–10.
114. Kuhn R. The psychotropic effect of carbamazepine in non-epileptic adults, with particular reference to the drug mechanism of action. In: Birkmayer WE, editor. Epileptic seizures, behaviour, and pain. Baltimore (MD): University Park Press; 1976. p. 268–74.
115. Butler D, Messiha FS. Alcohol withdrawal and carbamazepine. Alcohol 1986; 3(2):113–29.
116. Singh G. Do no harm–but first we need to know more: the case of adverse drug reactions with antiepileptic drugs. Neurol India 2011;59(1):53–8.
117. Wellington K, Goa KL. Oxcarbazepine: an update of its efficacy in the management of epilepsy. CNS Drugs 2001;15(2):137–63.
118. Keck PE Jr, McElroy SL. Clinical pharmacodynamics and pharmacokinetics of antimanic and mood-stabilizing medications. J Clin Psychiatry 2002;63(Suppl 4):3–11.
119. Schik G, Wedegaertner FR, Liersch J, et al. Oxcarbazepine versus carbamazepine in the treatment of alcohol withdrawal. Addict Biol 2005;10(3):283–8.
120. Croissant B, Loeber S, Diehl A, et al. Oxcarbazepine in combination with Tiaprid in inpatient alcohol-withdrawal–a RCT. Pharmacopsychiatry 2009;42(5):175–81.
121. Lu BY, Coberly R, Bogenschutz M. Use of oxcarbazepine in outpatient alcohol detoxification. Am J Addict 2005;14(2):191–2.
122. Ponce G, Rodríguez-Jiménez R, Ortiz H, et al. Oxcarbazepine in the prevention of epileptic syndromes in alcohol detoxification. Rev Neurol 2005;40(10):577–80 [in Spanish].
123. Croissant B, Scherle T, Diehl A, et al. Oxcarbazepine in alcohol relapse prevention–a case series. Pharmacopsychiatry 2004;37(6):306–7.
124. Croissant B, Diehl A, Klein O, et al. A pilot study of oxcarbazepine versus acamprosate in alcohol-dependent patients. Alcohol Clin Exp Res 2006;30(4):630–5.
125. Martinotti G, Romanelli R, Di Nicola M, et al. Oxcarbazepine at high dosages for the treatment of alcohol dependence. Am J Addict 2007;16(3):247–8.

126. Martinotti G, Di Nicola M, Romanelli R, et al. High and low dosage oxcarbazepine versus naltrexone for the prevention of relapse in alcohol-dependent patients. Hum Psychopharmacol 2007;22(3):149–56.

127. Loscher W. Basic pharmacology of valproate: a review after 35 years of clinical use for the treatment of epilepsy. CNS Drugs 2002;16(10):669–94.

128. Lambie DG, Johnson RH, Vijayasenan ME, et al. Sodium valproate in the treatment of the alcohol withdrawal syndrome. Aust N Z J Psychiatry 1980;14(3): 213–5.

129. Rosenthal RN, Perkel C, Singh P, et al. A pilot open randomized trial of valproate and phenobarbital in the treatment of acute alcohol withdrawal. Am J Addict 1998;7(3):189–97.

130. Myrick H, Brady KT, Malcolm R. Divalproex in the treatment of alcohol withdrawal. Am J Drug Alcohol Abuse 2000;26(1):155–60.

131. Reoux JP, Saxon AJ, Malte CA, et al. Divalproex sodium in alcohol withdrawal: a randomized double-blind placebo-controlled clinical trial. Alcohol Clin Exp Res 2001;25(9):1324–9.

132. Longo LP, Campbell T, Hubatch S. Divalproex sodium (Depakote) for alcohol withdrawal and relapse prevention. J Addict Dis 2002;21(2):55–64.

133. Eyer F, Schreckenberg M, Hecht D, et al. Carbamazepine and valproate as adjuncts in the treatment of alcohol withdrawal syndrome: a retrospective cohort study. Alcohol Alcohol 2011;46(2):177–84.

134. Goldstein DB. Sodium bromide and sodium valproate: effective suppressants of ethanol withdrawal reactions in mice. J Pharmacol Exp Ther 1979;208(2):223–7.

135. Hillbom ME. The prevention of ethanol withdrawal seizures in rats by dipropylacetate. Neuropharmacology 1975;14(10):755–61.

136. Le Bourhis B, Aufrere G. Effects of sodium dipropylacetate on the ethanol withdrawal syndrome in rats. Subst Alcohol Actions Misuse 1980;1(5–6):527–35.

137. Noble EP, Gillies R, Vigran R, et al. The modification of the ethanol withdrawal syndrome in rats by di-n-propylacetate. Psychopharmacologia 1976;46(2): 127–31.

138. McLean MJ. Gabapentin in the management of convulsive disorders. Epilepsia 1999;40(Suppl 6):S39–50 [discussion: S73–4].

139. Bonnet U, Banger M, Leweke FM, et al. Treatment of alcohol withdrawal syndrome with gabapentin. Pharmacopsychiatry 1999;32(3):107–9.

140. Cho SW, Cho EH, Choi SY. Activation of two types of brain glutamate dehydrogenase isoproteins by gabapentin. FEBS Lett 1998;426(2):196–200.

141. Kelly KM. Gabapentin. Antiepileptic mechanism of action. Neuropsychobiology 1998;38(3):139–44.

142. Taylor CP. Emerging perspectives on the mechanism of action of gabapentin. Neurology 1994;44(6 Suppl 5):S10–6 [discussion: S31–2].

143. Taylor CP. Mechanisms of action of gabapentin. Rev Neurol (Paris) 1997; 153(Suppl 1):S39–45.

144. Taylor CP, Gee NS, Su TZ, et al. A summary of mechanistic hypotheses of gabapentin pharmacology. Epilepsy Res 1998;29(3):233–49.

145. Watson WP, Robinson E, Little HJ. The novel anticonvulsant, gabapentin, protects against both convulsant and anxiogenic aspects of the ethanol withdrawal syndrome. Neuropharmacology 1997;36(10):1369–75.

146. McLean MJ. Clinical pharmacokinetics of gabapentin. Neurology 1994;44(6 Suppl 5):S17–22 [discussion: S31–2].

147. Bailey CP, Molleman A, Little HJ. Comparison of the effects of drugs on hyper-excitability induced in hippocampal slices by withdrawal from chronic ethanol consumption. Br J Pharmacol 1998;123(2):215–22.

148. Mariani JJ, Rosenthal RN, Tross S, et al. A randomized, open-label, controlled trial of gabapentin and phenobarbital in the treatment of alcohol withdrawal. Am J Addict 2006;15(1):76–84.

149. Myrick H, Malcolm R, Randall PK, et al. A double-blind trial of gabapentin versus lorazepam in the treatment of alcohol withdrawal. Alcohol Clin Exp Res 2009; 33(9):1582–8.

150. Bozikas V, Petrikis P, Gamvrula K, et al. Treatment of alcohol withdrawal with ga-bapentin. Prog Neuropsychopharmacol Biol Psychiatry 2002;26(1):197–9.

151. Myrick H, Malcolm R, Brady KT. Gabapentin treatment of alcohol withdrawal. Am J Psychiatry 1998;155(11):1632.

152. Rustembegovic A, Sofic E, Tahirović I, et al. A study of gabapentin in the treat-ment of tonic-clonic seizures of alcohol withdrawal syndrome. Med Arh 2004; 58(1):5–6.

153. Krupitsky EM, Rudenko AA, Burakov AM, et al. Antiglutamatergic strategies for ethanol detoxification: comparison with placebo and diazepam. Alcohol Clin Exp Res 2007;31(4):604–11.

154. Becker HC, Myrick H, Veatch LM. Pregabalin is effective against behavioral and electrographic seizures during alcohol withdrawal. Alcohol Alcohol 2006;41(4): 399–406.

155. Di Nicola M, Martinotti G, Tedeschi D, et al. Pregabalin in outpatient detoxifica-tion of subjects with mild-to-moderate alcohol withdrawal syndrome. Hum Psy-chopharmacol 2010;25(3):268–75.

156. Martinotti G, di Nicola M, Frustaci A, et al. Pregabalin, tiapride and lorazepam in alcohol withdrawal syndrome: a multi-centre, randomized, single-blind compar-ison trial. Addiction 2010;105(2):288–99.

157. Rustembegovic A, Sofic E, Kroyer G. A pilot study of Topiramate (Topamax) in the treatment of tonic-clonic seizures of alcohol withdrawal syndromes. Med Arh 2002;56(4):211–2.

158. Myrick H, Taylor B, LaRowe S, et al. A retrospective chart review comparing tia-gabine and benzodiazepines for the treatment of alcohol withdrawal. J Psychoactive Drugs 2005;37(4):409–14.

159. Stuppaeck CH, Deisenhammer EA, Kurz M, et al. The irreversible gamma-aminobutyrate transaminase inhibitor vigabatrin in the treatment of the alcohol withdrawal syndrome. Alcohol Alcohol 1996;31(1):109–11.

160. De Sousa A. The role of topiramate and other anticonvulsants in the treatment of alcohol dependence: a clinical review. CNS Neurol Disord Drug Targets 2010; 9(1):45–9.

161. De Sousa AA, De Sousa J, Kapoor H. An open randomized trial comparing disulfiram and topiramate in the treatment of alcohol dependence. J Subst Abuse Treat 2008;34(4):460–3.

162. Johnson BA, Ait-Daoud N, Bowden CL, et al. Oral topiramate for treatment of alcohol dependence: a randomised controlled trial. Lancet 2003;361(9370): 1677–85.

163. Kenna GA, Lomastro TL, Schiesl A, et al. Review of topiramate: an antiepileptic for the treatment of alcohol dependence. Curr Drug Abuse Rev 2009;2(2): 135–42.

164. Rubio G, Martinez-Gras I, Manzanares J. Modulation of impulsivity by topiramate: implications for the treatment of alcohol dependence. J Clin Psychopharmacol 2009;29(6):584–9.
165. Swift RM. Topiramate for the treatment of alcohol dependence: initiating abstinence. Lancet 2003;361(9370):1666–7.
166. Ait-Daoud N, Malcolm RJ Jr, Johnson BA. An overview of medications for the treatment of alcohol withdrawal and alcohol dependence with an emphasis on the use of older and newer anticonvulsants. Addict Behav 2006;31(9):1628–49.
167. Linnoila M, Mefford I, Nutt D, et al. NIH conference. Alcohol withdrawal and noradrenergic function. Ann Intern Med 1987;107(6):875–89.
168. Pohorecky LA. Effects of ethanol on central and peripheral noradrenergic neurons. J Pharmacol Exp Ther 1974;189(2):380–91.
169. Donello JE, Padillo EU, Webster ML, et al. alpha(2)-Adrenoceptor agonists inhibit vitreal glutamate and aspartate accumulation and preserve retinal function after transient ischemia. J Pharmacol Exp Ther 2001;296(1):216–23.
170. Lakhlani PP, Lovinger DM, Limbird LE. Genetic evidence for involvement of multiple effector systems in alpha 2A-adrenergic receptor inhibition of stimulus-secretion coupling. Mol Pharmacol 1996;50(1):96–103.
171. Reis DJ. A possible role of central noradrenergic neurons in withdrawal states from alcohol. Ann N Y Acad Sci 1973;215:249–52.
172. Zhang Y, Kimelberg HK. Neuroprotection by alpha 2-adrenergic agonists in cerebral ischemia. Curr Neuropharmacol 2005;3(4):317–23.
173. Stern TA, Gross AF, Stern TW, et al. Current approaches to the recognition and treatment of alcohol withdrawal and delirium tremens: "old wine in new bottles" or "new wine in old bottles". Prim Care Companion J Clin Psychiatry 2010;12(3).
174. Kobilka BK, Matsui H, Kobilka TS, et al. Cloning, sequencing, and expression of the gene coding for the human platelet alpha 2-adrenergic receptor. Science 1987;238(4827):650–6.
175. Lomasney JW, Lorenz W, Allen LF, et al. Expansion of the alpha 2-adrenergic receptor family: cloning and characterization of a human alpha 2-adrenergic receptor subtype, the gene for which is located on chromosome 2. Proc Natl Acad Sci U S A 1990;87(13):5094–8.
176. Regan JW, Kobilka TS, Yang-Feng TL, et al. Cloning and expression of a human kidney cDNA for an alpha 2-adrenergic receptor subtype. Proc Natl Acad Sci U S A 1988;85(17):6301–5.
177. Fagerholm V, Scheinin M, Haaparanta M. alpha2A-adrenoceptor antagonism increases insulin secretion and synergistically augments the insulinotropic effect of glibenclamide in mice. Br J Pharmacol 2008;154(6):1287–96.
178. Ma D, Hossain M, Rajakumaraswamy N, et al. Dexmedetomidine produces its neuroprotective effect via the alpha 2A-adrenoceptor subtype. Eur J Pharmacol 2004;502(1–2):87–97.
179. Takada K, Clark DJ, Davies MF, et al. Meperidine exerts agonist activity at the alpha(2B)-adrenoceptor subtype. Anesthesiology 2002;96(6):1420–6.
180. Fagerholm V, Rokka J, Nyman L, et al. Autoradiographic characterization of alpha(2C)-adrenoceptors in the human striatum. Synapse 2008;62(7):508–15.
181. Moura E, Afonso J, Hein L, et al. Alpha2-adrenoceptor subtypes involved in the regulation of catecholamine release from the adrenal medulla of mice. Br J Pharmacol 2006;149(8):1049–58.
182. Reis DJ, Granata AR, Joh TH, et al. Brain stem catecholamine mechanisms in tonic and reflex control of blood pressure. Hypertension 1984;6(5 Pt 2):II7–15.

183. Scheinin M, omasney JW, Hayden-Hixson DM, et al. Distribution of alpha 2-adrenergic receptor subtype gene expression in rat brain. Brain Res Mol Brain Res 1994;21(1–2):133–49.

184. Aoki C, Go CG, Venkatesan C, et al. Perikaryal and synaptic localization of alpha 2A-adrenergic receptor-like immunoreactivity. Brain Res 1994;650(2):181–204.

185. Buzsaki G, Kennedy B, Solt VB, et al. Noradrenergic control of thalamic oscillation: the role of alpha-2 receptors. Eur J Neurosci 1991;3(3):222–9.

186. Hemmingsen R, Clemmesen L, Barry DI. Blind study of the effect of the alpha-adrenergic agonists clonidine and lofexidine on alcohol withdrawal in the rat. J Stud Alcohol 1984;45(4):310–5.

187. Brunning J, Mumford JP, Keaney FP. Lofexidine in alcohol withdrawal states. Alcohol Alcohol 1986;21(2):167–70.

188. Cushman P Jr, Forbes R, Lerner W, et al. Alcohol withdrawal syndromes: clinical management with lofexidine. Alcohol Clin Exp Res 1985;9(2):103–8.

189. Braz LG, Camacho Navarro LH, Braz JR, et al. Clonidine as adjuvant therapy for alcohol withdrawal syndrome in intensive care unit: case report. Rev Bras Anestesiol 2003;53(6):802–7 [in Portuguese].

190. Baumgartner GR, Rowen RC. Clonidine vs chlordiazepoxide in the management of acute alcohol withdrawal syndrome. Arch Intern Med 1987;147(7):1223–6.

191. Baumgartner GR, Rowen RC. Transdermal clonidine versus chlordiazepoxide in alcohol withdrawal: a randomized, controlled clinical trial. South Med J 1991; 84(3):312–21.

192. Dobrydnjov I, Axelsson K, Berggren L, et al. Intrathecal and oral clonidine as prophylaxis for postoperative alcohol withdrawal syndrome: a randomized double-blinded study. Anesth Analg 2004;98(3):738–44 [Table of contents].

193. Manhem P, Nilsson LH, Moberg AL, et al. Alcohol withdrawal: effects of clonidine treatment on sympathetic activity, the renin-aldosterone system, and clinical symptoms. Alcohol Clin Exp Res 1985;9(3):238–43.

194. Nutt D, Glue P. Monoamines and alcohol. Br J Addict 1986;81(3):327–38.

195. Walinder J, Balldin J, Bokstrom K, et al. Clonidine suppression of the alcohol withdrawal syndrome. Drug Alcohol Depend 1981;8(4):345–8.

196. Wilkins AJ, Jenkins WJ, Steiner JA. Efficacy of clonidine in treatment of alcohol withdrawal state. Psychopharmacology (Berl) 1983;81(1):78–80.

197. Rovasalo A, Tohmo H, Aantaa R, et al. Dexmedetomidine as an adjuvant in the treatment of alcohol withdrawal delirium: a case report. Gen Hosp Psychiatry 2006;28(4):362–3.

198. Dyck JB, Maze M, Haack C, et al. The pharmacokinetics and hemodynamic effects of intravenous and intramuscular dexmedetomidine hydrochloride in adult human volunteers. Anesthesiology 1993;78(5):813–20.

199. Scheinin H, Aantaa R, Anttila M, et al. Reversal of the sedative and sympatholytic effects of dexmedetomidine with a specific alpha2-adrenoceptor antagonist atipamezole: a pharmacodynamic and kinetic study in healthy volunteers. Anesthesiology 1998;89(3):574–84.

200. Jaatinen P, Riihioja P, Haapalinna A, et al. Prevention of ethanol-induced sympathetic overactivity and degeneration by dexmedetomidine. Alcohol 1995;12(5): 439–46.

201. Riihioja P, Jaatinen P, Haapalinna A, et al. Effects of dexmedetomidine on rat locus coeruleus and ethanol withdrawal symptoms during intermittent ethanol exposure. Alcohol Clin Exp Res 1999;23(3):432–8.

202. Riihioja P, Jaatinen P, Oksanen H, et al. Dexmedetomidine alleviates ethanol withdrawal symptoms in the rat. Alcohol 1997;14(6):537–44.

203. Riihioja P, Jaatinen P, Oksanen H, et al. Dexmedetomidine, diazepam, and pro-pranolol in the treatment of ethanol withdrawal symptoms in the rat. Alcohol Clin Exp Res 1997;21(5):804–8.

204. Baddigam K, Russo P, Russo J, et al. Dexmedetomidine in the treatment of with-drawal syndromes in cardiothoracic Surgery patients. J Intensive Care Med 2005;20(2):118–23.

205. Bamgbade OA. Dexmedetomidine for peri-operative sedation and analgesia in alcohol addiction. Anaesthesia 2006;61(3):299–300.

206. Cooper L, Castillo D, Martinez-Ruid R, et al. Adjuvant use of dexmedetomidine may reduce the incidence of endotracheal intubation caused by benzodiaze-pines in the treatment of delirium tremens. Paper presented at the American So-ciety of Anesthesiology. Miami, October 23, 2005.

207. Darrouj J, Puri N, Prince E, et al. Dexmedetomidine infusion as adjunctive ther-apy to benzodiazepines for acute alcohol withdrawal. Ann Pharmacother 2008; 42(11):1703–5.

208. Finkel JC, Elrefai A. The use of dexmedetomidine to facilitate opioid and benzo-diazepine detoxification in an infant. Anesth Analg 2004;98(6):1658–9 [Table of contents].

209. Kandiah P, Jacob S, Pandya D, et al. Novel use of dexmedetomidine in 7 adults with Resistant Alcohol Withdrawal in the ICU, in Society of Critical Care Medicine (SCCM). 2009.

210. Maccioli GA. Dexmedetomidine to facilitate drug withdrawal. Anesthesiology 2003;98(2):575–7.

211. Prieto MN, et al, American Society of Anesthesiology. Dexmedetomidine: a novel approach to the management of alcohol withdrawal in the ICU. Anesthesiology 2007.

212. Balldin J, Berggren U, Eriksson E, et al. Guanfacine as an alpha-2-agonist inducer of growth hormone secretion–a comparison with clonidine. Psychoneur-oendocrinology 1993;18(1):45–55.

213. Arnsten AF, Cai JX, Goldman-Rakic PS. The alpha-2 adrenergic agonist guanfa-cine improves memory in aged monkeys without sedative or hypotensive side effects: evidence for alpha-2 receptor subtypes. J Neurosci 1988;8(11): 4287–98.

214. Parale MP, Kulkarni SK. Studies with alpha 2-adrenoceptor agonists and alcohol abstinence syndrome in rats. Psychopharmacology (Berl) 1986;88(2):237–9.

215. Fredriksson I, Jayaram-Lindström N, Wirf M, et al. Evaluation of guanfacine as a potential medication for alcohol use disorder in long-term drinking rats: behav-ioral and electrophysiological findings. Neuropsychopharmacology 2015;40(5): 1130–40.

216. Reid JL, Zamboulis C, Hamilton CA. Guanfacine: effects of long-term treatment and withdrawal. Br J Clin Pharmacol 1980;10(Suppl 1):183S–8S.

217. Maldonado JR, Sher Y, Das S, et al. Prospective validation study of the Predic-tion of Alcohol Withdrawal Severity Scale (PAWSS) in medically ill inpatients: a new scale for the prediction of complicated alcohol withdrawal syndrome. Alcohol Alcohol 2015;50(5):509–18.

218. Maldonado AL, Martinez F, Osuna E, et al. Alcohol consumption and crimes against sexual freedom. Med Law 1988;7(1):81–6.

219. Sullivan JT, Sykora K, Schneiderman J, et al. Assessment of alcohol withdrawal: the revised clinical institute withdrawal assessment for alcohol scale (CIWA-Ar). Br J Addict 1989;84(11):1353–7.

220. Wetterling T, Kanitz RD, Besters B, et al. A new rating scale for the assessment of the alcohol-withdrawal syndrome (AWS scale). Alcohol Alcohol 1997;32(6): 753–60.

221. Adinoff B. Double-blind study of alprazolam, diazepam, clonidine, and placebo in the alcohol withdrawal syndrome: preliminary findings. Alcohol Clin Exp Res 1994;18(4):873–8.

222. Billioti de Gage S, Begaud B, Bazin F, et al. Benzodiazepine use and risk of dementia: prospective population based study. BMJ 2012;345:e6231.

223. Billioti de Gage S, Moride Y, Ducruet T, et al. Benzodiazepine use and risk of Alzheimer's disease: case-control study. BMJ 2014;349:g5205.

224. Ciraulo DA, Sands BF, Shader RI. Critical review of liability for benzodiazepine abuse among alcoholics. Am J Psychiatry 1988;145(12):1501–6.

225. Forg A, Hein J, Volkmar K, et al. Efficacy and safety of pregabalin in the treatment of alcohol withdrawal syndrome: a randomized placebo-controlled trial. Alcohol Alcohol 2012;47(2):149–55.

226. Holbrook AM, Crowther R, Lotter A, et al. Diagnosis and management of acute alcohol withdrawal. CMAJ 1999;160(5):675–80.

227. Khan A, Levy P, DeHorn S, et al. Predictors of mortality in patients with delirium tremens. Acad Emerg Med 2008;15(8):788–90.

228. Lizotte RJ, Kappes JA, Bartel BJ, et al. Evaluating the effects of dexmedetomidine compared to propofol as adjunctive therapy in patients with alcohol withdrawal. Clin Pharmacol 2014;6:171–7.

229. Muller CA, Schafer M, Schneider S, et al. Efficacy and safety of levetiracetam for outpatient alcohol detoxification. Pharmacopsychiatry 2010;43(5):184–9.

230. Shaw JM, Kolesar GS, Sellers EM, et al. Development of optimal treatment tactics for alcohol withdrawal. I. Assessment and effectiveness of supportive care. J Clin Psychopharmacol 1981;1(6):382–9.

231. Stock CJ, Carpenter L, Ying J, et al. Gabapentin versus chlordiazepoxide for outpatient alcohol detoxification treatment. Ann Pharmacother 2013;47(7-8): 961–9.

232. Weich S, Pearce HL, Croft P, et al. Effect of anxiolytic and hypnotic drug prescriptions on mortality hazards: retrospective cohort study. BMJ 2014;348: g1996.

233. Wong A, Smithburger PL, Kane-Gill SL. Review of adjunctive dexmedetomidine in the management of severe acute alcohol withdrawal syndrome. Am J Drug Alcohol Abuse 2015;41(5):382–91.

234. Wetterling T, Weber B, Depfenhart M, et al. Development of a rating scale to predict the severity of alcohol withdrawal syndrome. Alcohol Alcohol 2006;41(6): 611–5.

Psychiatric Aspects of Lung Disease in Critical Care

Yelizaveta Sher, MD

KEYWORDS

- Psychiatric aspects of pulmonary disease • Critical care • Anxiety • Depression
- Intensive care unit • Demoralization • Neuropsychiatric symptoms
- Psychiatric aspects of lung disease

KEY POINTS

- Psychiatric conditions are common in patients with chronic lung disease and new psychiatric symptoms arise with pulmonary decompensation in critical care units.
- Substance use disorders (SUDs) are associated with the development of multiple acute and chronic pulmonary conditions, significantly contributing to morbidity and mortality of patients with lung disease.
- Differential for anxiety in intensive care unit (ICU) patients with lung disease includes underlying pulmonary or another medical condition, medications, assistive devices in ICU, and primary psychiatric conditions.
- Clinicians must be aware of potential neuropsychiatric side effects of medications used in patients with lung disease in the ICU, including steroids, immunosuppressants, beta-blockers, and antibiotics.
- Clinicians managing psychiatric symptoms in patients with lung disease must be aware of psychotropic drug properties (eg, half-life, mechanism of action), concerns (eg, QTc), side effects (eg, withdrawal, toxicity, acute reactions), and drug–drug interactions.

INTRODUCTION

Lung disease is highly associated with psychiatric disorders. These psychiatric disorders can occur as risk factors to lung disease (eg, tobacco use disorder in patients with chronic obstructive pulmonary disorder [COPD]), as a co-occurring condition (eg, cystic fibrosis [CF] and depression); as a result of a pulmonary condition (eg, panic attacks in patients with worsening respiratory disease), or as a treatment side effect (eg, steroid-induced mania). Respiratory conditions and respiratory failure are among the most common indications for admission to critical care units. Timely and appropriate recognition and management of psychiatric conditions in these patients can have significant positive effects on patient outcomes. Thus, it is crucial for intensivists

Disclosure Statement: The author has nothing to disclose.
Department of Psychiatry and Behavioral Sciences, Stanford University Medical Center, 401 Quarry Road, Suite 2320, Stanford, CA 94305, USA
E-mail address: ysher@stanford.edu

to be aware of the incidence and manifestations of psychiatric disorders in their patients, psychological and neuropsychiatric effects of the treatments in critical care, and management strategies to treat psychological and neuropsychiatric symptoms of patients with pulmonary conditions in an intensive care unit (ICU).

EPIDEMIOLOGY OF PSYCHIATRIC ILLNESS IN CHRONIC LUNG DISEASE

Psychiatric conditions are prevalent among patients suffering from chronic lung disease. Adults with asthma have a 50% higher likelihood of having a depressive or anxiety disorder compared with healthy population.[1] Depression and anxiety have been recognized as important comorbidities in patients with CF. A multisite study across 154 CF centers in Europe and the United States found elevated symptoms of depression in 10% of adolescents and 19% of adults; and elevated symptoms of anxiety in 22% of adolescents and 32% of adults.[2] These incidences were 2 to 3 times higher than those observed in community samples. Anxiety and depression were associated with decreased pulmonary function, increased number of hospitalizations, elevated health care costs, and diminished quality of life (QoL).[2] A meta-analysis of 8 controlled studies found a significantly increased prevalence of depression in 27.1% patients with COPD, as compared with 10.0% in controls.[3] Patients with COPD are 10 times more likely to have panic disorder (PD).[4] Depression and anxiety have negative consequences on outcomes in subjects with COPD. In a meta-analysis of 16 studies, the relative risk of mortality in COPD subjects with depression or anxiety was 1.83 and 1.27, respectively, as compared with COPD subjects without psychiatric comorbidities.[5] In addition, depression and anxiety were associated with a greater incidence of COPD exacerbations, hospitalizations for exacerbations, and hospital length of stay.[5] Approximately one-third of patients with pulmonary arterial hypertension (PAH) suffer from mental disorders, with 1 study demonstrating 15.9% incidence of major depressive disorder (MDD) and 10.4% incidence of PD.[6] The prevalence of psychiatric disorders in PAH increases with the degree of functional impairment and it is associated with worse QoL.[6]

Lung cancer is the third most common form of cancer among all malignancies in the United States and is the leading cause of cancer deaths.[7] Depression and anxiety are present in one-third of patients recently diagnosed with non-small cell lung carcinoma and are associated with decreased QoL, poor treatment adherence, and worse prognosis.[8] Subjects with lung cancer and depression were found to have decreased median survival of 6.8 months compared with nondepressed subjects surviving a median of 14 months (hazard ratio [HR] 1.9).[8]

Substance Use Disorders and Pulmonary Disease

Substance use disorders (SUDs) are associated with the development of multiple acute and chronic pulmonary conditions, significantly contributing to morbidity and mortality.[9] The pulmonary damage can occur with either systemic or inhalational route of drug administration and is mediated either via direct toxic effect of the substance or the presence of impurities and contaminants in the various substances. Toxicity may be immediate after exposure (eg, acute lung injury or hypersensitivity reaction) or delayed (eg, reactive airways dysfunction syndrome, or cancer).

Tobacco use disorder remains the most common risk factor for the development of COPD and lung cancer.[10] First-hand and second-hand tobacco exposure are detrimental to any pulmonary condition.[10] Prolonged marijuana smoking is associated with lung cancer and may result in respiratory symptoms suggestive of obstructive lung disease.[9] In addition, marijuana smoking is associated with allergic bronchopulmonary fungal disease, with species of *Aspergillus*, *Mucor*, *Penicillium*, and thermophilic actinomycetes having all been cultured from samples of marijuana.[11]

Patients with idiopathic PAH are much more likely to have abused methamphetamine and cocaine.[9,12] Inhalation of crack cocaine is also associated with crack lung, an acute pulmonary syndrome occurring up to 48 hours after cocaine inhalation and characterized by radiologic evidence of alveolitis and histologic findings of diffuse alveolar damage and hyaline membranes.[9]

Opioids, including heroin and prescription pain medications, may suppress the respiratory drive and are associated with deaths due to respiratory failure. In fact, opioid overdose is a common reason for ICU admission. In a retrospective study of 178 subjects admitted to ICU with opioid overdose, the most frequent opioids of abuse were oxycodone and hydrocodone and the most commonly coingested substances were benzodiazepines, followed by methamphetamines.[13] Most of these subjects (84.8%) required mechanical ventilation and 10% died in hospital. Aspiration pneumonia is likely the most common pulmonary complication of opioid drug abuse, related to central nervous system (CNS) depression.[9] In heroin users, aspiration pneumonia secondary to CNS depression was the second most common reason for ICU admissions, significantly contributing to deaths from acute respiratory distress syndrome (ARDS) and sepsis.[14]

Patients with alcohol-use disorders are also more susceptible to respiratory infections and lung injury, and are 2 to 4 times more likely to develop ARDS.[15]

Nitrous oxide, used as an anesthetic, is abused as an inhalant due to its euphoric effects. Its abuse leads to functional deactivation of vitamin B12, producing elevations in methylmalonyl-CoA and homocysteine.[16] Elevated homocysteine is a risk factor for venous thromboembolic disease,[17] which can lead to pulmonary embolism and present as a medical emergency.

Thus, patients with pulmonary disorders hospitalized in critical care units present with an elevated baseline risk for psychiatric disorders and SUDs. Appropriate screening, recognition, and treatment are required to provide comprehensive care to these patients.

ANXIETY IN CRITICALLY ILL PATIENTS WITH LUNG DISEASE

Feelings of anxiety, fear, and sadness can be part of a normal response to significant psychological stress of hospitalization in ICU. However, when these symptoms cause significant distress, further impair the underlying medical condition, or interfere with needed care, they need to be appropriately identified and addressed.

The differential diagnosis for anxiety conditions in ICU patients with pulmonary conditions is substantial, including comorbid long-standing anxiety disorders, emergence of new anxiety disorders, manifestations of a medical condition, medication side effects, or as a response to the use of assistive treatment (ie, ventilation, extracorporeal membrane oxygenations [ECMO]) side effect. In addition, patients might be withdrawing from substances of abuse, such as after abruptly stopping alcohol due to an unplanned ICU hospitalization, or from CNS-depressant agents administered by medical personnel for sedation or pain management while in the ICU setting, when these agents are suddenly discontinued (**Fig. 1**).

Comorbid Anxiety Disorders and Pathophysiology of Comorbidity

The most common comorbid anxiety disorders include generalized anxiety disorder (GAD), PD, post-traumatic stress disorder (PTSD), and specific phobias, as described in the Diagnostic and Statistical Manual of Mental Disorders, 5th edition (DSM-5).[18]

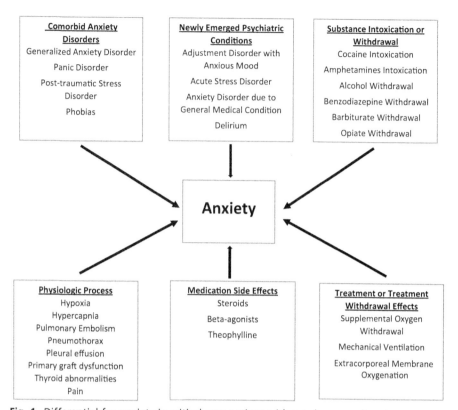

Fig. 1. Differential for anxiety in critical care patient with a pulmonary disorder.

GAD is characterized by excessive anxiety and worry about multiple domains in life for at least 6 months, associated with such somatic symptoms as restlessness, muscle tension, fatigue, and insomnia.[18] PD is characterized by the presence of unexpected panic attacks, manifested by intense anxiety lasting for several minutes, associated with feelings of doom, extreme fear, and a sympathetic physiologic response, including respiratory symptoms in a subset of patients. Some patients might have pre-morbid PTSD, characterized by a predisposing traumatic episode, followed by intrusive memories, hypervigilance, and avoidance behaviors. A history of trauma or PTSD might be a risk factor for these patients to have a lower threshold to experience retraumatization when exposed to the pain and discomfort associated with the ICU environment, experiencing further psychological distress. Premorbid phobias, such as the phobia of needles or seeing blood, can be precipitated or exacerbated in ICU.

Several hypotheses help explain comorbidity between respiratory conditions and anxiety, in particular PD. These hypotheses may also explain increased psychological sensitivity of these patients to acute respiratory symptoms, further placing them at risk of anxiety exacerbation. According to a physiologic model, patients with COPD and PD are sensitive to mild variations in carbon dioxide (CO_2) and pH. Increase in CO_2 and thus decrease in pH lead to the activation of particular brain areas, such as locus ceruleus, hypothalamus, and ventrolateral medulla, involved in ventilatory control, as well as activation of defensive behavior, as in the development of panic attacks.[4] On the other hand, hyperventilation can lead to lowering of P_{CO_2} resulting in respiratory alkalosis. This can precipitate sensation of dyspnea and panic attacks in predisposed individuals.[19]

In addition, per cognitive behavior model, patients with COPD and PD have been shown to demonstrate heightened symptom perception and misinterpretations of physical sensations as compared with COPD patients without PD but with similar respiratory condition severity.[20] When patients with COPD experience dyspnea, already an uncomfortable and frightening phenomenon, the experience of anxiety will further increase their respiratory rate, leading to hyperventilation and further exacerbating the sensation of dyspnea. Thus, patients with comorbid COPD and anxiety will likely misinterpret the meaning of their pulmonary symptoms and physiologic sensations, further worsening the cycle.

Not only are patients with comorbid pulmonary conditions and anxiety more physiologically sensitive to CO_2 changes, but they are also more likely to catastrophically interpret their physiologically elicited symptoms.

Behavioral sensitization as a result of near drowning or near suffocation experiences may also play a role in the development of PD. In fact, 19.3% to 33% of patients with PD have a history of traumatic suffocation as compared with only 6.7% of the normal controls.[4] COPD and other respiratory conditions can certainly be interpreted as traumatic suffocation events by predisposed individuals and trigger the development or exacerbation of PD.[19]

Acute Anxiety Disorders Emerging in Pulmonary Patients in the Intensive Care Unit

Patients can also develop new anxiety disorders in the critical care unit. The newly emergent anxiety disorders include adjustment disorders with anxious mood, acute stress disorders, and anxiety due to another medical condition, as described in DSM-5.[18]

The ICU experience can be very physiologically and psychologically challenging and frightening, and patients can develop anxious mood or panic attacks in response to this environment. The lack of control associated with the illness process and the high acuity of the critical care setting helps create a sense of helplessness and further contributes to the development of anxiety symptoms. Education, reassurance, and validation are helpful in treatment of acute anxiety (eg, adjustment disorder). Teaching patients simple behavioral interventions may also ease their anxiety and decrease the use of medications.

If patients develop symptoms of anxiety only in response to or in context of their medical condition, such as developing panic attacks with worsening respiratory function in context of endstage CF or acute respiratory failure due to asthma with resulting anxiety, the condition is considered to be an anxiety disorder due to another medical condition. The short-term use of psychotropic medications and behavioral interventions might be helpful for these patients, in addition to addressing the underlying medical condition.

Medical Conditions Manifesting as Anxiety in Pulmonary Patients in the Intensive Care Unit

The differential diagnosis of anxiety disorder among patients with pulmonary and other medical conditions in the critical care setting can be rather extensive. Hypoxia, hypercapnia, and hyperventilation can physiologically trigger anxious sensations, presenting as an anxiety disorder. Patients with pulmonary embolism, pneumothorax, pleural effusion, worsening lung infection, and atelectasis can all experience dyspnea and/or air hunger, which may be accompanied with the development of anxiety. In lung transplant patients, primary graft dysfunction can be accompanied by anxiety. It is important to actively search for medical causes of newly emerging or acutely exacerbated anxiety in medical patients in ICU. Anxiety can be a harbinger of a dangerous medical process that must be recognized and addressed in a timely fashion.

MOOD DISORDERS IN CRITICALLY ILL PATIENTS WITH LUNG DISEASE

Depressed mood can be a concerning symptom in critically ill patients with pulmonary conditions. Patients who are depressed are less likely to participate in their care and this can significantly hinder their recovery. The differential diagnosis for depressed mood in critical care patients includes mood disorders, demoralization, delirium, intracranial processes (eg, cerebrovascular accidents), endocrine disorders (eg, thyroid disease), and medication or substance effects and withdrawal (**Fig. 2**).

Major depressive episode (MDE) is characterized by at least 2 weeks of persistent depressed mood or loss of interest or pleasure, accompanied by at least 4 other symptoms (changes in appetite, changes in sleep, psychomotor agitation or retardation, fatigue, feelings of worthlessness or guilt, difficulty with concentration, or persistent thoughts of death or suicidal ideations).[18] The changes in mood or behavior are not better accounted for by a medical condition or substance effect, and cause significant distress or impairment in psychosocial functioning. MDE can occur in context of a major mood disorder, which consists of 1 or more depressive episodes, or bipolar affective disorder, which is defined by occurrence of at least 1 manic or hypomanic episode.[18]

When symptoms of a mood disorder occur only in context of a medical illness, it is designated as mood disorder due to another medical condition. Patients might also have an adjustment disorder with depressed mood, struggling with a particular stressor, such as new medical diagnosis, with their mood symptom constellation not meeting criteria for MDE either by a number of symptoms or their duration.

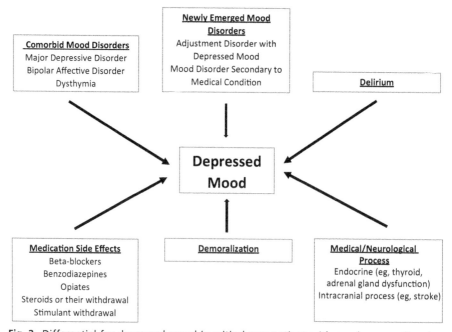

Fig. 2. Differential for depressed mood in critical care patient with a pulmonary disorder.

A frequent masquerade of depression in the hospital is delirium. In fact, in 1 study, consult psychiatry diagnosed delirium in 41% of elderly patients whom primary teams asked to evaluate for depression.[21] Patients with delirium often exhibit depressive symptoms, such as low mood, worthlessness, and thoughts of death, which can lead to diagnostic misunderstanding.[21] A hypoactive motoric subtype of delirium, characterized by quiet confusion, psychomotor retardation, subdued affect, and participation withdrawal, is more likely to look like depression to an untrained eye but is in fact much more common in critically ill patients compared with the hyperactive subtype of delirium.[22,23] In contrast with depression, patients with delirium have waning and waxing attention, likely acute or subacute decompensation of their mental status and cognitive functioning, and often exhibit positive primitive reflexes, which can be helpful in arriving at the correct diagnosis.

Demoralization is also common but frequently unrecognized in the ICU setting. Demoralization affects approximately one-third of medically ill patients,[24] and it is often characterized by a sense of helplessness and futility.[24] Patients feel disempowered, unable to function at their previous level, and often develop a sense of incompetence, futility, and hopelessness about the future. They might experience a sense of having failed their own and/or others' expectations. Demoralized patients view themselves as a burden to others. Over time, patients lose their will to go on, refuse to cooperate with needed care or treatment requiring participation or effort (eg, physical therapy), and eventually actively express a desire to stop treatment.[25] Patients on ventilator support may be restrained by their attachment to multiple lines and machines, affected by medications, and distanced from their caregivers by intense technology in the ICU setting.[25] They might feel completely helpless and alienated. In addition, data suggest, demoralization can also affect patient's family members and even their nursing staff. Demoralization often coexists with clinical depression but is a separate entity and may warrant different interventions. Although the key element in depression is anhedonia, demoralization is characterized by helplessness and incompetence, which should be targeted in treatment.[24] Treatment of demoralization incorporates continuity of care, promotion of empathic contact with caregivers, active symptom management, exploration of patient's meaning in life and hope, balancing grief and hope, cognitive restructuring of negative beliefs, and spiritual or religious support.[24]

DELIRIUM IN CRITICALLY ILL PATIENTS WITH LUNG DISEASE

Patients with pulmonary disorders in critical care are at increased risk for development of delirium, a neuropsychiatric condition marked by an acute change in attention accompanied by changes in cognition (eg, memory deficit, disorientation, language, visuospatial ability, or perception).[18] Patients can present with changes in their affect and appear restless and anxious, especially those experiencing the hyperactive type of delirium, or may appear depressed and withdrawn, common in the hypoactive type of delirium (see previous discussion). (See José R. Maldonado's article, "Acute Brain Failure: Pathophysiology, Diagnosis, Management and Sequelae of Delirium," in this issue.)

Patients with chronic pulmonary conditions have several specific risk factors for the development of delirium, including older age; problems with oxygenation, common to lung disease; and the use of various pharmacologic agents (eg, anticholinergic medications, steroids, sympathomimetics, opioids, antibiotics). Cognitive impairment is common in pulmonary conditions, likely due to persistent hypoxia, as well as comorbid cardiovascular risk factors. For example, patients with COPD have significantly increased prevalence of cognitive dysfunction, correlated with the severity of their illness.[26] Among patients awaiting lung transplantation, 47% have cognitive impairment.[27]

Once delirium develops, not only it is distressing to patients and their families but it also represents an independent risk factor associated with increased morbidity and mortality.[28] A prospective observational study of subjects with acute respiratory failure requiring noninvasive positive pressure ventilation indicated that the development of delirium was independently associated with earlier death within 1 year (HR 4.4, 95% CI 2.6–7.4).[29]

However, several specific etiologic factors should be considered in pulmonary patients in ICU compared with other delirium pathophysiology, differentials, and treatment in critical care.

Hypoxia, hypercapnia, and acidosis are frequent contributors to delirium etiologic factors in patients with pulmonary conditions. Mild impairments in oxygenation can be associated with poor judgment, inattention, and motor incoordination. As the condition progresses, moderate impairment of oxygenation may be associated with more pronounced memory deficits, whereas significant deficits in oxygenation may lead to significant impairment in cognitive functioning or even loss of consciousness.[30] Hypercapnia, usually associated with hypoxia and acidosis, can present with inattention, forgetfulness, drowsiness, and psychomotor slowing, and may eventually lead to loss of consciousness.[30] Other contributors to delirium may include electrolyte abnormalities, hepatic or renal insufficiency, infections, toxic effects of medications or recreational substances, or withdrawal from substances.

One particular cause of delirium in patients treated with immunosuppressant agents, in particular calcineurin inhibitors, is posterior reversible encephalopathy syndrome (PRES). PRES is a neuropsychiatric complication characterized by mental status changes, seizures, headache, autonomic instability, and visual changes. The use of immunosuppressant agents may be associated with endothelial dysfunction, eventually causing a breakdown of the blood-brain barrier, leading to cerebral edema.[31] PRES is diagnosed when characteristic clinical symptoms are supported by typical MRI findings demonstrating cerebral edema. PRES has been reported in patients who have undergone lung transplantation.[32] In addition, other immune disease processes that might affect pulmonary functioning (ie, Wegener granulomatosis, arthritis) and other processes commonly encountered in the ICU (eg, infection, inflammatory state, hyponatremia, hypomagnesemia, hypercalcemia, renal and hepatic dysfunction) can be additional contributing factors to this condition.[31]

Another specific cause of encephalopathy, associated with lung cancer, is limbic encephalitis. In fact, lung cancer is the most common cancer associated with paraneoplastic neurologic syndromes, typically associated with small cell lung cancer and including Lambert-Eaton myasthenic syndrome, cerebellar ataxia, sensory neuropathy, limbic encephalitis, encephalomyelitis, autonomic neuropathy, retinopathy, and opsomyoclonus.[33] In addition, patients can present with syndrome of inappropriate antidiuretic hormone secretion, often characterized by confusion, behavioral changes, and hyponatremia. Finally, cognitive changes from brain metastases and neuropsychiatric effects of chemotherapy should be considered in patients with lung cancer.

PULMONARY MEDICATIONS LEADING TO NEUROPSYCHIATRIC SYMPTOMS

Frequently, medications used in the treatment of pulmonary or comorbid medical conditions may be associated with various neuropsychiatric symptoms (**Table 1**).

Steroid agents, commonly used to treat inflammatory or autoimmune processes and administered in large boluses after lung transplantation, may be associated

Table 1
Neuropsychiatric side effects of pulmonary medications

Medications	Neuropsychiatric Side Effects
Steroids	Anxiety, insomnia, restlessness, cognitive dysfunction, delirium, mania, psychosis; depression long-term and when tapering off
Beta2-agonists Albuterol Levalbuterol Salmeterol	Anxiety, tremor, insomnia
Mixed alpha-agonists and beta-agonists Ephinephrine Ephedrine Phenylephrine Phenylpropanolamine	Anxiety, insomnia, tremor, psychosis
Methylxanthines Theophylline	Jitteriness, insomnia, anxiety, irritability, panic
Anticholinergics Atropine	Paranoia, hallucinations, memory loss, delirium agitation
Leukotriene inhibitors Montelukast	Dizziness, fatigue, asthenia, suicidal ideation
Acetazolamide	Confusion and malaise
Calcineurin inhibitors in transplant patients Tacrolimus Cellcept Sirolimus	Anxiety, tremor, anxiety, psychosis, delirium, PRES
Antibiotics Penicillins Cephalosporins (cefepime, ceftazidime) Antimycobacterials (isoniazid) Quinolones (ciprofloxacin) Macrolides (clartithromycin) Metronidazole Sulfonamides	Delirium, seizures, myoclonus Delirium, psychosis Delirium, cerebellar signs Psychosis

with a myriad of neuropsychiatric side effects.[34,35] There seems to be a correlation between the dose of steroid agent administered and the rate of occurrence and the severity of these symptoms. At lower doses, patients can experience anxiety, irritability, and insomnia. At higher doses, patients can develop delirium, mania, or psychosis. Depression can develop with longer term use of steroids or on tapering off the steroids. Additional potential risk factors for the development of neuropsychiatric side effects in response to steroid use include hypoalbuminemia, blood-brain barrier damage, prior neuropsychiatric symptoms due to steroids, psychiatric history, timing (especially during the first course of steroid therapy), female gender, and increasing age.[35]

Beta2-adrenergic agonists are also associated with restlessness, apprehension, anxiety, and tremors in dose-dependent fashion. Inhaled administration of beta2-agonists is associated with less neuropsychiatric risk as compared with systemic administration.[30] Methylxanthines are associated with tremor, anxiety, fear, and panic, in dose-dependent fashion. Nonprescription asthma preparations contain nonselective sympathomimetics (eg, epinephrine, phenylephrine), which can also cause anxiety as well as psychosis at higher doses. Anticholinergic medications contribute to delirium burden, whereas antileukotrienes can cause anxiety.[30,36]

Antibiotics can also be associated with the development of encephalopathy.[37] One group identified 3 syndromes of antibiotic-induced encephalopathy: encephalopathy accompanied by seizures or myoclonus within days after antibiotic administration (described after the use of cephalosporins and penicillin), encephalopathy character-ized by psychosis arising within days of antibiotic administration (described after the use of isoniazid, quinolones, macrolides, and procaine penicillin), and encephalopathy accompanied by cerebellar signs and MRI abnormalities emerging weeks after anti-biotic initiation (described after the use of metronidazole).[37]

ASSISTIVE RESPIRATORY TREATMENTS IN THE INTENSIVE CARE UNIT AND PSYCHOLOGICAL SYMPTOMS

Both the use of or withdrawal of various assistive respiratory therapies may be very anxiety producing for patients. Anxiety is very common in mechanically ventilated patients.[38] Patients who are mechanically ventilated struggle with loss of indepen-dence, inability to communicate, pain, and the overwhelming ICU environment. In one descriptive study, two thirds of the patients interviewed after surviving me-chanical ventilation in ICU, remembered their ventilation experience and described these memories as distressing. The cited causes of distress included of distress included pain, fear, anxiety, lack of sleep, feeling tense, inability to speak or communicate, lack of control, nightmares, and loneliness.[39] Experiencing spells of terror, feeling nervous when left alone, and poor sleeping patterns were associ-ated with stressful experience of endotracheal ventilation.[39] When the endotracheal tube is plugged, patients may experience a sense of choking and asphyxiation; similarly, the process of suctioning the endotracheal tube has been described as very distressing.[40] Most caregivers, including physicians, nurses, and respiratory therapists, underestimate the sensation of dyspnea in ventilated patients; yet this sensation significantly contributes to patients' anxiety and fear.[41] On the other hand, after prolonged intubation, patients may paradoxically be nervous about extubation, fearing their inability to breathe on their own.[30] In addition, too rapid ta-per or withdrawal of sedative medications may cause or exacerbate a patient's sense of anxiety.

Extracorporeal mechanical oxygenation (ECMO) is used in severely ill patients, whose risk of dying is greater than 50%. During ECMO, the patient's blood is pumped through an artificial lung, external to the body, which provides gas exchange and blood pressure support. The experience of ECMO, coupled with its administration in a very medically morbid situation, can be terrifying for some patients. In a qualitative study of 10 long-term ECMO survivors, subjects described their traumatic memories of rapid deterioration and crisis before the initiation of ECMO.[42] Patients treated with ECMO often experienced physical deconditioning, perceived threats of serious injury or death, psychological distress, and distressing symptoms associated with the devel-opment of delirium.[42]

In addition to addressing the physiologic contributors to patients' anxiety, physical and emotional distress, and pain, it is important to be psychologically present and available to these patients. Talking directly to the patient, informing them of the day's plan, and providing orientation and reassurance can be all very helpful. Behav-ioral strategies to ease anxiety can be useful as well. In fact, music therapy has been found to be therapeutic for alleviating anxiety in mechanically ventilated ICU patients.[43]

PSYCHIATRIC CONDITIONS AFTER THE INTENSIVE CARE UNIT

Patients with chronic and acute pulmonary conditions surviving their stay in ICU have an increased risk for developing new post-ICU psychiatric conditions. One-fifth of all ICU survivors develop PTSD related to the ICU experience.[44] The predictors for post-ICU PTSD include prior psychopathology, greater amount of ICU benzodiazepine use, and post-ICU recollections of ICU-related frightening and psychotic experiences.[44]

In a study of 629 ARDS survivors, evaluated 6 and 12 months after their discharge from the ICU, 66% of subjects exhibited significant psychiatric symptoms, with 36%, 42%, and 24% of subjects experiencing depression, anxiety, and PTSD at follow-up, respectively.[45] Younger age, female sex, unemployment, alcohol misuse, and greater opioid use in the ICU were significantly associated with the development of psychiatric symptoms, whereas illness severity and ICU length of stay were not.

In another study of 186 ICU-survivors with acute lung injury followed up to 2 years after their ICU stay, the prevalence of clinically elevated general anxiety, depression, and PTSD symptoms ranged from 38% to 44%, 26% to 33%, and 22% to 24%, respectively.[46] Fifty-nine percent of survivors had elevated symptoms in 2 or all 3 domains at 2-year follow-up. Better physical functioning during recovery was associated with subsequent remission of general anxiety and PTSD symptoms.

ICU diaries have been shown to be protective against post-ICU PTSD development.[47] They can be initiated by the critical care staff and filled out in collaboration with family members and friends.

Lung transplant recipients have increased incidence of mood and in particular anxiety disorders. In fact, 18% of lung transplant recipients have PD within 2 years of transplant compared with 8% of heart transplant recipients.[48]

USE OF PSYCHOTROPIC MEDICATIONS AMONG LUNG DISEASE PATIENTS IN THE CRITICAL CARE SETTING
Sedative Infusions

Continuous sedative infusions might be needed to provide comfort while patients are intubated as well as to treat patient's agitation, anxiety, and delirium. Dexmedetomidine, a selective alpha2-receptor agonist, has favorable benefit-risk profile for patients with respiratory conditions, given its anxiolytic properties, its minimal effects on respiratory drive, and reported deliriolytic properties.[49] It can ease anxiety and aid in the transition process during extubation of alert and awake patients. It can also be used in nonintubated patients, although respiratory status should be vigilantly monitored.

Other continuous sedative infusions used in the ICU environment include standard sedatives, such as propofol and benzodiazepine agents (ie, midazolam), and various opioid agents (eg, hydromorphone, fentanyl). These agents have all been associated with CNS and respiratory depression, and all carry the potential to increase the risk of delirium.[50] Furthermore, emerging evidence indicates that benzodiazepine agents and propofol use may carry an increased risk of health care–acquired infections in the ICU compared with dexmedetomidine, likely due to their immunomodulatory effects.[51]

Antipsychotics

Antipsychotics are used to treat agitation and delirium in the ICU. Moreover, they can be used to manage treatment-refractory anxiety in the acute care setting. Usually, sedating antipsychotics, such as quetiapine and olanzapine, are chosen for the management of anxiety but caution must be exercised when used in patients who retain carbon dioxide. Olanzapine is among the most anticholinergic of the novel antipsychotics and has a long half-life (ie, >30 hours). Relative to olanzapine, quetiapine is significantly less anticholinergic and has a short half-life (ie, 6 hours), which might be advantageous. Intravenous haloperidol has minimal anticholinergic activity and an intermediate half-life (ie, 20 hours), and can be rather helpful, especially in patients lacking an oral administration route or those extremely agitated requiring immediate tranquilization. For hypoactive delirium, a low dose of a nonsedating antipsychotic, such as haloperidol or risperidone, or a low to medium dose of aripiprazole can be considered. Of note, the abrupt discontinuation of anticholinergic antipsychotics may cause cholinergic rebound and impair the effectiveness of anticholinergic asthma medications.[36]

In the case of all antipsychotic agents, the QTc interval should be vigilantly monitored. Patients with asthma and COPD are particularly susceptible to cardiac arrhythmias, thus medications known to prolong the QTc (eg, ziprasidone) should be avoided. To date, aripiprazole and lurasidone have the fewest reports of antipsychotic agent-related QTc prolongation.[52]

All antipsychotic agent use may be associated with the development of extrapyramidal side effects. There have been rare cases of acute laryngeal dystonias, mostly associated with conventional antipsychotics,[53] but also reported with the use of the second-generation antipsychotic, ziprasidone.[54] Laryngeal dystonia may present as acute dyspnea within 24 hours of antipsychotic initiation or dose increase. This condition is usually treated with parenteral anticholinergic agents and the withdrawal of offending medications.[53]

If antipsychotics are used for acute indications in the ICU, clinicians should be very diligent about tapering off these medications or providing careful guidance as to how and when to taper them off in the near future.

Antidepressants

Antidepressant agents are generally used for the treatment of depression and anxiety; however, their primary effect may take 2 to 8 weeks. The selective serotonin reuptake inhibitors (SSRIs) are effective in the long-term treatment of anxiety and depression but caution should be used with paroxetine, due to significant anticholinergic and sedating potential, and fluvoxamine, due to significant drug–drug interactions. The abrupt discontinuation of paroxetine can precipitate cholinergic rebound, with associated worsening of bronchoconstriction. Both paroxetine and venlafaxine have been associated with significant symptoms of serotonin withdrawal on abrupt discontinuation, given their very short half-lives. Small trials have demonstrated benefit in the treatment of depression with SSRIs among patients with asthma[55] and COPD.[56] However, there is concern regarding potential worsening with the use of SSRIs among patients with PAH.[57]

The QTc should be reviewed before initiation of, and monitored during the use of, citalopram and all tricyclic antidepressant agents (TCAs).[52] Mirtazapine may be helpful for the more immediate alleviation of anxiety and insomnia, as well as for the long-term management of anxiety and depression, but should be avoided in patients who tend to retain carbon dioxide. The side effects of mirtazapine include weight gain and sedation.

Antianxiety Medications

Buspirone is a 5-hydroxytryptamine (5HT)-1 agonist that may be helpful in the management of anxiety and may be safe in patients with various pulmonary conditions.[36] Its use may improve exercise tolerance and dyspnea, yet the agent has a slow onset of action.

Benzodiazepine agents may reduce the respiratory drive and can significantly decrease the ventilatory response to hypoxia.[36] Clinicians should be mindful that their use may precipitate respiratory failure in patients with marginal respiratory reserve and should not be used in patients who retain carbon dioxide or patients with obstructive sleep apnea. Small doses of short half-life benzodiazepine agents, such as lorazepam, can be used in patients with COPD or asthma, when the patient's anxiety leads to a reduction in respiratory efficiency. ICU clinicians must be aware of the increased risk for delirium associated with benzodiazepine use.[58]

Other agents that can be considered for acute anxiety include gabapentin (a calcium channel blocker often used for the management of chronic pain) and hydroxyzine (an antihistaminic agent).

Drug–Drug Interactions

CF and tobacco use disorders can affect drug metabolism. The rate of gastrointestinal absorption is typically slowed in patients with CF due to abnormalities in ion transport.[36] Smoking induces CYP1A2, 2B6, and 2D6, which enhances the metabolism of these enzymes substrates, including olanzapine, duloxetine, TCAs, mirtazapine and theophylline,[36] among others.

Two antimicrobial agents, linezolid and isoniazid, are weak monoamine oxidase inhibitors (MAOIs) and, in combination with other serotonergic agents, can lead to hypertensive crisis and serotonin toxicity. Thus, SSRIs, serotonin-norepinephrine reuptake inhibitors, TCAs, St. John's Wort, and other MAOIs should be avoided in patients on these agents. It is important to be mindful that some opioid agents can have high serotonergic qualities and may add to the risk of serotonin toxicity.[59] Some investigators claim that mirtazapine does not increase intrasynaptic serotonin and thus may be safer when used with other serotonergic medications, if necessary.[60]

Lumacaftor/ivacaftor, a gene-modulating medication used in the management of CF, decreases the levels of SSRIs and antipsychotic agents, via CYP interactions.[61]

Certain respiratory conditions, CF in particular, may be associated with hepatic dysfunction and decreased platelets, thus the risk of bleeding should be considered before the use of SSRIs, which are known to affect platelet aggregation and increase bleeding risk.[62]

Rifampin is a cytochrome P450 3A4 substrate and may compete with many psychotropic medications, such as quetiapine, sertraline, fluoxetine, amitriptyline, bupropion, and trazodone.[63]

Finally, theophylline can decrease levels of lithium by up to 20% to 30%.[36]

SUMMARY

Acute lung disease is a frequent indication for admission to critical care units, while chronic lung disease is a common contributor. Patients with pulmonary disorders are at increased risk for chronic comorbid psychiatric and SUDs, as well as acute psychiatric decompensations. Anxiety and depression are common in these patient populations. Critically ill patients can be demoralized, fearful, depressed, and/or anxious in response to their medical condition, the acute life-threatening situation, or due to adverse effects of pharmacologic agents (eg, steroids or beta2-agonists) or assist device (ie, ECMO) treatment. Pulmonary patients are also at high risk for delirium. After their ICU experience, patients may be at increased risk for the development of PTSD and other anxiety and mood disorders. Skillful involvement and participation by ICU personnel is critical in the prevention, early detection, and management of these conditions and is paramount for patient's psychological wellbeing and recovery, as well as the long-term psychological and medical outcomes.

REFERENCES

1. Scott KM, Von Korff M, Ormel J, et al. Mental disorders among adults with asthma: results from the World Mental Health Survey. Gen Hosp Psychiatry 2007;29(2):123–33.
2. Quittner AL, Goldbeck L, Abbott J, et al. Prevalence of depression and anxiety in patients with cystic fibrosis and parent caregivers: results of the international depression epidemiological study across nine countries. Thorax 2014;69(12): 1090–7.
3. Matte DL, Pizzichini MM, Hoepers AT, et al. Prevalence of depression in COPD: a systematic review and meta-analysis of controlled studies. Respir Med 2016;117: 154–61.
4. Freire RC, Perna G, Nardi AE. Panic disorder respiratory subtype: psychopathology, laboratory challenge tests, and response to treatment. Harv Rev Psychiatry 2010;18(4):220–9.
5. Atlantis E, Fahey P, Cochrane B, et al. Bidirectional associations between clinically relevant depression or anxiety and COPD: a systematic review and meta-analysis. Chest 2013;144(3):766–77.
6. Harzheim D, Klose H, Pinado FP, et al. Anxiety and depression disorders in patients with pulmonary arterial hypertension and chronic thromboembolic pulmonary hypertension. Respir Res 2013;14:104.
7. Siegel RL, Miller KD, Jemal A. Cancer statistics, 2016. CA Cancer J Clin 2016; 66(1):7–30.
8. Arrieta O, Angulo LP, Nunez-Valencia C, et al. Association of depression and anxiety on quality of life, treatment adherence, and prognosis in patients with advanced non-small cell lung cancer. Ann Surg Oncol 2013;20(6):1941–8.
9. Megarbane B, Chevillard L. The large spectrum of pulmonary complications following illicit drug use: features and mechanisms. Chem Biol Interact 2013; 206(3):444–51.
10. Samet JM. Tobacco smoking: the leading cause of preventable disease worldwide. Thorac Surg Clin 2013;23(2):103–12.
11. Tomashefski JF, Felo JA. The pulmonary pathology of illicit drug and substance abuse. Curr Diagn Pathol 2004;10(5):413–26.
12. Chin KM, Channick RN, Rubin LJ. Is methamphetamine use associated with idiopathic pulmonary arterial hypertension? Chest 2006;130(6):1657–63.
13. Pfister GJ, Burkes RM, Guinn B, et al. Opioid overdose leading to intensive care unit admission: epidemiology and outcomes. J Crit Care 2016;35:29–32.
14. Grigorakos L, Sakagianni K, Tsigou E, et al. Outcome of acute heroin overdose requiring intensive care unit admission. J Opioid Manag 2010;6(3):227–31.
15. Yeligar SM, Chen MM, Kovacs EJ, et al. Alcohol and lung injury and immunity. Alcohol 2016;55:51–9.
16. Garakani A, Welch AK, Jaffe RJ, et al. Psychosis and low cyanocobalamin in a patient abusing nitrous oxide and cannabis. Psychosomatics 2014;55(6):715–9.
17. Ray JG. Meta-analysis of hyperhomocysteinemia as a risk factor for venous thromboembolic disease. Arch Intern Med 1998;158(19):2101–6.
18. American Psychiatric Association. Diagnostic and statistical manual of mental disorders (DSM-5). 5th edition. Washington, DC: American Psychiatric Association; 2013.

19. Pumar MI, Gray CR, Walsh JR, et al. Anxiety and depression-Important psychological comorbidities of COPD. J Thorac Dis 2014;6(11):1615–31.
20. Livermore N, Sharpe L, McKenzie D. Panic attacks and panic disorder in chronic obstructive pulmonary disease: a cognitive behavioral perspective. Respir Med 2010;104(9):1246–53.
21. Farrell KR, Ganzini L. Misdiagnosing delirium as depression in medically ill elderly patients. Arch Intern Med 1995;155(22):2459–64.
22. Peterson JF, Pun BT, Dittus RS, et al. Delirium and its motoric subtypes: a study of 614 critically ill patients. J Am Geriatr Soc 2006;54(3):479–84.
23. Pandharipande P, Cotton BA, Shintani A, et al. Motoric subtypes of delirium in mechanically ventilated surgical and trauma intensive care unit patients. Intensive Care Med 2007;33(10):1726–31.
24. Sansone RA, Sansone LA. Demoralization in patients with medical illness. Psychiatry 2010;7(8):42–5.
25. Roffey P, Thangathurai D. Demoralization syndrome: an evil ignored in the ICU setting. Psychosomatics 2013;54(1):98–9.
26. Schou L, Ostergaard B, Rasmussen LS, et al. Cognitive dysfunction in patients with chronic obstructive pulmonary disease–a systematic review. Respir Med 2012;106(8):1071–81.
27. Smith PJ, Rivelli S, Waters A, et al. Neurocognitive changes after lung transplantation. Ann Am Thorac Soc 2014;11(10):1520–7.
28. Ely EW, Shintani A, Truman B, et al. Delirium as a predictor of mortality in mechanically ventilated patients in the intensive care unit. JAMA 2004;291(14):1753–62.
29. Chan KY, Cheng LS, Mak IW, et al. Delirium is a strong predictor of mortality in patients receiving non-invasive positive pressure ventilation. Lung 2017;195(1):115–25.
30. Shapiro PA, Fedoronko DA, Epstein LA, et al. Psychiatric aspects of heart and lung disease in critical care. Crit Care Clin 2008;24(4):921–47, x.
31. Lamy C, Oppenheim C, Mas JL. Posterior reversible encephalopathy syndrome. Handb Clin Neurol 2014;121:1687–701.
32. Arimura FE, Camargo PC, Costa AN, et al. Posterior reversible encephalopathy syndrome in lung transplantation: 5 case reports. Transplant Proc 2014;46(6):1845–8.
33. Honnorat J, Antoine JC. Paraneoplastic neurological syndromes. Orphanet J Rare Dis 2007;2:22.
34. Dubovsky AN, Arvikar S, Stern TA, et al. The neuropsychiatric complications of glucocorticoid use: steroid psychosis revisited. Psychosomatics 2012;53(2):103–15.
35. Judd LL, Schettler PJ, Brown ES, et al. Adverse consequences of glucocorticoid medication: psychological, cognitive, and behavioral effects. Am J Psychiatry 2014;171(10):1045–51.
36. Thompson WL, Smolin YL. Respiratory disorders. In: Ferrando S, Levenson J, Owen JA, editors. Clinical manual of psychopharmacology in the medically ill. 1st edition. Washingon, DC: American Psychiatric Publishing, Inc; 2010. p. 213–36.
37. Bhattacharyya S, Darby RR, Raibagkar P, et al. Antibiotic-associated encephalopathy. Neurology 2016;86(10):963–71.
38. Chlan LL. Description of anxiety levels by individual differences and clinical factors in patients receiving mechanical ventilatory support. Heart Lung 2003;32(4):275–82.

39. Rotondi AJ, Chelluri L, Sirio C, et al. Patients' recollections of stressful experiences while receiving prolonged mechanical ventilation in an intensive care unit. Crit Care Med 2002;30(4):746–52.

40. Roffey P, Thangathurai D. Delayed endotracheal extubation and PTSD in ICU patients. Psychosomatics 2011;52(2):194.

41. Binks AP, Desjardin S, Riker R. ICU clinicians underestimate breathing discomfort in ventilated subjects. Respir Care 2017;62(2):150–5.

42. Tramm R, Ilic D, Davies AR, et al. Extracorporeal membrane oxygenation for critically ill adults. Cochrane Database Syst Rev 2015;(1):CD010381.

43. Lee CH, Lee CY, Hsu MY, et al. Effects of music intervention on state anxiety and physiological indices in patients undergoing mechanical ventilation in the intensive care unit: a randomized controlled trial. Biol Res Nurs 2017;19(2):137–44.

44. Davydow DS, Gifford JM, Desai SV, et al. Posttraumatic stress disorder in general intensive care unit survivors: a systematic review. Gen Hosp Psychiatry 2008; 30(5):421–34.

45. Huang M, Parker AM, Bienvenu OJ, et al. Psychiatric symptoms in acute respiratory distress syndrome survivors: a 1-year National multicenter study. Crit Care Med 2016;44(5):954–65.

46. Bienvenu OJ, Colantuoni E, Mendez-Tellez PA, et al. Cooccurrence of and remission from general anxiety, depression, and posttraumatic stress disorder symptoms after acute lung injury: a 2-year longitudinal study. Crit Care Med 2015; 43(3):642–53.

47. Jones C, Backman C, Capuzzo M, et al. Intensive care diaries reduce new onset post traumatic stress disorder following critical illness: a randomised, controlled trial. Crit Care 2010;14(5):R168.

48. Dew MA, DiMartini AF, DeVito Dabbs AJ, et al. Onset and risk factors for anxiety and depression during the first 2 years after lung transplantation. Gen Hosp Psychiatry 2012;34(2):127–38.

49. Barr J, Fraser GL, Puntillo K, et al. Clinical practice guidelines for the management of pain, agitation, and delirium in adult patients in the intensive care unit. Crit Care Med 2013;41(1):263–306.

50. Pandharipande P, Cotton BA, Shintani A, et al. Prevalence and risk factors for development of delirium in surgical and trauma intensive care unit patients. J Trauma 2008;65(1):34–41.

51. Caroff DA, Szumita PM, Klompas M. The relationship between sedatives, sedative strategy, and healthcare-associated infection: a systematic review. Infect Control Hosp Epidemiol 2016;37(10):1234–42.

52. Beach SR, Celano CM, Noseworthy PA, et al. QTc prolongation, torsades de pointes, and psychotropic medications. Psychosomatics 2013;54(1):1–13.

53. Christodoulou C, Kalaitzi C. Antipsychotic drug-induced acute laryngeal dystonia: two case reports and a mini review. J Psychopharmacol 2005;19(3):307–11.

54. Mellacheruvu S, Norton JW, Schweinfurth J. Atypical antipsychotic drug-induced acute laryngeal dystonia: 2 case reports. J Clin Psychopharmacol 2007;27(2): 206–7.

55. Brown ES, Howard C, Khan DA, et al. Escitalopram for severe asthma and major depressive disorder: a randomized, double-blind, placebo-controlled proof-of-concept study. Psychosomatics 2012;53(1):75–80.

56. Tselebis A, Pachi A, Ilias I, et al. Strategies to improve anxiety and depression in patients with COPD: a mental health perspective. Neuropsychiatr Dis Treat 2016; 12:297–328.

57. Sadoughi A, Roberts KE, Preston IR, et al. Use of selective serotonin reuptake inhibitors and outcomes in pulmonary arterial hypertension. Chest 2013;144(2): 531–41.
58. Pandharipande P, Shintani A, Peterson J, et al. Lorazepam is an independent risk factor for transitioning to delirium in intensive care unit patients. Anesthesiology 2006;104(1):21–6.
59. Rastogi R, Swarm RA, Patel TA. Case scenario: opioid association with serotonin syndrome: implications to the practitioners. Anesthesiology 2011;115(6):1291–8.
60. Gillman PK. A review of serotonin toxicity data: implications for the mechanisms of antidepressant drug action. Biol Psychiatry 2006;59(11):1046–51.
61. Orkambi [package insert]. Boston: Vertex Pharmaceuticals Incorporated; 2016. Available at: http://pi.vrtx.com/files/uspi_lumacaftor_ivacaftor.pdf. Accessed April 4, 2017.
62. Jeong BO, Kim SW, Kim SY, et al. Use of serotonergic antidepressants and bleeding risk in patients undergoing surgery. Psychosomatics 2014;55(3): 213–20.
63. Coffman K, Levenson JL. Lung disease. In: Levenson JL, editor. Textbook of psychosomatic medicine. 1st edition. Washington, DC: American Psychiatric Publishing; 2005. p. 445–64.

Psychiatric Aspects of Heart Disease (and Cardiac Aspects of Psychiatric Disease) in Critical Care

Peter A. Shapiro, MD[a,b]

KEYWORDS

- Depression • Anxiety • Delirium • Psychosis • Posttraumatic stress disorder
- Coronary artery disease • Heart failure • Critical care

KEY POINTS

- Strong emotional reactions are to be expected in patients admitted to cardiac critical care; only some of these are pathological.
- Important psychiatric issues associated with heart disease include anger and hostility, anxiety, depression, delirium and neurocognitive disorders, psychotic disorders, and posttraumatic stress disorder.
- All of these psychiatric issues affect and are affected by aspects of cardiac critical care. Heart surgery, transplantation, mechanical circulatory support, and defibrillators are associated with psychiatric morbidity.
- Depression is extremely common in patients with coronary disease and heart failure; treatment is helpful, but persistent depression is associated with increased morbidity and mortality.
- Some psychiatric drugs have significant cardiovascular effects.

PSYCHOLOGICAL RESPONSES TO CRITICAL CARE

This paper addresses the psychiatric aspects of heart disease and the cardiac aspects of psychiatric disease as they pertain in critical care. Because heart disease remains the leading cause of death in the United States, and affects about one-third of

This article is an update of an article previously published in Critical Care Clinics, Volume 24, Issue 4, October 2008.
Disclosure: Supported in part by the Nathaniel Wharton Fund, New York NY. The author has no financial or commercial interests to disclose.
Author Contributions: Dr P.A. Shapiro is solely responsible for all aspects of this article.
[a] Department of Psychiatry, Columbia University Medical Center, College of Physicians and Surgeons, Columbia University, 622 West 168 Street Box 427, New York, NY 10032, USA;
[b] Consultation-Liaison Psychiatry Service, New York-Presbyterian Hospital Columbia University Medical Center, 622 West 168 Street, New York, NY 10032, USA
E-mail address: pas3@cumc.columbia.edu

all adults over the age of 35, and many psychiatric disorders are associated with increased heart disease risk, it is inevitable that there is substantial comorbidity in cardiac critical care with psychiatric disorders.[1–4]

It is important to appreciate that people with no psychiatric problems may develop strong emotional adjustment reactions to critical heart disease that are not necessarily pathologic (**Box 1**). Hospitalization for acute coronary events, decompensated heart failure, or arrhythmias may be experienced as a crisis, with the illness perceived as a sudden and unexpected threat to survival, identity, and social role function. In these circumstances, some degree of fear, regression, hypervigilance, and sadness is to be expected. Patients may revisit past behavior that has contributed to illness, such as smoking or failure to adhere to the medication regimen, with feelings of guilt and regret. Denial of illness or of the significance of illness may occur as a defense against the conscious awareness of anxiety. If denial does not interfere with care, it is generally best left alone.

In addition to the illness, aspects of the cardiac critical care environment may provoke psychological problems. Constant cardiac monitoring, with recurring visual and auditory alarms, tethering to lines and wires, noise in the intensive care unit (ICU), and uncontrolled intrusions into sleep time and visiting time by medical, nursing, and ancillary staff are distressing and may contribute to sleep–wake cycle disruption and disorientation. Painful procedures, such as cardioversion and the placement of arterial and central venous lines, may be experienced as traumatic. Everyday experiences to which critical staff are inured are novel and of unknown significance to the patient; the value of explanation and guidance about what is happening cannot be overstated.

Crying and expressions of fear are not abnormal in these circumstances, but should not be ignored. Patients should be offered the opportunity to express feelings and have their experiences validated and normalized, rather than treated as pathologic. These reactions should only rarely provoke psychiatric consultation. Typically, the experience of acute critical illness is associated with increased dependence on others; the patient's comfort with dependence on care providers will be affected by his or her experience of early life relationships and subsequent attachment style.[5] Character style-based difficulty forming a trusting relationship may manifest in critical care settings with excessive dependence, independence, or emotional volatility; psychiatric consultation may help the patient and staff to set parameters for a workable relationship.

Box 1
Challenges to psychological adjustment to cardiac critical care

Patient factors

- Threat of death
- Threat to identity and role function
- Self-blame

Environment/care factors

- Noise
- Painful procedures
- Tethering to wires and lines; immobility
- Sleep disruption
- Loss of autonomy
- Treatment-specific effects

Patients with recurrent and chronic heart disease who require critical care may experience many of the same psychological adaptation issues as patients with acute disease described above. Because heart failure tends to follow a course of gradual deterioration punctuated by acute decompensations with incomplete recovery, sadness and fear with a preoccupation about death are more prominent features. Brief psychotherapy is possible for many dying patients, even in critical care environments, and has the potential to reduce depression and improve spiritual well-being. The possibility that heart transplantation or ventricular assist device therapy might provide an escape from death may provide hope, but also raises anxiety about being found acceptable as a candidate, and about the risks and difficulties associated with those treatments. Meeting other patients who have undergone such treatments and repeated opportunities to raise questions and discuss concerns can be helpful.

PSYCHIATRIC DISORDERS AND HEART DISEASE
Differential Diagnosis

The *Diagnostic and Statistical Manual of Psychiatric Disorders*, 5th edition,[6] makes a distinction between primary psychiatric disorders and disorders owing to the direct effects on the brain of other illnesses, medications, other substances, and substance withdrawal. In the cardiac critical care setting, this implies that the differential diagnosis of mood, anxiety, and psychotic symptoms must include an evaluation of anemia, fluid and electrolyte balance, renal and hepatic function, blood pressure and cardiac output, blood gases, concurrent medications and substance exposures, and possible infections (**Box 2**). Many medications used in cardiac intensive care have psychiatric side effects (**Table 1**).

Box 2
Workup for differential diagnosis of psychiatric disorders in cardiac disease

History, including screening questions (below) for current depression, anxiety, and posttraumatic stress disorder
   Have you been feeling sad, blue, or down in the dumps?
   Have you lost interest in things that you would normally be interested in?
   Have you been feeling anxious or fearful?
   Have you had an especially stressful or dangerous experience that continues to bother you?

Review of preexisting psychiatric disorder history

Review of current psychiatric symptoms

Review of medications

Review of substance use/withdrawal

Physical examination

Vital signs

Arterial hemoglobin O_2 saturation, blood gases

Mental status examination including cognitive function

Laboratory: complete blood count, electrolytes, serum glucose, renal, hepatic, thyroid, urinalysis, erythrocyte sedimentation rate, cultures

Chest radiograph

Brain imaging

Electroencephalograph

Table 1
Cardiac critical care medications causing psychiatric side effects

Medication	Psychiatric Effects
Angiotensin inhibitors and angiotensin receptor blockers	Mood elevation
Antiarrhythmic agents	Delirium
Benzodiazepines	Sedation, delirium
Beta-adrenergic blockers	Fatigue
Calcium channel blockers	Mood stabilizer effects
Corticosteroids	Mania, psychosis
Cyclosporine	Delirium
Digoxin	Visual hallucinations
Ketamine	Derealization, dissociation, amnesia, psychosis
Opiates	Sedation, delirium, psychosis
Propofol	Sedation, delirium
Tacrolimus	Delirium

Presented with a withdrawn, noninteractive patient who does not participate actively in care, cardiac intensive care staff sometimes have difficulty distinguishing hypoactive delirium from depression. Depressed patients often make poor effort, but do not have the fluctuating level of consciousness and altered sensorium characteristic of delirium. Although the gold standard for delirium diagnosis is an expert clinical evaluation, staff in the ICU may be aided by use of standardized assessment instruments such as the CAM-ICU (Confusion Assessment Method for the ICU)[7] or ICU Delirium Symptom Checklist.[8]

Thoughts of death are frequently expressed by critically ill patients; such thoughts alone are insufficient to diagnose depressive disorder. The desire to kill oneself, inappropriate guilt and loss of self-esteem, and persistent sad mood and loss of interest are more useful as markers of depressive illness. Nihilistic delusions, such as the belief that one is already dead, may occur in other psychotic disorders, delirium, and depression.

Anger, Hostility, and Stress

Anger, hostility, and chronic stress are associated with development of coronary disease and the incidence of myocardial infarction.[3,9,10] Acute, negatively valenced emotional arousal increases risk of myocardial infarction, and occurs as a triggering event in the hour before myocardial infarction in about 5% of myocardial infarctions.[11] Mental stress–induced myocardial ischemia, as indexed by transient ST segment depression, decreased left ventricular ejection fraction, or segmental wall motion abnormality, is common in patients who also have exercise-induced ischemia, and is associated with increased mortality risk.[12]

Psychotherapy and medication trials indicate that these effects can be attenuated. In the REMIT trial (Responses of Mental Stress Induced Myocardial Ischemia to Escitalopram Treatment), patients with coronary artery disease (CAD) with demonstrated mental stress–induced myocardial ischemia were randomized to treatment with placebo or escitalopram, up to 20 mg/d for 6 weeks.[13] Compared with subjects in the placebo group, those in the escitalopram group were about twice as likely (34% vs 18%; adjusted odds ratio, 2.62; 95% confidence interval, 1.06–6.44) to demonstrate absence of myocardial ischemia during mental stress testing after treatment. In a randomized, clinical trial enrolling 362 patients within 12 months of hospitalization for a coronary event, group cognitive–behavioral therapy (20 sessions over 1 year), focusing on stress management and anger reduction, led to reduced adverse outcomes: over a median follow-up of 94 months, fatal and nonfatal first recurrent CAD events were reduced by 41%, and recurrent myocardial infarction by 45%, in the intervention group, compared with the rates for the comparison group receiving usual care.[14]

Takutsubo Cardiomyopathy

Also known as "stress cardiomyopathy," "broken heart syndrome," or "apical ballooning syndrome," Takutsubo cardiomyopathy is characterized by acute left ventricular dysfunction precipitated by sudden emotional stress. The literature includes cases precipitated by seemingly benign stressors, such as surprise parties, as well as more negatively emotionally valenced stressors, such as being told of the unexpected death of a loved one[15,16] or the acute decompensation caused by a manic episode.[17] Although electrocardiograph changes may transiently resemble those of acute myocardial infarction, troponin elevation is minimal, and ventricular dysfunction resolves rapidly.

Anxiety

Anxiety disorders, including generalized anxiety, phobic anxiety, and panic disorder, have been associated with increased risk of coronary artery disease and with increased rates of cardiovascular events and mortality. Persons with type D personality, construed as high anxiety and/or depression symptoms ("negative affectivity"), along with inhibited expression of distress, also fit in this category.[4,18–21] Patients with anxiety disorders who require cardiac critical care can usually continue their maintenance pharmacotherapy with selective serotonin reuptake inhibitors and benzodiazepines. Circumstances may exacerbate symptoms and call for additional behavioral or psychotherapy interventions.

Panic disorder requires special consideration in cardiac critical care because symptoms of panic attacks often closely resemble those of an acute coronary syndrome (ACS), resulting in occasional admissions to cardiac intensive care to rule out myocardial infarction. Atypical quality of chest pain, younger age, and female sex, along with prior evidence of the absence of CAD, tend to discriminate panic disorder from myocardial ischemia.

Patients who have survived sudden cardiac death events have a high level of cardiac-specific anxiety and avoidant-protective behaviors. Eighteen percent have persistent worry even after normal testing. Presence of a heart murmur, younger age, history of implantable cardioverter-defibrillator shock, and history of generalized anxiety are associated with cardiac anxiety.[22]

Weaning from prolonged mechanical ventilation is a special circumstance that may evoke heightened anxiety. Pacing the patient's breathing and visualization exercises can facilitate weaning and extubation. Adjunctive benzodiazepine treatment may be helpful. Unrecognized delirium, sedative withdrawal reactions, sleep deprivation, cognitive impairment, inability to communicate, fear of being unable to breathe on one's own, depression, and absence of a trusting relationship with care providers may all contribute to difficulty with ventilator weaning.

Depression

Depression occurs in about 20% of patients with coronary heart disease and patients with heart failure. Self-reported elevated depressive symptoms are even more common. After cardiac surgery, delirium is often mistaken for depression. Many patients have transient, self-limited symptoms. Symptoms of depression such as low energy, low appetite, poor sleep often cannot be differentiated from symptoms resulting from postoperative sedation, pain, fatigue, and the ICU environment. Suicidal ideation, wishes to be dead, inappropriate guilt and loss of self-esteem, loss of interest and pleasure, and inability to anticipate pleasure in life are not normal symptoms during recovery from surgery and point toward a diagnosis of depression.

Depression after an ACS, after coronary artery bypass grafting, and in patients with heart failure, is associated with a substantial increased risk of subsequent morbidity and mortality, even after adjustment for other prognostic factors, and the effect persists for years.[23–27]

In addition, depression is associated with impaired physical function and health-related quality of life. Placebo-controlled, randomized trials support the efficacy of sertraline,[28] citalopram,[29] escitalopram,[30] and fluoxetine[31] for the treatment of depression in patients with coronary disease. A randomized trial of mirtazapine failed to find a benefit on its primary depression outcome measure, but did find benefit on secondary outcome measures.[32] None of these studies has demonstrated a significant beneficial effect of antidepressant treatment on cardiac outcomes and all-cause mortality, but all were underpowered to test this hypothesis. Recovery from depression predicts better survival,[33–36] suggesting that more effective depression treatments, or treatments that more precisely target mediators of the depression effect, may be of survival benefit.[37] In contrast with the studies in CAD, placebo-controlled, randomized trials of sertraline and escitalopram failed to find a benefit for treatment of depression in heart failure patients.[38,39] These negative results notwithstanding, serotonergic agents are considered to be first-line antidepressant treatment. Complex interventions using a variety of supportive psychotherapy interventions such as problem solving therapy, flexible psychotherapy, and medication using a team-based collaborative stepped care model care have demonstrated benefit for depression symptoms and suggestively promising improvement in cardiovascular outcomes.[40–43] In comparison with a health education intervention alone, the addition of cognitive–behavioral therapy for depression in patients with heart failure had beneficial effects on depression but not on heart failure self-care measures.[44] In aggregate, these studies suggest that the identification of depressed cardiac patients in the hospital and appropriate referral and treatment may be beneficial, but treatment need not start in the critical care setting.

Antidepressants may have cardiac effects and interactions that are relevant in the critical care setting. These are discussed elsewhere in this article.

Bipolar Affective Disorder

No trials have specifically studied treatment of bipolar disorder in patients with heart disease. There is at least 1 case report implicating the development of Takotsubo cardiomyopathy on an acute decompensation caused by a manic episode and acute social stressors. Lithium is a medication with a narrow therapeutic window; it depends on renal excretion, and blood levels may fluctuate dramatically in patients with heart failure if fluid balance is rapidly altered, risking lithium toxicity. Lithium can also cause sinus node dysfunction. Carbamazepine and oxcarbazine are occasionally used as mood stabilizers; both can cause hyponatremia. Antipsychotic medications are sometimes used as mood stabilizers for patients with bipolar disorder; they are discussed elsewhere in this article.

Posttraumatic Stress Disorder

Acute stress disorder and posttraumatic stress disorder (PTSD) are characterized by exposure to a dangerous traumatic event, followed by the onset of symptoms: intrusive reexperiencing, such as flashbacks, and nightmares; avoidance of stimuli associated with the traumatic event; negative alterations in mood and cognition; and heightened arousal and reactions to stimuli associated with the event.[6] More important than the objectively measured dangerousness of the trauma event as predictors of the likelihood of development of PTSD are intense fear, extreme distress during the event and feelings of helplessness and loss of control in the trauma experience.[45]

In recent years, PTSD has been recognized as a risk factor for the development of CAD, with hazard ratios of about 1.5- to 3-fold increased risk.[46] Proposed mechanisms linking PTSD to CAD events include altered hypothalamic–pituitary axis function and regulation of inflammatory responses, altered sympathoadrenal activity with high circulating catecholamines and reduced heart period variability, sleep disturbance, increased tobacco use, diminished adherence to medication, and reduced social support.

In turn, events taking place during care for ACS can be experienced as traumatic. For example, the experience of implanted defibrillator-delivered shock, especially multiple shocks, is widely recognized as potentially traumatic, and it has been estimated that about 5% of patients with an automatic implantable cardioverter defibrillator have elevated symptoms of PTSD. Other events linked to PTSD in cardiac critical care include waiting for treatment in a crowded emergency room, placement of arterial lines, and urgent intubation.[47] A meta-analysis of 24 studies with a total of more than 2300 subjects estimated the prevalence of ACS-induced PTSD to be about 12% to 16%.[47]

In a study of 247 patients with 42 months of follow-up, post-ACS PTSD was associated with a greater than 3-fold increased risk of the composite outcome of recurrent major adverse cardiac events and all-cause mortality.[48] A meta-analysis of incident PTSD after an ACS showed a greater than two-fold risk of recurrent cardiac events over 12 months of follow-up.[47] Strikingly, screening for PTSD is uncommon, and most patients do not receive treatment.[49]

Post-ACS PTSD as judged by self-report screening instruments is associated with a doubling of the risk of recurrent cardiovascular events and mortality.[47,48,50] Instruments such as the Impact of Events Scale—Revised, can be used to rate severity of symptoms and screen for possible cases of PTSD.[51] Treatments for PTSD include cognitive–behavioral therapy and medication (**Table 2**). Prazosin has been used to treat nightmares. Prophylaxis for PTSD might be accomplished by adequate sedation before painful procedures. It is not known whether increased explanation, education, and rehearsal, with the aim of increasing feelings of mastery and ability to cope, thereby reducing feelings of helplessness, can reduce incident PTSD in cardiac critical care settings.[45,52]

Psychosis

The differential diagnosis of psychosis in cardiac critical care should always begin with delirium and psychotic disorders owing to other medical problems and substances. Stroke, adverse effects of medication, and systemic illness can cause psychotic symptoms. Schizophrenia is the major primary psychotic disorder, with a lifetime population prevalence of about 1%, and schizophrenia poses some special concerns in cardiac care.

The incidence of heart disease, especially CAD, in persons with schizophrenia is higher than that in the general population; contributing factors are believed to include

Table 2 Managing posttraumatic stress disorder in cardiac critical care		
Stage	**Goal**	**Interventions**
Prevention	Decrease exposure to traumatic events, decrease feelings of helplessness, increase sense of control	Screening Education, preparation, coaching, rehearsal Sedation Premedication for painful procedures
Management	Reduce symptoms, improve feelings of mastery, correct cognitive distortions	Screening Debriefing, validation Cognitive behavioral psychotherapy Prazosin (for nightmares) Antipsychotic medication (for psychotic symptoms) Selective serotonin reuptake inhibitors Referral

the high rate of smoking in persons with schizophrenia, poor diet, lack of exercise, socioeconomic disadvantage, and stigma leading to reduced access to general medical and specialty care, and adverse effects of antipsychotic drugs leading to metabolic syndrome. Most patients with schizophrenia in cardiac intensive care can be maintained on antipsychotic medications, with appropriate electrocardiogram monitoring for QT interval prolongation and consideration of drug interactions (discussed further elsewhere in this article). Low potency, first-generation antipsychotic agents such as chlorpromazine have alpha-adrenergic blocking effects and may contribute to orthostatic hypotension.

Neither a schizophrenia diagnosis per se nor the presence of psychotic symptoms determines a patient's capacity to make decisions about medical treatment. Patients with schizophrenia who require invasive critical care interventions may be able to articulate treatment preferences, understand the medical situation, apply facts about the illness and proposed treatments to their situation, and make decisions in a rational manner. When clinicians are uncertain of the patient's capacity to make decisions, psychiatric consultation is warranted.

Clozapine is the most effective treatment for positive and negative symptoms of schizophrenia and has a beneficial effect on suicide rates in patients with schizophrenia. Although its use is limited by the risk of agranulocytosis, it is indicated for those patients who have not responded to adequate trials of 2 other antipsychotic agents. Another adverse effect of clozapine is cardiomyopathy, often with evidence of myocarditis, which occurs with an estimated lifetime incidence of 0.01% to 0.1%. An asymptomatic reduction in left ventricular ejection fraction may be much more common than clinical heart failure.[53,54] Symptoms of persistent tachycardia, shortness of breath, and fatigue progressing to overt heart failure occur weeks to years after initiation of treatment; a recent review found that the mean interval from initiation of clozapine to time of cardiomyopathy diagnosis was 14 months.[54] The mechanism of clozapine cardiomyopathy is unknown; proposed mechanisms include allergy-like hypersensitivity and inflammatory reactions and cholinergic receptor dysfunction. When cardiomyopathy develops, clozapine should be discontinued immediately. Typically, treatment is with standard heart failure therapy, along with cessation of clozapine; prognosis depends on the severity of left ventricular dysfunction at the time of diagnosis. Some patients require pressors and intensive care. Other antipsychotic agents can be substituted for clozapine even during heart failure treatment, without exacerbation of cardiomyopathy. After an episode of clozapine cardiomyopathy or myocarditis, clozapine rechallenge is not recommended, although there are a few case reports of rechallenge without adverse effect.[54]

Delirium and Cognitive Impairment

Delirium or acute brain failure is discussed at length in José Maldonado's article, "Acute Brain Failure: Pathophysiology, Diagnosis, Management and Sequelae of Delirium," in this issue, so the discussion here focuses on a few points relevant especially to cardiac intensive care. Delirium is the most important neuropsychiatric disorder in cardiac critical care, and is seen after coronary bypass and valve surgery, in patients with low cardiac output states, as an adverse effect of medication, as a consequence of cerebrovascular disease, and as an effect of infection and metabolic disarray. Manipulation of the aortic arch during cardiac surgery showers the cerebral circulation with microemboli. New onset of atrial fibrillation, for example, after mitral valve repair or replacement or after myocardial infarction, may reduce cardiac output and trigger delirium. Prolonged sedation with opiates, propofol, and benzodiazepines after cardiac surgery also increases risk.[55]

Delirium may pose acute management problems when patients climb out of bed, pull lines and tubes, and behave aggressively. The occurrence of delirium is associated with longer ICU and hospital durations of stay and heightened morbidity and mortality. Premorbid risk factors associated with delirium in cardiac intensive care settings include older age, prior alcohol use, and prior cerebrovascular disease, chronic renal insufficiency, and anemia. The widespread use of antipsychotic agents for sedation and management of agitation, and reduction of psychotic symptoms, carries risk of QT interval prolongation and cardiac arrhythmias, as discussed elsewhere in this article.

Persistent neurocognitive impairment may be a sequela of cardiac surgery. Early postoperative impairment may be evident in the ICU setting, even in patients who are not delirious. Such impairment is a sensitive but not a specific marker of long-term impairment, because most patients recover over a few weeks to months. However, preoperative deficits in more than 1 domain of cognitive function are surprisingly common, even in asymptomatic patients, and are associated with persistent postoperative deficits.[56]

Prolonged sedation for more than 24 hours with opiates, benzodiazepines, or propofol increases the risk of delirium.[55] Several studies have demonstrated that the use of dexmedetomidine in place of these agents is associated with a reduced incidence of delirium.[57,58] Additional strategies to reduce the incidence of delirium include early mobilization, avoiding opiates, and treating pain adequately with nonopiates.[55] (Delirium diagnosis and management in critical care are addressed in detail elsewhere in this issue of Critical Care Clinics.)

Alcohol Withdrawal

Alcohol withdrawal is a frequently overlooked diagnosis in intensive care. Patients may not accurately disclose the extent of recent alcohol intake at the time of admission, and early signs of withdrawal may be misattributed to anxiety. Neither a blood alcohol level of zero at the time of admission nor an elevated blood alcohol level at the time of symptom presentation precludes the possibility of alcohol withdrawal; individuals with high tolerance may experience withdrawal even with alcohol still present in their system. Symptoms of alcohol withdrawal include tremor, diaphoresis, headache, autonomic hyperactivity or instability, irritability, nervousness, sensitivity to light and noise, and nausea. Late signs include disorientation, hallucinations, and seizures.

Onset of withdrawal is typically within 24 to 48 hours of the last drink, but may be delayed by anesthesia. Therefore, patients admitted electively for cardiac surgery may develop withdrawal signs and symptoms many days after surgery. Untreated alcohol withdrawal progresses to delirium tremens in a minority of patients, but can be fatal. The management of alcohol withdrawal is discussed at length in José Maldonado's article, "Novel Algorithms for the Prophylaxis & Management of Alcohol Withdrawal Syndromes – Beyond Benzodiazepines," in this issue.

CARDIOVASCULAR EFFECTS OF PSYCHOTROPIC DRUGS

Many psychiatric medications have cardiac side effects (**Table 3**).[59] The text highlights a few points.

Antipsychotic drugs cause QT interval prolongation through inhibition of potassium channels that mediate ventricular myocyte repolarization. QT interval prolongation is associated with increased risk of torsades de pointes. In a recent large scale Swedish study, Danielsson and colleagues[60] found the antipsychotic drugs associated with the highest risk of malignant arrhythmias were haloperidol, risperidone, olanzapine, and quetiapine; aripiprazole seems to be the agent with least propensity to increase QT interval, and to have the lowest risk of torsades de pointes. Modifiable concurrent risk factors include hypokalemia and hypomagnesemia, concurrent use of other medications that themselves prolong the QT interval, and concurrent use of drugs that interfere with the metabolism of psychotropic drugs that prolong the QT interval.[61]

Selective serotonin reuptake inhibitors and other antidepressants also affect cardiac conduction. Among selective serotonin reuptake inhibitors, citalopram demonstrates a dose-related effect on QT prolongation sufficient for the Food and Drug Administration to require a boxed warning in its pharmaceutical labeling about risk

Table 3	
Selected cardiovascular effects of psychotropic medications	
Medication	**Effect**
Antipsychotic medications	Hypotension; orthostatic hypotension; QT interval prolongation, torsades de pointes
Bupropion	Increased blood pressure
Carbamazepine	Hyponatremia (SIADH)
Clozapine	Myocarditis, cardiomyopathy
Donepezil, galantamine, rivastigmine	Slowing of heart rate
Lithium	Sinus node dysfunction
Mirtazapine	Ventricular tachyarrhythmia
Oxcarbazine	Hyponatremia (SIADH)
SSRI antidepressants	Slowing of heart rate; increased bleeding risk; QT interval prolongation (citalopram); hyponatremia (SIADH)
Stimulants	Increased heart rate and blood pressure
Tricyclic antidepressants	Orthostatic hypotension; heart block; type I antiarrhythmic effects; proarrhythmic effects in overdose or in setting of ischemia
Venlafaxine	Increased blood pressure

Abbreviations: SIADH, syndrome of inappropriate antidiuretic hormone; SSRI, selective serotonin reuptake inhibitor.

of sudden cardiac death. Other selective serotonin reuptake inhibitors have weaker QT interval effects. Bupropion does not prolong the QT interval.[62]

Tricyclic antidepressants prolong the QRS interval and therefore the QT interval, via inhibition of sodium channels mediating the onset of ventricular myocyte depolarization. In overdose, tricyclic antidepressants may cause ventricular tachycardia–ventricular fibrillation. In the study by Danielsson and associates,[60] the antidepressant most associated with sudden death was mirtazapine.

Serotonin is stored in platelets, released upon platelet activation, and acts as an agonist for further platelet activation. Serotonin reuptake inhibitors interfere with platelet serotonin uptake and therefore tend to reduce thrombus formation in response to platelet-activating stimuli. The clinical significance of this effect is uncertain. In randomized trials such as the SADHART trial (Sertraline Antidepressant Heart Attack Randomized Trial) of sertraline versus placebo treatment in patients with depression after an ACS, subjects treated with placebo and sertraline had similarly low rates of adverse bleeding events.[28] No increase in the rate of adverse bleeding events after cardiac surgery has been observed with concurrent selective serotonin reuptake inhibitor use. However, doubling to tripling of the rate of bleeding events has been noted for patients taking selective serotonin reuptake inhibitors along with warfarin and combined warfarin and antiplatelet agents.[63–66]

SPECIAL SITUATIONS
Left Ventricular Assist Devices

The main psychiatric problems associated with left ventricular assist device treatment for heart failure are delirium, adjustment and mood disorders, and cognitive dysfunction.[67] Patients with heart failure who require ventricular assist device therapy frequently have preexisting cognitive impairment. Stroke after ventricular assist device placement is not infrequent, may be debilitating, and can lead to depression and cognitive impairment. Living with a ventricular assist device requires active management of the device and power supply, and protection of the skin entry site against infection. This can be extremely stressful for patients and family care providers. Infection, bleeding, device failure, and stroke are causes of readmission to cardiac critical care. Disconnection of the ventricular assist device from the power supply as a means of suicide and requests for treatment discontinuation as a means of hastening death have been reported. The postimplantation lifetime prevalence of depression in assist device patients is unknown. INTERMACs registry data (Interagency Registry for Mechanically Assisted Circulatory Support)[68] suggest a low 12-month incidence rate of psychiatric disorder in mechanical circulatory support patients (<1/100 patient-months) but psychiatric case ascertainment in the registry is not systematic.

Atrial Fibrillation

There is a bidirectional relationship of atrial fibrillation with psychological stress and psychiatric disorder. Acute emotional stress can precipitate the onset of atrial fibrillation. Thus, the experience of critical illness may itself stimulate onset of atrial fibrillation, and patients with medical risk factors for atrial fibrillation such as mitral valve disease, myocardial infarction, and heart failure, have risk compounded by the experience of being critically ill.

Reduced cardiac output in association with atrial fibrillation can lead to the onset of symptoms resembling depression or dementia—decreased energy, increased fatigue, apathy, and decreased mental acuity. In addition, cerebrovascular embolic events as a complication of atrial fibrillation can lead to delirium, cognitive impairment, psychomotor slowing, and depression. Complications of amiodarone treatment for rate and rhythm control in atrial fibrillation include hypothyroidism; edema, fatigue, and cognitive impairment may be mistakenly attributed to heart failure or a primary dementia.

Space does not permit discussion of heart transplantation here. The reader is referred to the article in Yelizaveta Sher and Paula Zimbrean's article, "Psychiatric Aspects of Organ Transplantation in Critical Care: An Update," in this issue.

SUMMARY

Strong emotional reactions are to be expected in patients admitted to cardiac critical care; only some of these are pathologic. Cardiac critical care and associated technologies such as mechanical ventilation, ventricular assist devices, and defibrillation, are associated with predictable psychiatric problems including anxiety, delirium, depression, and acute and PTSD. Many psychiatric problems in cardiac critical care occur as secondary complications of the medical status of the patient, which must be assessed carefully. Depression is extremely common in patients with coronary disease, in patients admitted with ACSs, and in coronary bypass surgery patients; treatment is helpful, but persistent depression is associated with elevated morbidity and mortality. Preexisting psychiatric disorders may predispose to heart disease, and they and their treatment may affect critical care management.

REFERENCES

1. Mozaffarian D, Benjamin EJ, Go AS, et al. Heart disease and stroke Statistics—2016 update: a report from the American Heart Association. Circulation 2016; 133:e38–360.
2. Rozanski A, Blumenthal JA, Davidson KW, et al. The epidemiology, pathophysiology, and management of psychosocial risk factors in cardiac practice. The emerging field of behavioral cardiology. J Am Coll Cardiol 2005;45:637–51.
3. Cohen BE, Edmondson D, Kronish IM. State of the art review: depression, stress, anxiety, and cardiovascular disease. Am J Hypertens 2015;28:1295–302.
4. Kent LK, Shapiro PA. Depression and related psychological factors in heart disease. Harv Rev Psychiatry 2009;17:377–88.
5. Maunder RG, Hunter JJ. Assessing patterns of adult attachment in medical patients. Gen Hosp Psychiatry 2009;31:123–30.
6. American Psychiatric Association. Diagnostic and statistical manual of mental disorders. 5th edition. Arlington (VA): American Psychiatric Association; 2013.
7. Ely EW, Inouye S, Bernard G, et al. Delirium in mechanically ventilated patients. JAMA 2001;286:2703–10.
8. Bergeron N, Dubois MJ, Dumont M, et al. Intensive care delirium screening checklist. Intensive Care Med 2001;27:859–64.
9. Chida Y, Steptoe A. The association of anger and hostility with future coronary heart disease: a meta-analytic review of prospective evidence. J Am Coll Cardiol 2009;53:936–46.
10. Rosengren A, Hawken S, Ôunpuu S, et al, for the INTERHEART investigators. Association of psychosocial risk factors with risk of acute myocardial infarction in 11 119 cases and 13 648 controls from 52 countries (the INTERHEART study): a case-control study. Lancet 2004;364:953–62.
11. Jiang W. Emotional triggering of cardiac dysfunction: the present and future. Curr Cardiol Rep 2015;17:1–10.

12. Sheps DS, McMahon RP, Becker L, et al. Mental stress-induced ischemia and all-cause mortality in patients with coronary artery disease: results from the Psychophysiological Investigations of Myocardial Ischemia study. Circulation 2002;105: 1780–4.

13. Jiang W, Velazquez EJ, Kuchibhatla M, et al. Effect of escitalopram on mental stress–induced myocardial ischemia: results of the REMIT trial. JAMA 2013; 309:2139–49.

14. Gulliksson M, Burell G, Vessby B, et al. Randomized controlled trial of cognitive behavioral therapy vs standard treatment to prevent recurrent cardiovascular events in patients with coronary heart disease: Secondary Prevention in Uppsala Primary Health Care Project (SUPRIM). Arch Intern Med 2011;171:134–40.

15. Wittstein IS. The broken heart syndrome. Cleve Clin J Med 2007;74(suppl 1): S17–22.

16. Wittstein IS, Thiemann DR, Lima JAC, et al. Neurohumoral features of myocardial stunning due to sudden emotional stress. N Engl J Med 2005;352:539–48.

17. Maldonado JR, Pajouhl P, Witteles R. Broken heart syndrome (Takotsubo cardiomyopathy) triggered by acute mania: a review and case report. Psychosomatics 2013;54(1):74–9.

18. Kawachi I, Colditz GA, Ascherio A, et al. Prospective study of phobic anxiety and risk of coronary heart disease in men. Circulation 1994;89:1992–7.

19. Kawachi I, Sparrow D, Vokonas PS, et al. Symptoms of anxiety and risk of coronary heart disease. The normative aging study. Circulation 1994;90:2225–9.

20. Weissman MM, Markowitz JS, Ouellette R, et al. Panic disorder and cardiovascular/cerebrovascular problems: results from a community survey. Am J Psychiatry 1990;147:1504–8.

21. Denollet J, Pedersen SS, Vrints CJ, et al. Usefulness of Type D personality in predicting five-year cardiac events above and beyond concurrent symptoms of stress in patients with coronary heart disease. Am J Cardiol 2006;97:970–3.

22. Rosman L, Whited A, Lampert R, et al. Cardiac anxiety after sudden cardiac arrest: severity, predictors and clinical implications. Int J Cardiol 2015;181:73–6.

23. Blumenthal JA, Lett HS, Babyak MA, et al, for the NORG Investigators. Depression as a risk factor for mortality after coronary artery bypass surgery. Lancet 2003;362:604–9.

24. Connerney I, Sloan RP, Shapiro PA, et al. Depression is associated with increased mortality 10 years after coronary artery bypass surgery. Psychosom Med 2010; 72:874–81.

25. van Melle JP, de Jonge P, Spijkerman TA, et al. Prognostic association of depression following myocardial infarction with mortality and cardiovascular events: a meta-analysis. Psychosom Med 2004;66:814–22.

26. Rutledge T, Reis VA, Linke SE, et al. Depression in heart failure: a meta-analytic review of prevalence, intervention effects, and associations with clinical outcomes. J Am Coll Cardiol 2006;48:1527–37.

27. Jiang W, Alexander J, Christopher E, et al. Relationship of depression to increased risk of mortality and rehospitalization in patients with congestive heart failure. Arch Intern Med 2001;161:1849–56.

28. Glassman AH, O'Connor CM, Califf RM, et al, for the Sertraline Antidepressant Heart Attack Randomized Trial (SADHART) Group. Sertraline treatment of major depression in patients with acute MI or unstable angina. JAMA 2002;288:701–9.

29. Lesperance F, Frasure-Smith N, Koszycki D, et al, for the Create Investigators. Effects of citalopram and interpersonal psychotherapy on depression in patients with coronary artery disease: the Canadian Cardiac Randomized Evaluation of

Antidepressant and Psychotherapy Efficacy (CREATE) trial. JAMA 2007;297: 367–79.

30. Kim JM, Bae KY, Stewart R, et al. Escitalopram treatment for depressive disorder following acute coronary syndrome: a 24-week double-blind, placebo-controlled trial. J Clin Psychiatry 2015;76:62–8.

31. Strik JJMH, Honig A, Lousberg R, et al. Efficacy and safety of fluoxetine in the treatment of patients with major depression after first myocardial infarction: findings from a double-blind, placebo-controlled trial. Psychosom Med 2000;62: 783–9.

32. Honig A, Kuyper AMG, Schene AH, et al, on behalf of the Mind-IT Investigators. Treatment of post-myocardial infarction depressive disorder: a randomized, placebo-controlled trial with mirtazapine. Psychosom Med 2007;69:606–13.

33. Dickens C, McGowan L, Percival C, et al. New onset depression following myocardial infarction predicts cardiac mortality. Psychosom Med 2008;70:450–5.

34. Parker GB, Hilton TM, Walsh WF, et al. Timing is everything: the onset of depression and acute coronary syndrome outcome. Biol Psychiatry 2008;64:660–6.

35. Glassman AH, Bigger JT Jr, Gaffney M. Psychiatric characteristics associated with long-term mortality among 361 patients having an acute coronary syndrome and major depression: seven-year follow-up of SADHART participants. Arch Gen Psychiatry 2009;66:1022–9.

36. Carney RM, Freedland KE. Treatment-resistant depression and mortality after acute coronary syndrome. Am J Psychiatry 2009;166:410–7.

37. Shapiro PA. Depression treatment and coronary artery disease outcomes: time for reflection. J Psychosom Res 2013;74:4–5.

38. Angermann CE, Gelbrich G, Stork S, et al. Effect of escitalopram on all-cause mortality and hospitalization in patients with heart failure and depression: the MOOD-HF randomized clinical trial. JAMA 2016;315:2683–93.

39. O'Connor CM, Jiang W, Kuchibhatla M, et al. Safety and efficacy of sertraline for depression in patients with heart failure: results of the SADHART-CHF (Sertraline Against Depression and Heart Disease in Chronic Heart Failure) trial. J Am Coll Cardiol 2010;56:692–9.

40. Rollman BL, Belnap BH, LeMenager MS, et al. Telephone-delivered collaborative care for treating post-CABG depression: a randomized controlled trial. JAMA 2009;302:2095–103.

41. Davidson KW, Rieckmann N, Clemow L, et al. Enhanced depression care for patients with acute coronary syndrome and persistent depressive symptoms: Coronary Psychosocial Evaluation Studies randomized controlled trial. Arch Intern Med 2010;170:600–8.

42. Davidson KW, Bigger JT, Burg MM, et al. Centralized, stepped, patient preference–based treatment for patients with post–acute coronary syndrome depression: CODIACS vanguard randomized controlled trial. JAMA Intern Med 2013; 173:997–1004.

43. Huffman JC, Mastromauro CA, Beach SR, et al. Collaborative care for depression and anxiety disorders in patients with recent cardiac events: the Management of Sadness and Anxiety in Cardiology (MOSAIC) randomized clinical trial. JAMA Intern Med 2014;174:927–35.

44. Freedland KE, Carney RM, Rich MW, et al. Cognitive behavior therapy for depression and self-care in heart failure patients: a randomized clinical trial. JAMA Intern Med 2015;175:1773–82.

45. Tulloch H, Greenman PS, Tassé V. Post-traumatic stress disorder among cardiac patients: prevalence, risk factors, and considerations for assessment and treatment. Behav Sci 2015;5:27–40.
46. Edmondson D, Kronish IM, Shaffer JA, et al. Posttraumatic stress disorder and risk for coronary heart disease: a meta-analytic review. Am Heart J 2013;166:806–14.
47. Edmondson D, Cohen BE. Posttraumatic stress disorder and cardiovascular disease. Prog Cardiovasc Dis 2013;55:548–56.
48. Edmondson D, Rieckmann N, Shaffer JA, et al. Posttraumatic stress due to an acute coronary syndrome increases risk of 42-month major adverse cardiac events and all-cause mortality. J Psychiatr Res 2011;45:1621–6.
49. Sundquist K, Chang BP, Parsons F, et al. Treatment rates for PTSD and depression in recently hospitalized cardiac patients. J Psychosom Res 2016;86:60–2.
50. von Känel R, Hari R, Schmid JP, et al. Non-fatal cardiovascular outcome in patients with posttraumatic stress symptoms caused by myocardial infarction. J Cardiol 2011;58:61–8.
51. Weiss DS, Marmar CR. The impact of event scale-revised. In: Wilson JP, Kean TM, editors. Assessing psychological trauma and PTSD: a practitioner's handbook (ch 15). New York: Guildford; 1995. Available at: www.getcbt.org. Accessed April 1, 2017.
52. Meister R, Princip M, Schmid JP, et al. Myocardial Infarction - stress PRevention INTervention (MI-SPRINT) to reduce the incidence of posttraumatic stress after acute myocardial infarction through trauma-focused psychological counseling: study protocol for a randomized controlled trial. Trials 2013;14:329.
53. Merrill DB, Dec GW, Goff DC. Adverse cardiac effects associated with clozapine. J Clin Psychopharmacol 2005;25:32–41.
54. Alawami M, Wasywich C, Cicovic A, et al. A systematic review of clozapine induced cardiomyopathy. Int J Cardiol 2014;176:315–20.
55. Barr J, Fraser GL, Puntillo K, et al, American College of Critical Care Medicine. Clinical practice guidelines for the management of pain, agitation, and delirium in adult patients in the intensive care unit. Crit Care Med 2013;41:263–306.
56. Habib S, Khan A, Afridi MI, et al. Frequency and predictors of cognitive decline in patients undergoing coronary artery bypass graft surgery. J Coll Physicians Surg Pak 2014;24:543–8.
57. Maldonado JR, Wysong A, van der Starre PJ, et al. Dexmedetomidine and the reduction of postoperative delirium after cardiac surgery. Psychosomatics 2009;50:206–17.
58. Pandharipande PP, Pun BT, Herr DL, et al. Effect of sedation with dexmedetomidine vs lorazepam on acute brain dysfunction in mechanically ventilated patients: the MENDS randomized controlled trial. JAMA 2007;298:2644–53.
59. Shapiro PA. Cardiovascular disorders. In: Levenson J, Ferranndo S, editors. Clinical manual of psychopharmacology in the medically ill. Arlington (VA): American Psychiatric Association; 2017. p. 233–70.
60. Danielsson B, Collin J, Jonasdottir Bergman G, et al. Antidepressants and antipsychotics classified with torsades de pointes arrhythmia risk and mortality in older adults - a Swedish nationwide study. Br J Clin Pharmacol 2016;81:773–83.
61. Beach SR, Celano CM, Noseworthy PA, et al. QTc prolongation, torsades de pointes, and psychotropic medications. Psychosomatics 2013;54:1–13.
62. Castro VM, Clements CC, Murphy SN, et al. QT interval and antidepressant use: a cross sectional study of electronic health records. BMJ 2013;346:f288.
63. Cochran KA, Cavallari LH, Shapiro NL, et al. Bleeding incidence with concomitant use of antidepressants and warfarin. Ther Drug Monit 2011;33:433–8.

64. Labos C, Dasgupta K, Nedjar H, et al. Risk of bleeding associated with combined use of selective serotonin reuptake inhibitors and antiplatelet therapy following acute myocardial infarction. Can Med Assoc J 2011;183:1835–43.

65. Schelleman H, Brensinger CM, Bilker WB, et al. Antidepressant-warfarin interaction and associated gastrointestinal bleeding risk in a case-control study. PLoS ONE 2011;6:e21447.

66. Wallerstedt SM, Gleerup H, Sundstrom A, et al. Risk of clinically relevant bleeding in warfarin-treated patients–influence of SSRI treatment. Pharmacoepidemiol Drug Saf 2009;18:412–6.

67. Rosenberger EM, Fox KR, DiMartini AF, et al. Psychosocial factors and quality-of-life after heart transplantation and mechanical circulatory support. Curr Opin Organ Transplant 2012;17:558–63.

68. Kirklin JK, Naftel DC, Pagani FD, et al. Seventh INTERMACS annual report: 15,000 patients and counting. J Heart Lung Transplant 2015;34:1495–504.

Psychiatric Disorders and Suicidality in the Intensive Care Unit

 CrossMark

Renee M. Garcia, MD

KEYWORDS

- Psychiatric disorders • Suicidality • Intensive care unit • Self-injury

KEY POINTS

- Suicidality assessments in those admitted to the intensive care unit, as in all other settings, consists of a comprehensive evaluation of the patient's clinical status, risk/protective factors, psychiatric history, and current degree of suicidality.
- The goal of identifying any primary psychiatric disorders is to enable appropriate treatment to be initiated and to ensure a safe environment until the patient can be transferred to an inpatient psychiatric unit.
- There are multiple challenges specific to an intensive care population.
- These challenges include the high risk of comorbid delirium, limitations in communication (ie, intubation, fatigue related to medical illness, sedative medications), and psychotropic medication issues (drug-drug interactions, limited routes of administration, reduction/elimination of deliriogenic medications, potential for medication withdrawal syndromes).

INTRODUCTION

Suicidality is a general term that describes the continuum of suicidal ideation, intent, self-injurious behavior, attempts, and completed suicide.[1] Suicidality across the entire spectrum is a public health concern with significant impact. Suicide was the tenth leading cause of death for all age groups[2] and the rate has increased since 2006.[2] Men complete suicide at 4 times the rate of women, and often use more violent, lethal means, with firearms being the most common method.[2] Women most commonly use poisoning as the method for suicide.[2] According to the Centers for Disease Control and Prevention (CDC), 9.3 million adults reported having suicidal thoughts in the past year.[2] The highest rate of suicidal ideation was found in adults aged 18 to 25 years (7.4%), then adults aged 26 to 49 years (4.0%), and adults aged more than 50 years (2.7%).

Disclosures: None.
Division of Psychosomatic Medicine, Department of Psychiatry & Behavioral Sciences, Stanford Hospital and Clinics, 401 Quarry Road, Stanford, CA 94305, USA
E-mail address: Rgarcia7@stanford.edu

Crit Care Clin 33 (2017) 635–647
http://dx.doi.org/10.1016/j.ccc.2017.03.005
0749-0704/17/© 2017 Elsevier Inc. All rights reserved.
criticalcare.theclinics.com

The national economic costs of both fatal and nonfatal suicide-related injuries in 2013 were estimated to be about $58.4 billion in medical and work loss.[2,3] One retrospective study estimated that 412,000 emergency department (ED) visits were attributed to attempted suicide and self-inflicted injuries, or 0.4% of total ED visits.[4] Approximately 31% of patients who presented to ED required an intensive care unit (ICU) admission.[4] The most common methods of self-injury were poisoning in 66.5%, cutting at 22.1%, and both hanging and firearms were rare at less than 1%.[5] Intentional poisoning requiring ICU admission should be considered a serious suicide attempt and the most commonly used drugs include tranquilizers, psychotropics, analgesics, antipyretics, antirheumatics, and unspecified substances.[4]

Patients admitted after a suicide attempt require numerous precautions to be instituted to ensure a safe environment. However, the ICU has a limited ability to make drastic adjustments to its environment because many items that can be used as means of self-harm are necessary for day-to-day workings. This article reviews the prevalence of suicide attempts in different psychiatric diagnoses, conducting a suicide assessment, the role of involuntary psychiatric holds, and the most common challenges encountered in the ICU setting.

Psychiatric Disorders

According to the World Health Organization, approximately 98% of people who have completed suicide had a diagnosable mental illness.[6] The risk for suicide varies for each psychiatric diagnosis and risk often increases with additional comorbidities.

Mood Disorders

Mood disorders include unipolar depression and both bipolar I and II disorders in all mood states (depressive, manic, mixed). Presence of a mood disorders increases risk for suicide significantly, and is the most frequently identified psychiatric diagnosis (20%–35%) of people who completed suicide[6] and in those who presented to ED with self-harm at 58.5%.[7] **Table 1** provides additional details regarding suicidality in mood disorders.

Psychotic/Thought Disorders

Psychotic spectrum disorders include schizophrenia, schizoaffective disorders, brief psychotic disorder, and unspecified psychotic disorders. Most studies group disorders that are not schizophrenia into another category of schizophrenia-like disorders. Schizophrenia carries an approximately 5.6% lifetime risk of suicide.[8] The highest risk of suicide occurs in the early course of the illness and is often a focus of suicide prevention strategies for this population.[8] One study assessing the risk of suicide after first hospitalization found the absolute risk in schizophrenia to be 5.85% to 7.34% for men and 4.03% to 5.98% for women, as well as 5.21% to 6.67% for men and 3.28% to 5.04% for women with schizophrenia-like illnesses.[9] See **Table 1** for additional details regarding suicidality in psychotic disorders.

Substance Use Disorders

Substance use disorders can span the range of illicit drug use, nicotine, prescription drugs, and alcohol use disorders. In 2010, 33.4% of patients who completed suicide had alcohol in their systems.[2] The comorbid presence of an alcohol use disorder increases risk almost 10 times compared with the general population.[10,11] People who inject drugs are approximately 14 times more likely to commit suicide.[10] Up to 40% of patients with substance use disorder seeking treatment report a positive history of prior suicide attempts and often enter treatment with increased risk for suicide

Table 1
Suicide risk and special considerations by psychiatric diagnosis

	Diagnosis	Risk of Suicide (%)[a]	Special Considerations
Mood disorders	Unipolar depression	Men: 5.7–7.8 Women: 3.1–4.7	• Found in estimated 30%–90% of completed suicides • 1 in 3 suicide attempts presenting to the ED have MDD
	BPD	Men: 6–10 Women: 3.5–6.6	• BPDII has higher associated risk of suicide than BPDI • Highest risk in mixed > depressed > manic • Increased risk thought to be caused by spending more time in high-risk phases • Family history of bipolar increases risk by 2×
Psychotic disorders	Schizophrenia	Men: 5.9–7.3 Women: 4–6	• More likely to use lethal and violent means • Highest risk is early in course of illness • Use of cocaine or methamphetamines increases risk for suicide by 8×
	Schizophrenialike disorders	Men: 5.2–6.7 Women: 3.3–5.0	
Substance use disorders	General hospital setting	Men: 2.2–3.0 Women: 1.4–2.0	• Any comorbid substance use disorder increases risk of attempted and completed suicide • Family history of alcoholism is associated with increased risk of suicidality • Alcohol use disorder increases risk ~10× to die by suicide • IV users are 14× more likely to commit suicide • Alcohol is involved in 25%–35% of all suicides and associated with more dangerous attempts
	Inpatient psychiatric setting	Men: 4.2–5.2 Women: 2.8–4	
PDs[b]	Borderline PD	60–70 attempt suicide 5–10 complete suicide	• Only DSM diagnosis with criteria of recurrent suicidality • High risk of self-injurious (nonsuicidal) behaviors: cutting, burning • Often have childhood history of trauma
	ASPD	11 attempt suicide 5 complete suicide	• More likely to die by violent means, including suicide • Risk of serious suicide attempt was 3.7× higher in ASPD than GP

Abbreviations: ASPD, antisocial personality disorder; BPD, bipolar disorder; DSM, Diagnostic and Statistical Manual of Mental Disorders; GP, general population; IV, intravenous; PD, personality disorder.
[a] Absolute Risk of Suicide.
[b] Risk over course of lifetime.

and depressive symptoms, in part caused by numerous stressors such as loss of relationships, employment, health, and financial stability.[9,10] See **Table 1** for additional details regarding suicidality in substance use disorders.

Personality Disorders

Personality disorders are pervasive mental disorders with a rigid, unhealthy, and maladaptive patterns of thinking, functioning, and behaving, which lead to significant impairments across many dimensions of life (relationships, work, social, and so forth). The nomenclature describing the personality disorder class has evolved over the many revisions of the Diagnostic and Statistical Manual of Mental Disorders (DSM) since its inception. Most recently, the current DSM5 eliminated the clusters with which clinicians previously categorized personality disorders. Most studies on personality disorders and suicidality used this framework, so most suicidality literature exists for the cluster B personality disorders, which include antisocial, borderline, narcissistic, and histrionic. See **Table 1** for additional details regarding suicidality in these personality disorders.

NEUROBIOLOGY OF SUICIDE

The underlying pathophysiologic mechanism behind suicidality remains poorly understood but what is known stems from studies involving various study designs, postmortem techniques, and in-vivo techniques. The serotonin neurotransmitter system and hypothalamus-pituitary-adrenal axis stress response have repeatedly been identified to have abnormalities in suicidal patients.[12] At the cellular level, postmortem studies have identified 3 patterns of cellular changes to be associated with people who carry a diagnosis of mood disorder, including cell loss of glia (astrocytes, oligodendrocytes), cell atrophy or lower neuronal density, and increased numbers of serotonin cells.

There have also been circuitry issues evaluated using functional neuroimaging and molecular studies with special focus on serotonin circuitry. Molecular studies have found that prefrontal localized hypofunction and impaired serotoninergic responsivity are proportional to the lethality of suicide behavior.[12] PET studies have shown a deficit in serotonin transporter expression and binding in postmortem studies of completed suicides. Structural MRI has also been used to evaluate abnormalities in nonfatal suicide attempters, including right-sided volume deficits of gray matter in certain cortical areas, greater volume in thalamus and right amygdala, and white matter hyperintensities coupled with increased bilateral volumes of frontal white matter tracts. These data point to the presence of impairments in structural connectivity within serotonin circuits.[12]

Early life adversity is thought to lead to epigenetic changes that may be associated with increased risk for suicidality, and has been shown to be a strong risk factor for suicide. A classic study conducted many years ago identified low cerebrospinal fluid concentrations of 5-hydroxyindoleacetic acid, a major metabolite of serotonin in the brain, in psychiatric patients after a suicide attempt. This finding was one of the first to point to a deficiency in serotonin release. HPA axis abnormalities have also been proposed as contributing to an altered stress response. Animal studies in rats have found DNA methylation of glucocorticoid receptor leading to decreased expression, resultant impaired feedback inhibition, and an excessive stress response. Patients who have completed suicide and have history of childhood adversity were found in postmortem studies to have increased DNA methylation of the glucocorticoid receptor promoter and less receptor gene expression in the hippocampus compared with those without childhood adversity.[12]

SUICIDE SAFETY ASSESSMENT IN THE INTENSIVE CARE UNIT

Completing a thorough suicide assessment is a complex process involving critical analysis of the patient's individual risk and protective factors, past psychiatric history, current level of suicidality, and ensuring that their environment is safe. This process is best facilitated through psychiatric consultation, ideally with a psychosomatic medicine psychiatrist who is accustomed to the ICU environment. Psychiatric consultants complete a full psychiatric evaluation, as able, with special focus on determining the underlying primary psychiatric disorder and current level of suicidality, identifying the risk and protective factors, and assessing the need for psychotropic medications.

Current State of Suicidality

Suicidality can be conceptualized to be on a continuum starting on one end with thoughts of hopelessness and not wanting to be alive ("What's the point?"), and progressing through to thoughts of self-harm, developing specific plans, intent to act on suicidal plan, and the final stage of attempting suicide, successful or not. Suicidal patients move through these phases dynamically with most patients remaining ambivalent to last moment about dying[13] and the eventual decision to perform a suicide attempt is often impulsive.[14]

In patients specifically admitted to the ICU after a suicide attempt, it is important to address whether active suicidal thoughts, plans, or intent are present. However, it is also essential that their feelings about surviving a suicide attempt must be explored and assessed. One study detailed the patient's perspective of waking up in the ICU after a failed suicide attempt and experiencing despair, shame, fear, sense of inferiority, guilt, and ambivalence about surviving.[15] It is reassuring when a patient expresses feelings of remorse about attempting suicide and denies the presence of active suicidality, but does not mitigate the need to safeguard the patient's environment and maintain close observation. The other extreme is when a patient is upset about having survived, expresses feelings of hopelessness and worthlessness, and confirms the presence of ongoing suicidality. In this situation, all safety measures and proactive psychiatric management should be instituted immediately.

Risk Factors

The goal of an individualized suicide assessment is to identify, treat, and manage patient-specific risk factors acutely.[16] There have been many factors that have been associated with increased suicide risk and, even though risk factors are not predictive, they are still positively correlated with future attempts and/or suicide. **Table 2** provides a detailed compilation of risks factors.

Protective Factors

As with risk factors, there have been certain psychosocial factors that have been associated with a decreased risk of suicide. Protective factors for some patients may be a risk factor for others, which emphasizes the importance of conducting an individualized suicide assessment. These factors commonly lead patients to feel socially connected and supported, and provide a base for future fulfillment in life, including parenthood, pregnancy, religion/spirituality, social support, access to care, and family cohesiveness.[14]

Precipitating and Perpetuating Factors

A crucial aspect to fully understanding a patient's mood state and motivation behind a suicide attempt is what psychosocial stressors, triggers, or losses may have

Table 2
Risk factors associated with suicide

Risk Factor	Specific Statistics
Presence of psychiatric disorder	• >90% of all suicides have a psychiatric disorder
Previous suicide attempt	• Most strongly associated risk factor for suicide • 19.8% of suicides had prior attempt • 12%–30% risk of another attempt in year after attempt • 1%–3% risk of completed suicide in year after attempt
Family history	• Having a first-degree relative who completed suicide increases risk 6×
Age	• Highest among people aged 18–29 y • Suicide accounts for ∼20% of all deaths in people aged 15–24 y • Suicide rates for women are highest in those aged 45–54 y • Suicide rates for men are highest in those aged >75 y
Gender	• Men 4× more likely to complete suicide than women • Men represent 79% of all suicides in United States
Suicide method	• Risk of completed suicide 3× higher in those with access to firearms • Men: 56.7% firearms, 25.3% asphyxiation • Women: 36.9% poisoning, 33.8% firearms
Race/ethnicity	• Suicide is second leading cause of death among American Indians/Alaska natives aged 15–34 y, or 2.5× the national average
Substance use disorders	• People with alcohol use disorder are ∼10× more likely to die by suicide • IV users are 14× more likely to commit suicide • Alcohol is involved in 25%–35% of all suicides and is associated with more dangerous attempts

Social factors	• Of those who completed suicide:
	  ○ 31.4% experienced intimate partner problems
	  ○ 26.6% experienced preceding crisis within 2 wk
	  ○ 21% experienced physical health problems
	  ○ 14.6% experienced professional or 13.8% financial problems

Behavioral factors	• Agitation and impulsivity were found in most suicide attempters • 69% of suicide attempters report making attempt in response to fleeting suicidal ideation without careful planning • 92% of suicide attempters report high anxiety at time of attempt
Marital status	• Married persons ≥25 y old had lowest rate of suicide • Increasing risk of suicide: widowed > divorced > never married
Occupation	• Unemployed/unskilled persons are at higher risk of suicide • Physicians considered to be high-risk occupation for suicide
Health status	• Chronic physical illness associated with increased suicide risk • Two or more medical illnesses doubled the risk for suicidal ideation or attempts • High-risk illness: CNS disorders, cancer, chronic pain, AIDS, fibromyalgia
Geography	• Metropolitan areas had lower rates of suicide

Abbreviations: AIDS, acquired immunodeficiency syndrome; CNS, central nervous system.

contributed to the patient's emotional distress and turmoil. Some of these factors may be modifiable, whereas other may not. Categorizing these identified issues allows more directed interventions targeted at what is most relevant and beneficial for the patient. For stressors that are unmodifiable (eg, chronic medical conditions), the focus then becomes equipping patients with set of coping strategies (eg, use of distraction techniques, communication skills) to help them manage or navigate more appropriately. The overall goal is to minimize the contribution of these factors to mood and, thus, risk of suicide.

Environmental Safety Assessment

The ICU, by definition, provides life-sustaining treatment that is unable to be managed at any lower level of care. Administration of these specialized interventions, depending on the extent of medical injury, can range from use of intubation with ventilator support, sedative and analgesics intravenously via central and peripheral lines, and end-organ support (eg, extracorporeal membrane oxygenation, continuous renal replacement therapy/intermittent hemodialysis), which cannot be conducted without lines connecting these supportive machines to the patient. In addition, the patient's physical state in the ICU can be expected to be limited by being critically ill and, depending on method of suicide attempted, possibly with orthopedic injuries requiring traction, casting, or surgical repair. All of these are common for medical care at an ICU level, but can be used for self-harm or attempting suicide; therefore, it is essential that measures are taken to reduce access to items that can be considered dangerous or can be used for self-harm.

The first step in securing a patient's safety is to ensure close monitoring or keeping the patient in the line of sight. In the ICU, the registered nurse (RN) is directly at the bedside most of the time because of the level of medical care that critically ill patients require. When RN/patient ratios decrease to less than 1:1, other means of supervision and prevention of self-harm need to be instituted for moments when the RN is not at bedside, such as 1:1 sitter, obtain covering nurse/staff, or (the less preferred option) using restraints. Direct supervision reduces available opportunities for patients to inflict self-harm via jumping from windows or balconies, asphyxiation with the use of lines or cords, ingestion of medications, or use of sharp objects to cut self. If the patient is in a condition such that a diet can be ordered safely, then food orders should be cut up before arrival or by staff to avoid the need for utensils more than a plastic spoon; an alternative is to serve finger foods that do not require cutlery. Critical analysis of the patient's clinical surroundings with the goal of identifying any potential means of self-harm must be done throughout the day.

Interdisciplinary communication is essential when managing any suicidal patient. This communication allows all staff to maintain a safe environment with removal of any dangerous objects and to contribute to any observational information regarding patients' behavior. Psychiatric treatment often entails close observation of social interactions, behaviors, and tendencies so it is important that all involved staff are in close communication. It also provides a context for any suicidal comments or utterances during care delivery. In the less frequent situation, the critically ill patient may be organized and mentally clear enough to use the well-known maladaptive coping mechanism of splitting staff. Splitting is when a patient uses division of people, objects, medications, and so forth into good and bad categories, with intense fixation on positive and negative attributes. Characterologically challenging patients, like those with drug-seeking behaviors, personality disorders, or traits, can lead to conflict among staff and between treatment team and patient by inducing many negative emotions.

Thereby, tight staff communication minimizes the chances for patients to use the behaviors.

Staff Attitudes Toward Patients Who Self-Harm

Many studies have examined the attitudes of general hospital staff toward patients who self-harm and have consistently found negative attitudes.[17] The most common feelings are of irritation and anger, but staff also experience feelings of anxiety, insecurity, and sympathy.[17] These negative attitudes and emotions have not improved significantly despite heightened suicide awareness in recent years. This fact is compounded by a decline in the number of psychiatric inpatient beds, leading to greater exposure of hospital staff to suicidal patients. Research studies investigated impacts on staff training on the care of suicidal patients and found that it did improve their knowledge and self-reported attitudes.[17] This literature base is what supported the specific requirement of the National Collaborating Centre for Mental Health (NCCMH)[18] for formal training of all clinical staff on the care of patients who self-harm. An improved knowledge base makes them aware of these negative emotions and prevents these from hampering the delivery of care.[19]

The Patient's Perspective

Waking up in an ICU is a frightening and daunting experience. Compounding that is the knowledge of having attempted suicide and never intending to be waking up. One study examined found that most patients experienced ambivalence about whether they wanted to continue to live or die in addition to feelings of shame, guilt, fear, inferiority, and anger.[15] These emotions can lead to many different reactions on waking up, ranging from unwillingness to talk, "drawing their blankets over their heads, keeping their eyes closed, and…turning their backs to personnel,"[15] to seeking support or help by reaching out to staff.

A study from 2009 examined the experiences of patients who self-harm to find that they often had negative reactions and perceptions of their medical care. Most commonly cited issues to be related to their level of involvement in medical decision making, inappropriate staff behavior, and poor knowledge base of staff regarding suicidality and self-harm.[20] This study also found that a more sympathetic approach was correlated with a more positive perception of care received.[20] Using an empathic approach is appropriate in most cases, focusing on trying to understand the patient's feelings and communicating clearly and directly to the patient that staff are there to help.[15]

Suicide Attempts and Completions in General Hospitals

The most serious outcome of treating a suicidal patient is a repeated suicide attempt or completion on the unit. One study in the Veterans Health Administration examined the incidence of attempts or completions, as well as conducting a root-cause analysis for each incident.[21] It identified 50 suicide attempts or completions in the general hospital: 5 completions and 45 attempts. There were 7 attempts and no completions in the ICU. The most common admitting diagnosis was alcohol detoxification, mirroring the high prevalence rates of alcohol use disorders in suicide. The most common method was cutting with a sharp object, followed by overdose and hanging,[21,22] which reinforces the importance of preventing access to means of self-harm. A root-cause analysis was conducted for each of these events, with the most prevalent being poor communication among staff (ie, suicidality not communicated to all members of the team or during handoffs).[23]

There is not much of a literature base exploring the differences between the suicidal patients on a psychiatric unit versus those hospitalized on a medical or surgical unit.

However, some correlated factors have been identified between medical/surgical patients and suicidality, including agitation, impulsivity, high anxiety levels, chronic pain, and number of medical illnesses.[21–24] Agitation preceding a suicide attempt in the hospital was often observed and should serve as a warning sign.[22] It is important to recognize it and determine the underlying cause (ie, unidentified depression/anxiety, delirium) so that appropriate treatment can be initiated. In one Finish study, it was identified that up to 12% of suicide attempters in the hospital met criteria for delirium.[22]

The overall rates of suicide on medical units, surgical units, or ICUs is notably low, with many studies reporting 0.5% to 1% of suicides occurring in this setting.[21–25] Based on current literature, there are 3 high-risk populations on medical/surgical units: patients admitted after a suicide attempt who require medical care before transfer to a psychiatric unit; demented or delirious patients with associated agitation and impulsivity; patients with a newly diagnosed medical illness or those with chronic illnesses with health-related anxiety/worry.[21,25]

INVOLUNTARY PSYCHIATRIC HOLDS IN THE INTENSIVE CARE UNIT

Historically, mentally ill patients were confined to institutions for long, unspecified amounts of time. Legislation regarding mental health treatment in the 1960s went along with similar legislation at the time, the civil rights movement.[26] In the early 1960s, both the District of Columbia and California instituted involuntary, or civil, commitment laws moving toward the current dangerousness model (ie, danger to self or others in those with a mental disorder) with remaining states following suit.[26,27] Then, in 1975, the US Supreme Court ruled in O'Connor v. Donaldson that the primary purpose of involuntary commitment must be active treatment, not just confinement or so-called custodial care. If treatment is not being provided and patients are not a danger to themselves or others, then there is no constitutional basis for confinement.[27]

The situation of a patient who is admitted to the ICU after a suicide attempt is less straightforward because these patients do meet criteria for involuntary commitment but do not legitimately have access to the intended intensive psychiatric treatment as result of their more pressing medical needs. Intensive psychiatric treatment involves daily psychiatric assessment with focus on ascertaining an accurate diagnosis, proactive psychotropic medication management, and multiple forms of therapy: recreational, occupational, individual, group, and milieu therapies.

There are multiple variables that factor into the decision as to when an involuntary hold is placed, including the patient's current level of suicidality, access and physical ability to inflict self-harm, and severity of medical injuries with the focus on anticipated length of stay in the ICU or medical unit. Most patients requiring ICU level of care are limited in their ability physically to inflict legitimate self-harm and, in the context of not having access to intensive psychiatric treatment, it could be argued that it is unnecessary to place a hold if psychiatric consultation is obtained, a suicide assessment is performed (to best of ability), and all safety measures are in place. This argument is more feasible if the patient is expressing remorse about the suicide attempt and is accepting of medical and psychiatric care. However, certain patients are not cooperative, demanding to leave against medical advice (albeit not reasonable or feasible), actively attempting to sabotage their care, showing overt agitation with or without aggression, or refusal of psychiatric treatment. It is these cases in which involuntary hold placement is indicated in an ICU setting so that confinement to hospital is ensured and an opportunity to reattempt suicide is eliminated.

One particularly challenging situation arises when a suicidal patient is refusing psychiatric medications, which are often administered, if medically appropriate and safe, to target and treat the underlying primary psychiatric disorder. These cases require placement of an involuntary hold so that the psychiatric consultant can petition the mental health court for a medication capacity hearing. This hearing allows psychotropic medications to be administered despite the patient's refusal, if the patient is deemed to lack medical decision-making capacity to consent to medications. This process is common in patients with psychotic symptoms and delusion-based beliefs that influence their willingness to take medications. Even if a court order is granted, the available medications that can be administered involuntarily are limited by route of administration because patients often refuse to take medications orally. In these situations, it is crucial that ICU team members and psychiatric consultants are in communication daily with a clearly delineated medical and psychiatric treatment plan.

LIMITATIONS OF SUICIDE ASSESSMENTS

Despite all the knowledge on the risk factors, protective factors, and trends in attempted and completed suicide, clinicians continue to struggle with limitations in suicide assessments for many reasons. There are no current objective tests for suicidality despite improvements in growing knowledge regarding serotonin dysfunction, which forces clinicians to rely on the patient's subjective report regarding level of suicidality. Hence, collateral information is an important part of any thorough psychiatric assessment. A study reported that 80% of suicide completers denied suicidal thoughts in the last verbal communication.[28] According to the American Psychiatric Association (APA), it is impossible for clinicians to predict whether patients will attempt or complete suicide, largely because of the rarity of suicide and resultant statistical challenges with low base rates.[29] In addition, the current use of subjective report, risk, and protective factors in suicide assessment has consistently resulted in high false-positives.[30] As a result, research has explored other means of reducing high false-positives via creation of multiple standardized assessments, scales, and tools, including a computer-based implicit association tests, which has some growing data.

OUTCOMES OF SUICIDE ATTEMPTS

There are currently no studies specifically examining the outcomes of suicide attempts that required ICU admission, but there have been a few that studied the outcomes of those presenting to the ED after a suicide attempt or self-injury. The most recent study evaluated suicide-related ED presentations from 2006 to 2013 via the Nationwide Emergency Department Sample. There was a total in-hospital mortality of 1%, with 0.4% dying in the ED and 0.6% dying after admission.[5,31] One-third of suicide attempters and patients who self-harm were directly hospitalized, and one-third of those were admitted to the ICU.[4,5] No current studies are available that detail the outcomes specifically of those requiring ICU care after they leave the unit; however, the rates of suicide attempts and suicide completions following a suicide attempt range from 12% to 30% and 1% to 3%, respectively.

SUMMARY

Suicidality assessments in patients admitted to the ICU, as in all other settings, consist of a comprehensive evaluation of the patient's clinical status, risk/protective factors, psychiatric history, and current degree of suicidality, with the goals of identifying any primary psychiatric disorders so that appropriate treatment can be initiated and ensuring a safe environment until patients can be transferred to an inpatient psychiatric unit. However, there are multiple challenges specific to an intensive care population, including high risk of comorbid delirium, limitations in communication (eg, intubation, fatigue related to medical illness, sedative medications), and psychotropic medication issues (drug-drug interactions, limited routes of administration, reduction/elimination of deliriogenic medications, potential for medication withdrawal syndromes).

Psychiatric consultants are crucial to the management of suicidal patients on any medical unit, surgical unit, or ICU. Their expertise transcends the suicide assessment to provide diagnostic clarity and thorough psychotropic medication assessment. Psychotropic medications are notorious for their complex mechanisms of actions; in addition there are drug-drug interactions with numerous other medication classes (antibiotics, antiarrhythmic, potential for serotonin toxicity or neuroleptic malignant syndrome with concurrent use of serotoninergic/dopaminergic medications) and effects on impaired organ systems (organs compromised by suicidal act or inherent potential for organ toxicity). Daily psychiatric assessment is required of any suicidal patient so close communication with consultants is paramount. Psychiatrists also facilitate patients' dispositions when they are medically cleared for transfer to inpatient psychiatric hospitals for further stabilization and treatment.

An important aspect to keep in mind is that most patients who self-harm and attempt suicide in the general hospital do so by access to means in their environment; therefore, ensuring that all staff are privy to this is essential for maintaining a safe environment. Also, suicide risk in medical/surgical patients has been associated with high anxiety levels, agitation, and pain, which should be treated proactively to minimize contribution to ongoing suicidality. In addition, staff should be mindful of that suicidal patients often have negative perceptions of the medical care received after a suicide attempt, as well as their own reactive emotions or insecurities to the suicidal patient; both of these factors may present as obstacles to the provision of medical care.

REFERENCES

1. Meyer RE, Salzman C, Youngstrom EA, et al. Suicidality and risk of suicide–definition, drug safety concerns, and a necessary target for drug development: a consensus statement. J Clin Psychiatry 2010;71(8):1–21.
2. Centers for Disease Control and Prevention. National Center for Health Statistics. 2016. Available at: http://www.cdc.gov/nchs/products/databriefs/db241.htm. Accessed November 3, 2016.
3. Shepard DS, Gurewich D, Lwin AK, et al. Suicide and suicidal attempts in the United States: costs and policy implications. Suicide Life Threat Behav 2016; 46(3):352–62.
4. Carmargo CA, Doshi A, Boudreaux ED, et al. National study of US emergency department visits for attempted suicide and self-inflicted injury, 1997-2001. Ann Emerg Med 2005;46(4):369–75.
5. Canner JK, Giuliano K, Selvarajah S, et al. Emergency department visits for attempted suicide and self harm in the USA: 2006–2013. Epidemiol Psychiatr Sci 2016;25:1–9.
6. Bertolote JM, Fleischmann A. Suicide and psychiatric diagnosis: a worldwide perspective. Geneva (Switzerland): Department of Mental Health and Substance Dependence, World Health Organization; 2002.
7. Hawton K, Saunders K, Topiwala A, et al. Psychiatric disorders in patients presenting to hospital following self-harm: systematic review. J Affect Disord 2013; 151:821–30.

8. Bostwick JM,, Pankratz VS, Bostwick JM, et al. Lifetime risk of suicide in schizophrenia. Arch Gen Psychiatry 2005;62:247–53.

9. Nordentoft M, Mortensen PB, Pedersen CB. Absolute risk of suicide after first hospital contact in mental disorder. Arch Gen Psychiatry 2011;68(10): 1058–64.

10. Yuodelis-Flores C, Ries RK. Addiction and suicide: a review. Am J Addict 2015; 24:98–104.

11. Zaheer J, Links PS, Liu E. Assessment and emergency management of suicidality in personality disorders. Psychiatr Clin North Am 2008;31:527–43.

12. Mann JJ, Heeringen K. The neurobiology of suicide. Lancet Psychiatry 2014;1: 63–72.

13. Cornelius JR, Salloum IM, Day NL, et al. Patterns of suicidality and alcohol use in alcoholics with major depression. Alcohol Clin Exp Res 1996;20(8):1451–5.

14. Maldonado JM. Suicide risk assessment and management. Clinical manual of emergency psychiatry. Chapter 2. Virginia: American Psychiatric Publishing, Inc; 2015. p. 33–68.

15. Wolk-Wasserman D. The intensive care unit and their suicide attempt patient. Acta Psychiatr Scand 1985;71:581.

16. Simon RI. Imminent suicide: the illusion of short-term prediction. Suicide Life Threat Behav 2006;36(3):296–301.

17. Saunders K, Hawton K, Fortune S, et al. Attitudes and knowledge of clinical staff regarding people who self-harm: a systematic review. J Affect Disord 2012;139: 205–16.

18. National Collaborating Centre for Mental Health. Clinical guideline self-harm: the short-term physical and psychological management and secondary prevention of self-harm in primary and secondary care. London: National Institute for Clinical Excellence; 2004.

19. Murakami S. Managing the suicidal patient in the intensive care unit. Irwin and Rippe's intensive care medicine. Chapter 200. Philadelphia: Lippincott Williams & Wilkins; 2008. p. 2100–2.

20. Taylor TL, Hawton K, Fortune S, et al. Attitudes towards clinical services among people who self-harm: systematic review. Br J Psychiatry 2009;194:104–10.

21. Mills PD, Watts BV, Hemphill RR. Suicide attempts and completions on medical-surgical and intensive care units. J Hosp Med 2014;9(3):182–5.

22. Bostwick JM, Rackley SJ. Completed suicide in medical/surgical patients: who is at risk? Curr Psychiatry Rep 2007;9:242–6.

23. Mills PD, Watts BV, DeRosier JM, et al. Suicide attempts and completions in the emergency department in Veterans Affairs Hospitals. Emerg Med J 2012;29(5): 399–403.

24. Botega NJ, de Azevedo RC, Mauro ML, et al. Factors associated with suicide ideation among medically and surgically hospitalized patients. Gen Hosp Psychiatry 2010;32:396–400.

25. Tishler CL, Reiss NS. Inpatient suicide: preventing a common sentinel event. Gen Hosp Psychiatry 2009;31:103–9, 105.

26. Testa M, West SG. Civil commitment in the United States. Psychiatry (Edgmont) 2010;7(10):30–40.

27. Goldman A. Continued overreliance on involuntary commitment: the need for a less restrictive alternative. J Leg Med 2015;36(2):233–51.

28. Babeva K, Hughes JL, Asarnow J. Emergency department screening for suicide and mental health risk. Curr Psychiatry Rep 2016;18:100.

29. American Psychiatric Association (APA) guidelines on suicidal behavior (APA, 2003).
30. Fowler JC. Suicide assessment in clinical practice: pragmatic approaches for imperfect assessments. Psychotherapy 2012;49(1):81–90.
31. Dubovsky SL, Dubovsky AN. Mood disorders and the outcome of suicidal thoughts and attempts. Crit Care clinic 2008;24:857–74.

Posttraumatic Stress Disorder Phenomena After Critical Illness

Oscar Joseph Bienvenu, MD, PhD[a],*, Ted-Avi Gerstenblith, MD[b]

KEYWORDS

- Respiratory distress syndrome • Adult • Critical illness • Critical care
- Posttraumatic stress disorders

KEY POINTS

- Experiencing critical illness and intensive care can be extremely stressful.
- Roughly 1 in 5 critical illness survivors have clinically significant posttraumatic stress disorder symptoms in the year after intensive care.
- Patient-friendly documenting of events during the period of critical illness and intensive care seems to help patients and their family members to later process what occurred and be less distressed.

INTRODUCTION

With advances in critical care medicine, more patients are surviving critical illnesses, sometimes making miraculous recoveries. However, many survivors cannot be considered "well" at the time they leave the intensive care unit (ICU) or acute care hospital.[1] That is, many survivors have reduced physical functioning,[2,3] cognitive impairments,[4,5] and other psychiatric morbidity,[6–8] and these problems may be long-lasting.[9,10] In this article, we focus on one aspect of psychiatric morbidity in critical illness survivors, posttraumatic stress disorder (PTSD) phenomena. To illustrate some points, we present a case, told in the second person (*in italics*), because it is helpful to imagine what being critically ill can be like from the patient's perspective (*imagine you are a patient with no medical training*).

The authors report no relevant commercial or other financial relationships to disclose.
[a] Department of Psychiatry and Behavioral Sciences, Johns Hopkins University School of Medicine, 600 North Wolfe Street - Meyer 115, Baltimore, MD 21287, USA; [b] Department of Psychiatry and Behavioral Sciences, Johns Hopkins University School of Medicine, 600 North Wolfe Street - Meyer 106, Baltimore, MD 21287, USA
* Corresponding author.
E-mail address: obienve1@jhmi.edu

Crit Care Clin 33 (2017) 649–658
http://dx.doi.org/10.1016/j.ccc.2017.03.006
criticalcare.theclinics.com

WHAT IS STRESSFUL ABOUT CRITICAL ILLNESS?

You are 52 years old and healthy. You have a good job, a close family, and lots of friends. One day you get a "cold," with a nagging cough. You try over-the-counter remedies, which seem to help a bit, but you get sicker, with subjective fever and pain when you cough. Your spouse notices you look really unwell in the morning and talks you into an urgent appointment with the primary care physician you see rarely, although you will have to miss an important meeting at work. Your doctor calls an ambulance when she checks your vitals and sees that your temperature is very high, your pulse is fast, your blood pressure is low, and you are breathing rapidly but still seem hungry for air. On the way to the emergency room, the paramedic puts a tight-fitting mask on you to administer oxygen and starts an intravenous line to administer fluids. You feel panicky and sense you are dying. In the emergency room, staff are concerned, attaching devices, drawing blood, getting radiographs, and asking you and your spouse whether it is okay to put a tube down your throat to help you breathe. Your spouse insists you were perfectly healthy a week ago and to do all that is needed to keep you alive. The nurse gives you some intravenous medication, and everything gets hazy, some of it nightmarish.

Critically ill patients who need intensive care face potentially severe physical and psychic stressors (**Box 1**), including critical illnesses themselves, associated

---

Box 1
Common stressors in the critically ill

- *Respiratory failure.* Hypoxemia and carbon dioxide disturbances can be quite anxiogenic.

- *Invasive procedures.* Having an endotracheal tube or tracheostomy can be quite unnatural and uncomfortable, and deep suctioning is markedly noxious. In addition, many patients need arterial lines, central intravenous lines, chest tubes, and urinary catheters for proper care and monitoring, as well as physical restraints for safety. If patients are not fully alert to the purpose of these procedures, it is easy to imagine why patients might think they are being tortured purposefully, raped, and imprisoned.

- *Inflammation.* Sepsis can involve massive activation of the inflammatory cascade throughout the body, affecting a number of vital organs, including the brain.

- *Hypothalamic–pituitary–adrenal axis activation.* With systemic inflammation, blood vessels become "leaky," and the adrenal glands can be relatively unresponsive to the brain's release of adrenocorticotropic hormone, resulting in less production of cortisol than would normally be expected.

- *High catecholamines levels.* Especially without adequate endogenous cortisol, the adrenal medullae respond with catecholamine release to maintain blood pressure, and critical care clinicians commonly administer these stress mediators for the same purpose.

- *Delirium.* Although intensivists are increasingly aware of the importance of delirium as a risk marker for mortality and long-term cognitive impairment, many clinicians do not appreciate the perceptual disturbances that can co-occur with this manifestation of acute brain dysfunction. Patients can have great difficulty telling what is real versus a nightmare-like distortion, and frightening visual hallucinations and beliefs involving persecution seem to be common when delirium occurs in the context of life-threatening illness.

- *Communication barriers.* Endotracheal tubes, deep sedation, delirium, and muscle weakness can prevent patients from communicating verbally or writing legibly. If patients are stable enough to use speaking valves with tracheostomies, communication can remain limited.

- *Reduced autonomy.* Critically ill patients are often entirely dependent on others, for survival, but also to address their basic needs. Their reduced ability to communicate complicates this reliance on others.

physiologic disturbances, necessary treatments, and difficulty processing what is occurring.[11] **Box 1** lists common stressors in the critically ill.

When you are extubated and more awake, waiting to be transferred from the ICU to a hospital floor, your spouse and medical team tell you that you have been there for 10 days, that you had pneumonia complicated by sepsis (a severe bodily reaction to infection) and acute respiratory distress syndrome or ARDS (the doctor explains that your lungs were like a wet sponge and took a while to recover). You are told that you received intravenous antibiotics, fluids, pain medication, sedative medication to keep you from fighting the breathing machine, another medication to calm you when you were agitated (the staff were concerned you might pull out lines and tubes and had you physically restrained as well at times), and liquid nutrients through a tube that still goes in through your nose to your stomach (you want it OUT, and you want some water, but the nurse explains that you need to pass a swallowing test before you are able to eat and drink normally). You feel weak and uncomfortable, your throat is sore, and it is difficult to process what you are being told, sometimes repeatedly (eg, that you have been "delirious"). Your nurse removes your urinary catheter, and you are helped to void. You go along with what you are told, participate in exercises with the rehabilitation staff, and thank the doctors, nurses, and others for saving your life. However, you feel very uneasy and cannot reconcile your memories with those of the people around you. You speak to your spouse when the two of you are alone and start to process that you have not been abducted, taken to South America, and ritually tortured in elaborate ceremonies (this seemed so REAL!). You learn that, not only was your daughter not murdered, she is alive and well and in school today (your spouse shows you a get well card your daughter made herself). Your spouse is tired and stressed but overjoyed that you are improving; however, your spouse seems to be confused and concerned when you ask about the tribesmen who hurt you. Afterward, you are reluctant to say anything about the frightening experiences you remember so vividly, and you try not to mention them.

ARE POSTTRAUMATIC STRESS PHENOMENA REALLY A PROBLEM AFTER CRITICAL ILLNESS?

After transfer to a medical floor and further rehabilitation, you are able to get around sufficiently to go home and continue to rehabilitate there. However, your memory is not great, nor is your physical endurance, and you cannot return to work right away. You no longer enjoy television shows that feature hospitals, you make excuses not to visit with friends, you avoid your daughter when she has a cold (you are afraid of getting sick again), and you keep thinking about your critical illness (eg, the ambulance ride to the hospital, the emergency room, and the ritual torture that must not have occurred, right?), although you try to push these thoughts out of your mind. It is very difficult to sleep, and when you are able to sleep you have nightmares involving drowning, torture, and danger to yourself and your loved ones. You try to avoid talking with your spouse about what is going on in your mind, because your spouse is stressed with work (had to miss a lot of days when you were in intensive care), caring for your daughter, and the new responsibility of caring for you. You overhear your spouse speaking on the phone about confusing medical bills and financial worries. Thankfully, your sister and in-laws have been able to pitch in and help your family with day-to-day activities and keep up morale in the rest of your household.

In the mid-to-late 2000s, several skeptical groups of clinical researchers simultaneously reviewed what was known about PTSD and PTSD symptoms after critical illness,[12–15] our interest piqued by what pioneers in the field were reporting.[16–19]

Although it was clear there was still much to be learned, all of these skeptical groups concluded that PTSD phenomena were in fact a real potential problem after critical illness,[12–15] as with other life-threatening events like intense military combat and rape.[13] Our clinical experiences with critical illness survivors only added to this conviction.[20–22]

Recently, Parker and colleagues[6] conducted a systematic review and metaanalysis of posttraumatic stress phenomena in critical illness survivors, given the increasing number of relevant studies (36 unique cohorts, 4260 patients).[18,23–61] Several findings deserve mention. First, although prevalence estimates varied across settings, assessment methods, and threshold scores on questionnaire measures, the pooled prevalence of clinically significant PTSD symptoms was at least 20% in the year after a critical illness. Second, risk markers for post-critical illness PTSD included pre-critical illness psychiatric morbidity (eg, common mental illnesses like anxiety and depressive conditions), in-ICU benzodiazepine administration, and early memories of frightening experiences in the ICU. Note that these factors seem to be correlated within persons, which is why we choose the term "risk marker" instead of "risk factor"—whether or not prior psychiatric morbidity long predates the critical illness, patients might receive higher benzodiazepine doses in the ICU because of their high levels of arousal in the context of critical illness and intensive care, and patients with a history of anxiety and depressive conditions might be particularly susceptible to frightening experiences in the context of critical illness.[26] Third, European studies suggested that ICU diaries may help to prevent lasting posttraumatic stress phenomena in survivors. Finally, as expected,[15] PTSD symptoms were associated with substantial decrements in quality of life.

Notably, Parker and colleagues[6] excluded studies of survivors of specific critical illnesses. Thus, it remains unclear whether ARDS and/or septic shock survivors have higher prevalences of PTSD than the broader group of critical illness survivors.[12] This possibility was suggested by results in small but otherwise methodologically rigorous studies conducted by a research group in Germany who used experienced clinicians administering structured interviews to diagnose PTSD and related syndromes, with follow-up after many years.[19,62,63]

SO PSYCHIATRIC ILLNESS IS A "RISK MARKER" FOR PSYCHIATRIC ILLNESS?

Eventually, family members notice your excessive use of an alcohol-based disinfectant on your hands, as well as your reluctance to return to the hospital for outpatient physical therapy. You overhear them say "hypochondriac," and you are ashamed when you realize they must be talking about you. Your spouse gently asks you if you think it would be worthwhile to "get help again." [Years ago you saw a Dr Brown, who is a psychologist or a psychiatrist—you cannot remember the difference—in the context of moving, changing jobs, and difficulty in the marriage. You had been tense and irritable, with difficulty focusing at your new job and trouble sleeping, and speaking with Dr Brown helped you, maybe especially her advice that you reach out to old friends who had gone through similar life changes. You also recall that Dr Brown recommended that you take time each day to do some aerobic exercise, and you and your spouse had taken long walks together as often as you could. Neither of you have been able to do so lately.]

A naïve view of mental illness and distress as a single entity would be as silly as equating all diseases and physiologic perturbations involving the lungs. Obviously, having a history of anxiety or depression does not mean the patient has a history of PTSD (although this would be important to know). Nevertheless, knowing about a prior history of psychiatric illness can be important to help identify patients who may benefit from closer monitoring during a critical illness, or at least during recovery from critical illness. Prior psychiatric history is a known risk factor for PTSD after other life-threatening stressors, as well; critical illnesses are not unique in this regard.[64]

An obvious problem with knowing whether or not a critically ill patient has a history of psychiatric morbidity is that the patient may not be able to communicate clearly, and some family members may not be aware of a patient's prior difficulties with anxiety or depression, at least the most common and less severe forms (most patients with these conditions are not admitted to psychiatric hospitals; they are treated on an outpatient basis, often by primary care physicians). Nevertheless, clinicians often do collect such information eventually during the course of a hospitalization, and it is becoming increasingly clear that the information is useful prognostically, as is early post-critical illness mental distress.[15,46,65]

WHAT ARE INTENSIVE CARE UNIT DIARIES?

You make an appointment to see Dr Brown next week (thankfully, her office is nowhere near the hospital). In addition, your spouse remembers that an ICU nurse recommended that your family keep a journal of what happened while you were critically ill and delirious—including what was going on with you medically and what was going on at home. Your spouse finds the notebook, which includes dated entries for most of the time you were in the ICU, and you are astounded. As you look at the entries, you feel intense anxiety, so you put it down. Later, you pick it up again, and you start to ask questions about it. When you see Dr Brown, you catch her up a bit on your life, and you mention your recent difficulties. Dr Brown is curious to learn more about your critical illness and what you recall. She surprises you by asking whether or not you remember people trying to harm you, and you burst into tears. Dr Brown says she has experience treating delirious patients when she was a psychiatric resident doing consults on medical and surgical units, and she has recently read about the vivid, frightening memories patients can have from the time they were delirious and critically ill. You promise to bring the notebook in next week, and you leave her office feeling understood and strangely hopeful. As time goes on, with Dr Brown's encouragement, you discuss your critical illness, fears of sudden death, and even your memories of what you learn are delirium-associated, nightmare-like distortions of reality and persecutory delusions. You find that you sleep much better, and the nightmares gradually begin to fade. You feel more confident, and you worry less about contracting an infectious disease. You even return to the ICU, where some of the staff remember you and comment on how well you look.

ICU diaries differ from most personal diaries in that they are written in the second person, typically by medical staff and/or family members. Also, unlike medical charts, ICU diaries are written in patient-friendly language. ICU diaries originated in Europe, where many ICUs have follow-up clinics run by ICU clinicians; these clinicians recognized post-critical illness psychiatric morbidity earlier than most of us in North America, where multidisciplinary ICU follow-up clinics are a relatively recent phenomenon.[66–68] Clinicians focusing on these issues also realized a need to help patients fill in gaps in their memories (given deep sedation and delirium owing to medications and organ failure during critical illness) and incorporate factual information into their autobiographical memories (eg, why they might recall being stabbed, tortured, imprisoned, experimented upon, etc). ICU diaries can also help patients to understand how ill they actually were (eg, why they might be so weak), what care they received (many patients recall being alone and helpless), and why they may have scars from lines and tubes. They can also facilitate communication with family members and other clinicians, and patients can look at them when they are ready. (For a wealth of information and literature regarding ICU diaries, visit ICU-diary.org.)

What evidence is there that ICU diaries prevent or lessen long-term PTSD symptoms in critical illness survivors? To our knowledge, the only large-scale (n = 352), multisite, randomized, clinical trial was conducted in 6 European countries.[34] The study could be considered an effectiveness trial, because all of the participating sites had experience with ICU diaries, although there was study coordination and an attempt to standardize the intervention. Patients in both groups completed a baseline PTSD symptom questionnaire at the 1-month follow-up. Those in the intervention group had their ICU diaries handed over afterward, typically in person, by a research nurse or doctor who could explain diary contents (the clinicians gave no explicit advice regarding what to do with the diary). Patients in both groups completed outcome assessments at 3 months. Clinicians writing in the diary only needed a few minutes per day to make entries, slightly more on the day of ICU admission. For the primary outcome, PTSD related to the critical illness and intensive care, the intervention group fared better than the control group. Specifically, only 5% of the patients in the intervention group met the diagnostic criteria for critical illness-related PTSD at the 3-month follow-up, compared to 13% of the patients in the control group. Notably, the patients who had the most symptoms at 1-month follow-up had the greatest benefit from the intervention. Patients in the intervention group read the diary a median of 3 times, and 84% said a family member, friend, colleague, or clinician read the diary. Patients reported what was most helpful was reading text, although many patients also reported benefitting from accompanying photographs. Despite the promise of this large clinical trial and other smaller, less methodologically rigorous studies, the field has a lot to learn about the potential benefits of ICU diaries (eg, the mechanism by which they may be helpful; what therapeutic ingredients might be necessary).[69] In addition, the results of the large study by Jones and colleagues[34] emphasize that having a diary is no guarantee that patients will successfully process what they have gone through, at least by the 3-month follow-up. Nevertheless, ICU diaries are a low-risk, low-tech, and relatively inexpensive intervention compared with most ICU interventions, and they seem to provide a great tool for patients to recover psychologically that can supplement other psychiatric care. We hope that the fear of lawsuits and other barriers to staff participation in ICU diaries in North America are gradually overcome, for the psychological benefit of our patients.

REFERENCES

1. Iwashyna TJ. Survivorship will be the defining challenge of critical care in the 21st century. Ann Intern Med 2010;153(3):204–5.
2. Herridge MS, Cheung AM, Tansey CM, et al. One-year outcomes in survivors of the acute respiratory distress syndrome. N Engl J Med 2003;348(8):683–93.
3. Herridge MS, Tansey CM, Matté A, et al. Functional disability 5 years after acute respiratory distress syndrome. N Engl J Med 2011;364(14):1293–304.
4. Hopkins RO, Suchyta MR, Beene K, et al. Critical illness acquired brain injury: neuroimaging and implications for rehabilitation. Rehabil Psychol 2016;61(2): 151–64.
5. Hopkins RO, Wade D, Jackson JC. What's new in cognitive function in ICU survivors? Intensive Care Med 2017. http://dx.doi.org/10.1007/s00134-016-4550-x.
6. Parker AM, Sricharoenchai T, Raparla S, et al. Posttraumatic stress disorder in critical illness survivors: a metaanalysis. Crit Care Med 2015;43(5):1121–9.

7. Rabiee A, Nikayin S, Hashem MD, et al. Depressive symptoms after critical illness: a systematic review and meta-analysis. Crit Care Med 2016;44(9): 1744–53.
8. Nikayin S, Rabiee A, Hashem MD, et al. Anxiety symptoms in survivors of critical illness: a systematic review and meta-analysis. Gen Hosp Psychiatry 2016; 43:23–9.
9. Needham DM, Davidson J, Cohen H, et al. Improving long-term outcomes after discharge from intensive care unit: report from a stakeholders' conference. Crit Care Med 2012;40(2):502–9.
10. Elliott D, Davidson JE, Harvey MA, et al. Exploring the scope of post-intensive care syndrome therapy and care: engagement of non-critical care providers and survivors in a second stakeholders meeting. Crit Care Med 2014;42(12): 2518–26.
11. Bienvenu OJ, Gellar J, Althouse BM, et al. Post-traumatic stress disorder symptoms after acute lung injury: a 2-year prospective longitudinal study. Psychol Med 2013;43(12):2657–71.
12. Griffiths J, Fortune G, Barber V, et al. The prevalence of post traumatic stress disorder in survivors of ICU treatment: a systematic review. Intensive Care Med 2007;33(9):1506–18.
13. Jackson JC, Hart RP, Gordon SM, et al. Post-traumatic stress disorder and posttraumatic stress symptoms following critical illness in medical intensive care unit patients: assessing the magnitude of the problem. Crit Care 2007;11(1):R27.
14. Davydow DS, Desai SV, Needham DM, et al. Psychiatric morbidity in survivors of the acute respiratory distress syndrome: a systematic review. Psychosom Med 2008;70(4):512–9.
15. Davydow DS, Gifford JM, Desai SV, et al. Posttraumatic stress disorder in general intensive care unit survivors: a systematic review. Gen Hosp Psychiatry 2008; 30(5):421–34.
16. Weinert CR, Gross CR, Kangas JR, et al. Health-related quality of life after acute lung injury. Am J Respir Crit Care Med 1997;156(4 Pt 1):1120–8.
17. Schelling G, Stoll C, Haller M, et al. Health-related quality of life and posttraumatic stress disorder in survivors of the acute respiratory distress syndrome. Crit Care Med 1998;26(4):651–9.
18. Jones C, Griffiths RD, Humphris G, et al. Memory, delusions, and the development of acute posttraumatic stress disorder-related symptoms after intensive care. Crit Care Med 2001;29(3):573–80.
19. Kapfhammer HP, Rothenhäusler HB, Krauseneck T, et al. Posttraumatic stress disorder and health-related quality of life in long-term survivors of acute respiratory distress syndrome. Am J Psychiatry 2004;161(1):45–52.
20. Bienvenu OJ, Williams JB, Yang A, et al. Posttraumatic stress disorder in survivors of acute lung injury: evaluating the Impact of Event Scale-Revised. Chest 2013;144(1):24–31.
21. Schelling G, Kapfhammer HP. Surviving the ICU does not mean that the war is over. Chest 2013;144(1):1–3.
22. Jackson JC, Jutte JE, Hunter CH, et al. Posttraumatic stress disorder (PTSD) after critical illness: a conceptual review of distinct clinical issues and their implications. Rehabil Psychol 2016;61(2):132–40.
23. Cuthbertson BH, Hull A, Strachan M, et al. Post-traumatic stress disorder after critical illness requiring general intensive care. Intensive Care Med 2004;30(3): 450–5.

24. Girard TD, Shintani AK, Jackson JC, et al. Risk factors for post-traumatic stress disorder symptoms following critical illness requiring mechanical ventilation: a prospective cohort study. Crit Care 2007;11(1):R28.

25. Griffiths J, Gager M, Alder N, et al. A self-report-based study of the incidence and associations of sexual dysfunction in survivors of intensive care treatment. Intensive Care Med 2006;32(3):445–51.

26. Jones C, Bäckman C, Capuzzo M, et al. Precipitants of post-traumatic stress disorder following intensive care: a hypothesis generating study of diversity in care. Intensive Care Med 2007;33(6):978–85.

27. Jones C, Skirrow P, Griffiths RD, et al. Rehabilitation after critical illness: a randomized, controlled trial. Crit Care Med 2003;31(10):2456–61.

28. Nickel M, Leiberich P, Nickel C, et al. The occurrence of posttraumatic stress disorder in patients following intensive care treatment: a cross-sectional study in a random sample. J Intensive Care Med 2004;19(5):285–90.

29. Perrins J, King N, Collings J. Assessment of long-term psychological well-being following intensive care. Intensive Crit Care Nurs 1998;14(3):108–16.

30. Rattray JE, Johnston M, Wildsmith JA. Predictors of emotional outcomes of intensive care. Anaesthesia 2005;60(11):1085–92.

31. Samuelson KA, Lundberg D, Fridlund B. Stressful memories and psychological distress in adult mechanically ventilated intensive care patients: a 2-month follow-up study. Acta Anaesthesiol Scand 2007;51(6):671–8.

32. Scragg P, Jones A, Fauvel N. Psychological problems following ICU treatment. Anaesthesia 2001;56(1):9–14.

33. Sukantarat K, Greer S, Brett S, et al. Physical and psychological sequelae of critical illness. Br J Health Psychol 2007;12(Pt 1):65–74.

34. Jones C, Bäckman C, Capuzzo M, et al. Intensive care diaries reduce new onset post traumatic stress disorder following critical illness: a randomised, controlled trial. Crit Care 2010;14(5):R168.

35. Garrouste-Orgeas M, Coquet I, Périer A, et al. Impact of an intensive care unit diary on psychological distress in patients and relatives*. Crit Care Med 2012; 40(7):2033–40.

36. Sackey PV, Martling CR, Carlswärd C, et al. Short- and long-term follow-up of intensive care unit patients after sedation with isoflurane and midazolam–a pilot study. Crit Care Med 2008;36(3):801–6.

37. Strøm T, Stylsvig M, Toft P. Long-term psychological effects of a no-sedation protocol in critically ill patients. Crit Care 2011;15(6):R293.

38. Jackson JC, Girard TD, Gordon SM, et al. Long-term cognitive and psychological outcomes in the awakening and breathing controlled trial. Am J Respir Crit Care Med 2010;182(2):183–91.

39. Treggiari MM, Romand JA, Yanez ND, et al. Randomized trial of light versus deep sedation on mental health after critical illness. Crit Care Med 2009;37(9):2527–34.

40. Cuthbertson BH, Rattray J, Campbell MK, et al. The PRaCTICaL study of nurse led, intensive care follow-up programmes for improving long term outcomes from critical illness: a pragmatic randomised controlled trial. BMJ 2009;339: b3723.

41. van der Schaaf M, Beelen A, Dongelmans DA, et al. Functional status after intensive care: a challenge for rehabilitation professionals to improve outcome. J Rehabil Med 2009;41(5):360–6.

42. Paparrigopoulos T, Melissaki A, Tzavellas E, et al. Increased co-morbidity of depression and post-traumatic stress disorder symptoms and common risk

factors in intensive care unit survivors: a two-year follow-up study. Int J Psychiatry Clin Pract 2014;18(1):25–31.

43. Wade DM, Howell DC, Weinman JA, et al. Investigating risk factors for psychological morbidity three months after intensive care: a prospective cohort study. Crit Care 2012;16(5):R192.

44. Azoulay E, Kouatchet A, Jaber S, et al. Noninvasive mechanical ventilation in patients having declined tracheal intubation. Intensive Care Med 2013;39(2): 292–301.

45. Davydow DS, Kohen R, Hough CL, et al. A pilot investigation of the association of genetic polymorphisms regulating corticotrophin-releasing hormone with posttraumatic stress and depressive symptoms in medical-surgical intensive care unit survivors. J Crit Care 2014;29(1):101–6.

46. Davydow DS, Zatzick D, Hough CL, et al. A longitudinal investigation of posttraumatic stress and depressive symptoms over the course of the year following medical-surgical intensive care unit admission. Gen Hosp Psychiatry 2013; 35(3):226–32.

47. Bugedo G, Tobar E, Aguirre M, et al. The implementation of an analgesia-based sedation protocol reduced deep sedation and proved to be safe and feasible in patients on mechanical ventilation. Rev Bras Ter Intensiva 2013;25(3):188–96.

48. Schandl A, Bottai M, Hellgren E, et al. Gender differences in psychological morbidity and treatment in intensive care survivors–a cohort study. Crit Care 2012;16(3):R80.

49. Twigg E, Humphris G, Jones C, et al. Use of a screening questionnaire for posttraumatic stress disorder (PTSD) on a sample of UK ICU patients. Acta Anaesthesiol Scand 2008;52(2):202–8.

50. Wallen K, Chaboyer W, Thalib L, et al. Symptoms of acute posttraumatic stress disorder after intensive care. Am J Crit Care 2008;17(6):534–43.

51. Myhren H, Ekeberg Ø, Stokland O. Health-related quality of life and return to work after critical illness in general intensive care unit patients: a 1-year follow-up study. Crit Care Med 2010;38(7):1554–61.

52. Myhren H, Ekeberg O, Tøien K, et al. Posttraumatic stress, anxiety and depression symptoms in patients during the first year post intensive care unit discharge. Crit Care 2010;14(1):R14.

53. Myhren H, Tøien K, Ekeberg O, et al. Patients' memory and psychological distress after ICU stay compared with expectations of the relatives. Intensive Care Med 2009;35(12):2078–86.

54. Weinert CR, Sprenkle M. Post-ICU consequences of patient wakefulness and sedative exposure during mechanical ventilation. Intensive Care Med 2008; 34(1):82–90.

55. da Costa JB, Marcon SS, Rossi RM. Posttraumatic stress disorder and the presence of recollections from an intensive care unit stay. J Bras Psiquiatr 2012;61(1): 13–9.

56. Schandl AR, Brattström OR, Svensson-Raskh A, et al. Screening and treatment of problems after intensive care: a descriptive study of multidisciplinary follow-u. Intensive Crit Care Nurs 2011;27(2):94–101.

57. Granja C, Gomes E, Amaro A, et al. Understanding posttraumatic stress disorder-related symptoms after critical care: the early illness amnesia hypothesis. Crit Care Med 2008;36(10):2801–9.

58. Badia-Castelló M, Trujillano-Cabello J, Serviá-Goixart L, et al. Recall and memory after intensive care unit stay. Development of posttraumatic stress disorder. Med Clin (Barc) 2006;126(15):561–6.

59. Richter JC, Waydhas C, Pajonk FG. Incidence of posttraumatic stress disorder after prolonged surgical intensive care unit treatment. Psychosomatics 2006; 47(3):223–30.
60. Rattray J, Johnston M, Wildsmith JA. The intensive care experience: development of the ICE questionnaire. J Adv Nurs 2004;47(1):64–73.
61. Van Ness PH, Murphy TE, Araujo KL, et al. Multivariate graphical methods provide an insightful way to formulate explanatory hypotheses from limited categorical data. J Clin Epidemiol 2012;65(2):179–88.
62. Schelling G, Briegel J, Roozendaal B, et al. The effect of stress doses of hydrocortisone during septic shock on posttraumatic stress disorder in survivors. Biol Psychiatry 2001;50(12):978–85.
63. Stoll C, Kapfhammer HP, Rothenhäusler HB, et al. Sensitivity and specificity of a screening test to document traumatic experiences and to diagnose posttraumatic stress disorder in ARDS patients after intensive care treatment. Intensive Care Med 1999;25(7):697–704.
64. Brewin CR, Andrews B, Valentine JD. Meta-analysis of risk factors for posttraumatic stress disorder in trauma-exposed adults. J Consult Clin Psychol 2000; 68(5):748–66.
65. Davydow DS. Posttraumatic stress disorder in critical illness survivors: too many questions remain. Crit Care Med 2015;43(5):1151–2.
66. Lasiter S, Oles SK, Mundell J, et al. Critical care follow-up clinics: a scoping review of interventions and outcomes. Clin Nurse Spec 2016;30(4):227–37.
67. Khan BA, Lasiter S, Boustani MA. Critical care recovery center: an innovative collaborative care model for ICU survivors. Am J Nurs 2015;115(3):24–31.
68. Huggins EL, Bloom SL, Stollings JL, et al. A clinic model: post-intensive care syndrome and post-intensive care syndrome - family. AACN Adv Crit Care 2016; 27(2):204–11.
69. Aitken LM, Rattray J, Hull A, et al. The use of diaries in psychological recovery from intensive care. Crit Care 2013;17(6):253.

Psychiatric Aspects of Organ Transplantation in Critical Care: An Update

Yelizaveta Sher, MD[a],*, Paula Zimbrean, MD[b]

KEYWORDS

- Psychiatric • Organ transplantation • Critical care • Update

KEY POINTS

- Transplant patients face challenging medical journeys, with many detours to the intensive care unit.
- Before and after transplantation they have significant psychological and cognitive comorbidities, which decrease their quality of life and potentially compromise their medical outcomes.
- Critical care staff are essential in these journeys.
- Being cognizant of relevant psychosocial and mental health aspects of transplant patients' experiences can help critical care personnel to take comprehensive care of these patients.

INTRODUCTION

Intensive care unit (ICU) teams play an integral part in the medical journeys of transplant patients. They stabilize patients prior and after transplant surgery and provide care to patients with rejections or other complications. Appreciating psychosocial and psychiatric aspects of these patients' journeys is crucial to provide comprehensive care. Few advancements have been published since the excellent review on this topic was written in 2009 by DiMartini and colleagues.[1] Thus, this review aims to inform the reader with the most up-to-date information on the psychosocial aspects of transplant patients in the ICU, including pretransplant evaluation, psychological considerations of assist devices in the ICU, peri-transplant mood and cognitive disorders, and relevant psychopharmacology.

This article is an update of an article previously published in *Critical Care Clinics*, Volume 24, Issue 4, October 2008.
Disclosure Statement: The authors have nothing to disclose.
[a] Department of Psychiatry and Behavioral Sciences, Stanford University Medical Center, 401 Quarry Road, Suite 2320, Stanford, CA, 94305, USA; [b] Departments of Psychiatry and Surgery (Transplant), Yale New Haven Hospital, 20 York Street, Fitkin 611, New Haven, CT 06511, USA
* Corresponding author.
E-mail address: ysher@stanford.edu

EPIDEMIOLOGY OF TRANSPLANTATION

Based on the Organ Procurement and Transplantation Network data as of November 2016, 119,857 patients were waiting on the transplant list in the United States.[2] Many patients wait on the transplant list before an appropriate organ is identified, and others die before ever receiving such an organ. Living donation has become an option for many candidates, improving survival. Yet, there are more patients in need of a life-saving donation than donors available. To date, every 10 minutes one patient is added to the transplant list, and 22 patients die every day waiting on the transplant list.[2]

Following the tremendous surgical and medication improvements in the last decades, patients' survival after transplantation has continued to improve. As of December 2012, 83.4% of deceased and 92.0% of live-donor kidney recipients survive more than 5 years.[2] Similarly, 74.3% of patients receiving a liver from decreased donors and 81.3% of patients receiving a liver from live donors survive more than 5 years. Although 76.8% of heart recipients survive beyond 5 years, only 55.2% of all lung recipients live beyond 5 years.

PRETRANSPLANT PERIOD
Psychosocial Transplant Evaluation

Patients considered for transplantation require psychosocial evaluation focused on cognitive, psychological, behavioral, and social aspects of their life, which may influence the success of transplantation. The primary goal of this evaluation is to recognize patients' strengths and to identify their vulnerabilities with the goal of designing a multimodal plan to maximize patients' candidacy and ensure posttransplant success. Studies have shown that psychosocial evaluation can predict posttransplant morbidity and mortality.[3–6] Psychosocial risk factors most recognized as correlated with posttransplant morbidity and mortality include lack of functional social support and nonadherence to the posttransplant regimen. Other factors that may adversely influence the outcome of transplantation include uncontrolled psychiatric disorders and substance use disorders (SUDs).

Several psychosocial rating tools have been created to standardize such assessments and to ensure fairness in patient selection. Older tools include the Transplant Evaluation Rating Scale, adapted from the Psychosocial Levels System,[7] and the Psychosocial Assessment of Candidates for Transplantation.[8] The most recently developed tool is the Stanford Integrated Psychosocial Assessment for Transplantation.[4,5] Dedicated transplant social workers are usually the first clinicians to conduct such evaluations, usually leaving the most complex cases to the transplant psychiatrists. In addition to direct patient evaluation, a comprehensive transplant evaluation seeks to obtain collateral information from family caregivers and health care providers.

When patients are evaluated for transplantation in the ICU, the critical care staff can provide a crucial role in the evaluation process. Through their own interactions, during their customary provision of care, the staff is able to observe how patients and caregivers deal with the extreme stress of ICU hospitalization and each other (eg, observe family structure and dynamics). This information is important to build on, as patients will require strong and reliable caregivers after transplantation to ensure their well-being and success.

Waiting Period

The waiting period can be extremely challenging for many patients. Recipients often feel in a state of limbo, with their lives frozen into survival mode, waiting for the call with mixed emotions (ie, fear and excitement). In a qualitative study of transplant recipients, the time waiting for the transplant was described as the time haunted by death.[9] Transplant patients describe their notion of life taken away, their shock at the situation, and their sense that "no real choice" was given to them.[9] Yet, they must work through their complex feelings, for example, garnering most motivation to go forward, while quietly preparing for the worst. Although most of the waiting period is used to prepare for the transplant and waiting for a suitable donor, this is a golden opportunity to assist patients, caregivers, and members of the transplant team address end-of-life issues.[1]

Some patients present for the transplant surgery from home, finally having received the call, with a mixture of excitement and fear. Other patients experience multiple dry runs during which they have been called to come to the hospital just to find out that the offered organs are unsuitable for transplantation. This period is usually filled with strong negative emotions of fear, disappointment, and frustration. They may be followed by subsequent anxiety and disbelief about the next time they are called to the hospital for transplantation.

Not uncommonly, patients wait for their organ in the critical care setting. Often, these patients are the sickest of all and the most in need for the life-saving operation. Their condition is usually tenuous, as a new infection or failure of another organ may make them medically ineligible for transplantation. The staff taking care of such patients bear a lot of emotional stress and may have a lot of mixed feelings (ie, countertransference) and yet often provide the most support to these most vulnerable patients and their families.

Psychological Considerations in Assistive Devices in Intensive Care Unit

Ventricular assist devices for heart transplant candidates

Implantable assist devices (eg, left ventricular assist device [LVAD]) are often used in patients with heart failure to provide adequate systemic blood flow.[10] They are used as a bridge to transplantation (BTT), a bridge to recovery, or, increasingly, destination therapy (DT). In fact, in 2014, DT accounted for 45.7% of all implanted LVADs, BTT accounted for 30.3%, while bridge to potential transplant candidacy (ie, with LVAD recipient addressing modifiable medical or psychosocial contraindications to become a suitable heart transplant candidate) accounted for 23.2%.[11]

LVADs have revolutionized the treatment of heart failure and made the road to transplantation possible for many patients. Over the last decades, the machines have become smaller, more affordable, and durable, progressing cumbersome and adverse event-prone pulsatile-flow ventricular assist devices (VADs) to continuous-flow VADs. However, these patients continue to experience significant physical, cognitive, and psychological challenges. Reported side effects for continuous-flow LVADs/biventricular VADs include bleeding (7.8 events per 100 patient months during the first 12 months), infection (7.28 events), and stroke (1.61 events).[11] Psychiatric complications are reported as 0.93 events per 100 patient months.[11]

Similar to patients undergoing transplantation evaluation, LVAD candidates require a psychosocial evaluation. Thus, again, critical care staff may provide vital information regarding the patients' and their caregivers' state of mind and offer an insight into their relationship. LVAD candidates found to be at a high psychosocial risk during the initial evaluation for VAD implantation, experienced significantly fewer out-of-hospital days after discharge as compared to low-risk patients.[12] Additionally, depression has been found to increase the risk of infections[13] and the incidence of hospital readmissions[14] after LVAD implantation.

Even though up to 75% of patients with heart failure experience cognitive deficits, data suggest that cognition stabilizes or improves somewhat after implantation of continuous-flow LVADs.[15] However, studies with older models of VADs have shown that patients who were bridged to transplantation with VADs retained more cognitive impairment (CI) and had more difficulties with social functioning, as compared with patients with heart transplant who were not bridged.[16]

Overall, LVAD patients usually experience an improvement in their quality of life (QoL) compared with the preimplantation period. However, VAD patients may experience significant psychological challenges, given the challenges posed by the unique characteristics of the VAD procedure: alterations in body image, securing battery power for the device, loss of independence, managing transplant expectations, limitations of physical activity (eg, swimming, driving), personal care (eg, bathing), and effects on intimacy.[17] Emotional distress and adjustment disorders have been described after device implantation.[14] At least one suicide after LVAD implantation has also been documented.[18]

One study demonstrated that two-thirds of LVAD patients required mental health interventions, consisting of supportive psychotherapy, pharmacotherapy, or both.[19] Yet, the use of psychotropic agents requires great care because of the increased risk of bleeding (associated with serotonergic antidepressants) as well as myocardial scarring leading to prolonged QTc interval (associated with antipsychotics, tricyclic antidepressants, and citalopram).[10]

Extracorporeal membrane oxygenation in lung transplant patients

Extracorporeal membrane oxygenation (ECMO) is used in severely ill patients whose risk of dying is greater than 50%.[20] During ECMO, patients' blood is actively pumped through an external artificial lung, providing gas exchange and blood pressure support.[20] Adverse events can include hemorrhage, extremity ischemia, pump failure, oxygenator failure, and thrombus formation. Increasingly, ECMO is used as a bridge to lung transplantation and for the support of primary graft dysfunction after transplantation. When used as BTT, one of its goals is to allow patients to continue a degree of physical activity, preserve strength, and avoid deconditioning. In the experience of one center, of the 43 patients on BTT ECMO, 25 patients continued to ambulate with physical therapy before transplantation. Of the 23 (53.5% of total) patients successfully bridged to transplant, 20 survived and were discharged (87.0% of patients who underwent transplant), with a 1-year survival similar to patients not bridged with ECMO.[21]

Although providing obvious survival benefits, the additional instrumentation carries an added psychological burden. More than 40% of patients surviving ECMO in the ICU go on to develop posttraumatic stress disorder (PTSD) symptoms, a number that is twice as high as other ICU survivors.[22] In a qualitative study of 10 long-term ECMO survivors (that included transplant patients), patients identified their rapid deterioration and clinical crisis before ECMO initiation as a traumatic memory.[22] More than 50% of patients described experiencing distressing symptoms of delirium.[22] Again, the critical care staff can play an important role in identifying those experiencing emotional distress and providing psychological support for those in need. Psychiatric consultation should be sought out if further support is needed.

PSYCHIATRIC DISORDERS IN TRANSPLANT PATIENTS
Depression and Anxiety

Depression and anxiety are common and frequently comorbid in patients experiencing chronic medical illness. Although up to a quarter of patients with heart disease have at least one episode of major depressive disorder (MDD) during their lifetime, even greater numbers have subsyndromal symptoms.[23] Increased symptoms of depression have been found in 10% of adolescents and 19% of adults in a large epidemiologic study of patients with cystic fibrosis (CF), whereas increased anxiety has been identified in 22% of adolescents and 32% of adults with CF.[24] A meta-analysis of patients with chronic obstructive pulmonary disease (COPD) (8 controlled studies, n = 5552 subjects) found depression in 27.1% of patients, compared with 10% of controls.[25]

In fact, in a study evaluating patients undergoing lung transplant evaluation, 41.5% and 61.0% of patients were found to have current and lifetime prevalence of psychiatric disorders, respectively. In this sample, 11.8% of patients had a mood disorder and 39.8% experienced clinical anxiety.[26] Similarly, 39.4% of patients referred for liver transplantation evaluation were found to be depressed.[27]

Although many patients experience a honeymoon period after a successful transplantation, depression and anxiety often resume after surgery. Among 178 lung transplant recipients and 126 heart transplant recipients followed up to 2 years after transplantation, 18% and 8% of patients were diagnosed with panic disorder, 22% and 14% with adjustment disorder with anxiety, and 30% and 26% with MDD, respectively.[28]

Some patients may develop PTSD related to the transplant experience (PTSD-T) and ICU stay.[29] In a study of heart and lung transplant recipients, 14% to 15% of patients experienced PTSD-T mostly within the first year after transplant.[28] ICU personnel may be especially helpful in identifying patients at risk for PTSD-T and possibly initiating interventions aimed at prevention. Some predictors for the development of ICU-related PTSD-T include prior psychopathology, greater ICU benzodiazepine administration, and post-ICU memories of in-ICU frightening and/or psychotic experiences.[30] These predictors can be more easily identified by the ICU staff than any other member of the team. Some studies indicate that ICU diaries in critical illness survivors may be helpful in the prevention of post-ICU PTSD development.[31] In some studies, ICU nurses and physicians initiate the diaries with contribution from patients and their family members.[32]

The development of depression and anxiety after transplantation decreases patients' QoL and can also have negative effects on morbidity and mortality. In a meta-analysis of 27 studies (n = 53,158 heart, liver, kidney, lung, and pancreas recipients), depression increased patients' relative risk of mortality and death-censored graft loss risk.[33] In another study, early posttransplant depression among lung transplant recipients was associated with bronchiolitis obliterans syndrome, graft loss, and increased mortality.[34]

Suicidality

Some of the most challenging clinical cases in the critical care environment include patients presenting with fulminant hepatic failure after an acetaminophen overdose, often intentional. In many cases, a careful and comprehensive psychosocial evaluation cannot be performed because of the critical state, the emergent timeframe, a compromised mental status, or patients' tenuous medical status. Psychosocial providers find these cases challenging and may differ on their recommendations across different centers.[35] However, good outcomes have been reported in small retrospective studies of patients presenting with fulminant hepatic failure due to intentional acetaminophen overdose.[36] Still, these patients remain at higher risk for future self-harm and should receive a careful mental health assessment and, if needed, substance abuse treatment on discharge from the hospital.

Critical care staff taking care of these patients and interacting with potential caregivers can provide invaluable information about patients' mental status and family dynamics and help teams make appropriate assessments and decisions regarding transplant candidacy. They can help educate patients and their families and provide supportive and nonjudgmental education regarding long-term risks and the importance of rigorous mental health follow-up.[35]

Severe Mental Illness

Previously, severe mental illness was considered a relative or even absolute contraindication to transplantation in many programs.[37] Yet, published case reports and small studies have demonstrated that patients with psychotic or mood disorders can do well after transplantation.[38,39] However, it is important for critical care and hospital staff to be able to recognize patients with psychosis or mood disorder and be prepared to assist in the care of these patients. This assistance includes being able to respect patients' personal and psychological boundaries, explain why and what is going on with patients, and be skilled in verbal de-escalation techniques. Of special challenge in the immediate postoperative period and critical care setting is being ability to recognize and distinguish delirium from an exacerbation of another underlying psychiatric disorder in patients experiencing mental status change. Nevertheless, taking into consideration pharmacodynamics and kinetic issues, antipsychotics are usually the first-choice agent to help manage the behavioral manifestations of these conditions in the critical care setting.

Cognitive Impairment and Delirium

CI is common in end-stage chronic illness. Patients with end-stage renal disease (ESRD) may experience hypertension, cardiovascular disease, uremia, and other metabolic derangements that may contribute to CI. Fluid and volume shifts, electrolyte abnormalities, and hypoxia contribute to CI in patients undergoing hemodialysis. In a study of 338 subjects on hemodialysis, 13.9% of subjects had mild CI, 36.1% had moderate CI, and 37.3% had severe CI.[40]

Patients with liver disease may experience hepatic encephalopathy (HE) and persistent CI. Some of the etiologies of liver disease may also carry an increased risk for HE, for example, patients with liver cirrhosis due to alcoholic liver disease (ALD) are more likely to have HE (43% cumulative incidence at 2 years) compared with patients with viral liver cirrhosis (23% incidence at 2 years).[41] Although CI usually improves after liver transplantation, patients with pretransplant CI tend to have worse posttransplant cognitive recovery, QoL, and physical functioning.[42]

Patients with end-stage lung disease frequently experience CI due to hypoxia. In fact, a study found that 47% of lung transplant recipients had CI before the transplant.[43] Low cardiac outputs, comorbid cerebrovascular disease, and vascular complications due to mechanical circularity supports are all factors that contribute to CI in heart transplant candidates.

These impairments make it more challenging for patients to care for themselves, process new information, follow instructions, and understand ICU structure, all of which places them at higher risk for delirium. When delirium develops during the posttransplant period, it can significantly complicate the rate of postsurgical recovery. Studies have found that some transplant recipients experiencing ICU delirium describe feeling disorganized, experiencing nightmares and perceptual disturbances, feeling paranoid, all leading to a terrifying lack of control and mistrust of hospital personnel and perceiving a sense of physical threat. Overtime, patients may feel embarrassed about their experience and behavior while delirious.[9]

A study of patients after orthotopic liver transplantation (OLT) (n = 281) found that 10% experienced delirium in the ICU.[44] In this sample, risk factors included intraoperative transfusion (odds ratio [OR] 1.15), pretransplant dialysis (OR 12.12), and increased Acute Physiology and Chronic Health Evaluation II score (OR per unit increase 1.10). Delirium was also associated with a 2-fold increased risk for longer hospital stays, a 4-fold risk of dying in the hospital, and 3-fold risk of death within 1 year after transplantation. Another study demonstrated 11% incidence of agitated delirium in liver transplant recipients.[45] A prospective study of lung transplant recipients (n = 63) found a 37% incidence of delirium within the first postoperative week.[46] Development of delirium was associated with preoperative CI[46] and reduced perfusion pressure during the lung transplantation surgery.[47] The presence and duration of delirium were further associated with increased postoperative length of hospital stay.[46] In an earlier study, post–lung transplant delirium was also associated with increased duration of ventilator support.[48]

These findings demonstrate the importance of instituting a system to formally screen all transplant recipients for the occurrence of delirium and, when appropriate, to implement prophylactic measures to decrease risk and duration of the syndrome. See José R. Maldonado's article, "Acute Brain Failure: Pathophysiology, Diagnosis, Management and Sequelae of Delirium," in this issue, for a detailed discussion of delirium screening and management in the critical care setting.

The confusion assessment method for the ICU and the Intensive Care Delirium Screening Checklist are the most-used and validated screening tools for monitoring delirium in the ICU. These tools are recommended for use by the Society of Critical Care Medicine.[49]

A positive screen should be followed by a thorough clinical evaluation to diagnose delirium, identify contributing causes, and design and implement an appropriate treatment plan. The differential diagnosis for postoperative delirium among transplant recipients includes primary graft dysfunction, infection, metabolic derangements, electrolyte imbalances, the ICU environment itself, various pharmacologic agents (ie, opiates, benzodiazepines, steroids, immunosuppressants, voriconazole, lidocaine), and renal insufficiency. Posterior reversible encephalopathy syndrome (PRES) is a rare but serious condition that may present with delirium and is further discussed later in this article.

Although there is robust evidence in support of nonpharmacologic interventions (ie, multicomponent interventions) for the prevention of delirium in non-ICU populations,[50] there is a lack of evidence in support of these modalities in the ICU setting, except for early mobilization, which is widely recognized as the best delirium prevention technique in any setting.[49]

Substance Use Disorders

SUDs may be the underlying cause for the disease process leading to end-organ failure and transplantation (eg, cocaine-induced cardiomyopathy, amphetamine-induced pulmonary hypertension) or may be a comorbid problem. Hepatitis C, usually secondary to intravenous (IV) substance use, and ALD are the cause of 60% of all liver transplantations.[51] COPD, often acquired or exacerbated by tobacco smoking, accounts for one-third of all lung transplantations. Transplant programs frequently require abstinence from all substances in patients with an SUD. Most programs adhere to the 6-month abstinence rule, even though there are limited data supporting this duration of abstinence as an optimal cutoff point for improved outcomes. Although this time frame may allow patients to gain insight into their SUD and/or attend appropriate rehabilitation treatments, true recovery from substance use takes months to years and requires commitment and support from the patients' extended psychosocial support system. On the other hand, patients may not have 6 months to engage in appropriate treatments or may be unable to truly benefit from a program because of CI.

A review of 54 transplant studies (50 liver, 3 kidney, and 1 heart), found that the average alcohol relapse rates (examined only in liver studies) were 5.6 cases per 100 patients per year (PPY) for relapse to any alcohol use and 2.5 cases per 100 PPY for relapse with heavy alcohol use.[52] Illicit drug relapse in all patients averaged 3.7 cases per 100 PPY. Average rates in tobacco use relapse and immunosuppressant and clinic appointment nonadherence were 2 to 10 cases per 100 PPY. Among liver transplant recipients, the presence of the following factors were associated with small but significant associations with alcohol use relapse after transplantation: poorer social support, family alcohol history, and pretransplantation abstinence of less than 6 months.[52]

Acute alcohol hepatitis

Recently, patients with acute alcoholic hepatitis (AH) refractory to medical management, with high 6-month mortality and no time to engage in rehabilitation treatment or to demonstrate 6-month sobriety, have been considered and received a transplant.[53,54] In a few small pilot programs, these patients have achieved favorable short-term survival rates, compared with patients with AH not offered OLT[53] or patients with ALD who achieved 6-month sobriety.[54] The overall alcohol relapse rates in transplant patients with AH have been reported to be similar to patients with ALD. However, more transplant patients with AH engaged in hazardous drinking once relapsed.[54] Of note, in one small study, the deaths of 2 transplant patients with AH were attributed to their alcohol relapse.[54] This patient population may evoke strong emotions in the critical care staff caring for them and raise ethical questions regarding organs and resource allocation. Thus, it is important for each institution to have clear guidelines regarding patient selection.

Patients with acute AH are at potential risk for alcohol withdrawal syndromes (AWSs) and should be diligently monitored for that possibility. AWSs present with autonomic instability, which includes hypertension, tachycardia, diaphoresis, tremors, and increased deep tendon reflexes. Often, these symptoms can be confused with hyperactive delirium or another medical process accompanied with high sympathomimetic activity. Alcohol withdrawal can manifest in alcohol withdrawal seizures within 48 to 72 hours of cessation of alcohol intake or progress to delirium tremens within 7 days of such cessation. Treatment of AWS in the critical care setting may include benzodiazepines with shorter half-lives and requiring only glucuronidation (eg, lorazepam) or alternative benzodiazepine-sparing modalities, such as alpha-2 agonists, which do not have the risk of delirium associated with benzodiazepines.[55,56] For more details regarding the use of the benzodiazepine-sparing protocol refer to José R. Maldonado's article, "Novel Algorithms for the Prophylaxis & Management of Alcohol Withdrawal Syndromes – Beyond Benzodiazepines," in this issue. Patients with ALD and AH are likely to be malnourished and, thus, at risk for the development of Wernicke encephalopathy. Therefore, thiamine supplementation should be instituted in these patients to prevent the development of this neurologic emergency.

Methadone maintenance therapy

Many patients with end-stage liver disease secondary to hepatitis C have a history of opioid use disorder, in particular heroin, and may benefit from methadone maintenance therapy (MMT). Although in the past programs required patients with opioid use disorder to taper off methadone before liver transplant consideration, this strategy has been recognized to place patients at greater risk of relapse on opioids and, thus, worsen their chances of survival. Thus, it is now recommended to continue MMT and to offer liver transplantation to patients otherwise meeting the appropriate medical and psychosocial criteria. Patients on MMT can do well after transplant and have comparable outcomes with other patients after liver transplantaton.[57,58] However, their intraoperative anesthesia and posttransplant analgesia requirements might be higher because of the development of tolerance.[57] Expert psychiatric or pain management consultation is most suited to optimize pain management in this patient population.

PSYCHOPHARMACOLOGY IN TRANSPLANT PATIENTS
Effects of Immunosuppressant Medications

Steroids
High-dose corticosteroids are often used to facilitate immunosuppression in combination with other agents during the acute posttransplant period. Furthermore, patients who present with acute rejections are customarily treated with pulsed corticosteroid doses.

Corticosteroid use can be associated with a variety of neuropsychiatric side effects, including anxiety, insomnia, irritability, mania, depression, psychosis, delirium, and suicidality. Although 13% to 62% of patients experience only mild side effects, 3% to 6% experience severe symptoms, such as delirium, psychosis, or full-blown mania.[59] In the national database UK study, the hazard ratio in exposed patients as compared with not-exposed controls was 6.89 for suicide or suicide attempt, 4.35 for mania, and 5.14 for delirium.[60] The most-validated risk factor for development of the steroid-induced neuropsychiatric side effects is the dose.[59–61] A now classic case-series study demonstrated that 1.3% of patients receiving at most 40 mg of prednisone per day developed psychiatric side effects; 4.6% of those receiving 41 to 80 mg/d developed psychiatric side effects; and 18.4% of those receiving 80 mg and greater per day developed such side effects.[59] Therefore, critically ill patients receiving high steroid doses are at the highest risk. Other possible risk factors include hypoalbuminemia, disruption of blood-brain barrier integrity, prior steroid-induced neuropsychiatric symptoms, a prior psychiatric history, timing (especially during the first course of steroid therapy), female sex, and increasing age.[62,63] Furthermore, neuropsychiatric manifestations can occur even while corticosteroids are been withdrawn, as in the case of rapid tapering in the early weeks following transplantation. Longer-acting steroid preparations are more likely to cause neuropsychiatric problems.[64]

Steroid-induced neuropsychiatric side effects may be alleviated by reduction or elimination of the offending agent, in most cases. Sometimes though, the timing of the evening dose can be changed in collaboration with the transplant team to help manage insomnia and sundowning. Sleep aid agents, such as benzodiazepines, may be effective in the short-term.[1] For agitation, delirium, or psychosis, antipsychotics are usually most effective when used short-term.[1,61,65] Lithium has been shown to be prophylactic against the development of steroid-induced psychosis[66]; anticonvulsant mood stabilizers, such as valproic acid (VPA), have been demonstrated to treat steroid-induced mania,[67] yet the use of these medications can be challenging in transplant recipients. Selective serotonin reuptake inhibitors (SSRIs) can be used to treat depression associated with longer-term use of steroids if necessary.[1]

Calcineurin-inhibiting immunosuppressants
Calcineurin-inhibiting immunosuppressants (CIIs), tacrolimus and cyclosporine, serve as the backbone of the immunosuppressive regimen. They exert their

immunosuppressive action by interfering with the activation and proliferation of cytotoxic T cells.[68] These agents are metabolized by cytochrome P450 (CYP) 3A4. Both inhibitors and inducers of the CYP3A4 and P-glycoprotein may alter CIIs levels[65,68] by affecting their metabolism. Both cyclosporine and tacrolimus inhibit 3A4, thus, affecting the levels of medications that depend on the same enzymes for their metabolism.[68]

The use of CIIs may be associated with significant adverse side effects, including nephrotoxicity, hypertension, hyperglycemia, and infections.[65] In addition, up to 40% to 60% of transplant recipients on CIIs may experience mild neuropsychiatric symptoms, such as tremulousness, headache, restlessness, insomnia, photophobia, peripheral sensory disturbances, anxiety, or agitation.[65] Moreover, during the acute postoperative state, 21% to 32% of CII users may experience moderate to severe neuropsychiatric side effects, such as CI, coma, seizures, focal neurologic deficits, dysarthria, cortical blindness, and delirium. The occurrence of these syndromes is usually associated with higher levels of immunosuppressants, disturbance of brain-blood barrier, hypocholesterolemia, and hypomagnesemia.[69] Other processes, such as infection, can further disrupt the blood-brain barrier and, thus, potentiate the neuropsychiatric side effects of immunosuppressants.

The pathophysiology of the CIIs' neurotoxic effects is poorly understood but is likely multifactorial. Possible mechanisms include calcineurin inhibition, alteration of sympathetic outflow, changes in N-methyl-d-aspartate and γ-aminobutyric acid neurotransmission, selective toxicity of glial cells, and induction of apoptosis of oligodendrocytes.[69]

Mild neuropsychiatric side effects can be managed by correction of any underlying metabolic disturbances or by decreasing the drug's blood level. More severe symptoms may require discontinuation of the offending agent, thus, needing to switch immunosuppressants (eg, from tacrolimus to cyclosporine) or discontinuation of CIIs altogether.[1] CII-induced seizures can be treated by reduction or discontinuation of the offending medication and/or the use of anticonvulsant agents, which are usually not required long-term.[1]

A rare but rather serious clinicoradiological complication of CIIs is PRES, a neuropsychiatric syndrome occurring in 1% to 3% of transplant recipients, associated with brain-blood barrier disruption caused by immunosuppressants' clinical action.[55,56] In addition to alterations in mental status, patients may experience seizures, headache, nausea and vomiting, and visual disturbances. If the condition is not properly diagnosed and treated, it can progress to ischemia, frank cerebral infarction, and occasionally death.[56] The occurrence of PRES is correlated with higher doses of immunosuppressant agents, but it can occur at therapeutic doses. The diagnosis is made by eliciting the characteristic clinical symptoms and the presence of classic radiographic changes. Typical findings on brain MRI include symmetric, posterior occipital, parietal, or temporal white matter edema; however, atypical locations in the frontal lobes, brainstem, and basal ganglia, as well as asymmetric lesions have all been described.[56] The treatment of PRES requires discontinuation of the offending agent (ie, changing the immunosuppressant), pharmacologic seizure control, and supportive measures.

Finally, a rare, severe, multifocal demyelinating sensorimotor polyneuropathy has been described in patients treated with CIIs, usually occurring within weeks after transplantation.[1]

Treatment of Psychiatric Conditions in Transplant Patients

Sedative drips

In the acute posttransplant setting, IV sedative may be required to provide comfort while patients are intubated or otherwise attached to various lifesaving technologies as well as to treat patients' anxiety, agitation, or delirium. Dexmedetomidine, a selective α2-receptor agonist with sedative and analgesic/opioid-sparing effects, is a preferred choice because of its beneficial benefit-risk profile.[70] It has anxiolytic properties, is minimally associated with respiratory depression, is devoid of anticholinergic activity, and is associated with decreased risk of delirium.[70] It can be titrated to provide comfort without excessive sedation. It can also be used to aid with the process of extubation; it can even be used in nonintubated individuals, although ongoing respiratory status monitoring would be required.[70] As expected, side effects include bradycardia and hypotension. In addition, there is emerging evidence that GABAergic agents (ie, benzodiazepines and propofol) carry an increased risk of health care acquired infections in ICU, as compared with dexmedetomidine, likely due to their further immunomodulatory effects.[71] Finally, dexmedetomidine has been successfully used to treat agitated delirium in a small retrospective study of liver transplant patients in the ICU.[45]

Antidepressants

Antidepressant agents, especially the SSRIs, are increasingly used to treat a variety of depressive and anxiety syndromes among transplant candidates and recipients. The onset of action for their clinical effects is about 4 to 8 weeks. It is important to be aware of some clinically important drug-drug interactions and adverse effects when using these medications. Paroxetine, fluoxetine, and fluvoxamine are 2D6 inhibitors, whereas sertraline's inhibition of 2D6 follows a dose-dependent fashion. Fluoxetine is also a 3A4 inhibitor, although its clinical relevance is not clear.[65] Paroxetine is the most anticholinergic of the SSRIs and is associated with sedation, weight gain, and cognitive side effects. Fluoxetine has a long half-life, thus, is not ideal for the use in medically ill patients. Fluvoxamine should be avoided because of multiple pertinent drug-drug interactions. Of all the SSRIs, citalopram causes the highest degree of QTc prolongation. In fact, the Food and Drug Administration has warned against its use in dosages greater than 40 mg per day.[72] Overall, escitalopram, sertraline, and citalopram (unless there is concern for QTc) are likely the best SSRI choices for transplant recipients.

Mirtazapine may be a good choice for some patients, especially in the acute ICU setting, given its beneficial profile for sleep and anxiety and its minimal drug-drug interaction profile. In addition, mirtazapine may have a quicker onset of antidepressant and anxiolytic action.[73] The side effects include sedation and weight gain.

The use of SSRIs and other serotonergic antidepressants can lead to the development of serotonergic toxicity, especially when combined with other serotonergic medications or drugs inhibiting metabolism of these antidepressants. In the ICU setting, the use of linezolid, a weak monoamine oxidase inhibitor (MAOI), and various opioid agents with serotonergic activity[74] are of potential concern. Some reports suggest that mirtazapine, which has not been shown to increase serotonin in the synaptic cleft, can be potentially combined with linezolid; but caution should be used.[75]

Bupropion can lower the seizure threshold in higher doses or in those experiencing electrolyte abnormalities. Bupropion may also cause restlessness, tremulousness, irritability, and insomnia; thus, it should be used with caution in the immediate peritransplant period.[1]

Antipsychotics

Antipsychotic agents are used to treat a variety of neuropsychiatric syndromes in the critical care setting, including delirium, agitation, psychosis, and any number of neuropsychiatric complications in transplant recipients. There are only a limited number of reports regarding the use of haloperidol, specifically in transplant recipients for the treatment of delirium.[45,76] Haloperidol is available in oral, intramuscular, and IV form and, thus, useful in the ICU setting, especially for the management of altered mental status associated with hyperactivity. Quetiapine, a second-generation antipsychotic (SGA), has been shown to be effective in the treatment of ICU delirium.[77] Even though quetiapine is only available for oral administration, it conveniently has sedative qualities and a short half-life. Risperidone, aripiprazole, and olanzapine are available in oral and rapidly disintegrating forms; however, gastrointestinal absorption is still required. Olanzapine has several drawbacks, primarily its long half-life and high anticholinergic activity. Aripiprazole is the least-sedating agent in this class and may be especially useful in the management of hypoactive delirium.

Quetiapine is metabolized by 3A4; thus, its levels are affected by coadministered immunosuppressants. All antipsychotics can potentially prolong the QTc interval, thus, increasing the risk for torsades de pointes.[72] Consequentially, these agents should be used with caution in critically ill patients, especially in the context of multiple other QTc-prolonging medications, such as tacrolimus, antibiotics, antifungals, and other agents. Aripiprazole and lurasidone have been shown to prolong the QTc interval the least.[72]

Mood stabilizers

Mood stabilizers may be required to treat comorbid psychiatric conditions, such as bipolar disorder, or to address newly emerged neuropsychiatric side effects of steroids and/or immunosuppressants.

Lithium administration may be challenging; it can be dangerous to use in the posttransplant setting because of large fluid volume shifts, in addition to its potential to cause nephrotoxicity by itself or combined with other medications, including diuretic use.[1] VPA should be avoided in patients with liver disease because of a small risk of hepatotoxicity.[1] In addition, VPA can cause thrombocytopenia and impair platelet aggregation.

Antianxiety medications

SSRIs are the first-line drug for the long-term management of impairing anxiety. However, it can take weeks for these agents to have their full effect. Therefore, for shortterm use and for use in the acute setting, there are several benzo-sparing anxiolytic agents that can be considered, including gabapentin (also used for the management of neuropathic pain) and hydroxyzine.

Benzodiazepines can be used sparingly for the management of acute anxiety but with caution because of their negative effect in the respiratory drive, anticholinergic activity, and delirium-inducing effects. If benzodiazepines are needed, the authors recommend the use of agents with a shorter half-life and those that do not depend on CYP metabolism, such as lorazepam.

LIVE DONORS

Among the 15,070 organ transplantations performed in 2015, a total of 5991 (39.7%) had a living donor.[2] Most living donors donate one kidney or a hepatic lobe, with other rare living organ donations consisting of a lung lobe, pancreas, intestine, and uterus. Donors can be blood related or not; they can be directed, nondirected, or part of a paired exchange.[78]

Living organ donation is a unique procedure because it requires that a healthy individual undergoes major surgery for the benefit of another person. In order to reduce the negative impact of the donation procedure on living donors, the donor candidates undergo very detailed physical and psychological evaluations aimed at identifying and minimizing any potential risks. Recently, the Live Donor Assessment Tool was created to standardize psychosocial assessment of live donation candidates.[79]

New surgical techniques, such laparoscopic or semirobotic surgery, have decreased the duration of the surgery for living donors and speeded up the recovery process.[80] Some kidney donors are discharged from the hospital within 3 days after surgery.[81] Major immediate postsurgical complications are rare, and full physical recovery is usually expected. A study of 42 living lung lobe donors indicated that donors usually return to their previous functional ability without restrictions.[82] Sixteen percent of living kidney donors experience perioperative adverse events; however, only 2.5% of them have a clinically significant complication.[83] Major postoperative surgical complications occur in 13.3% of living liver donors.[84] Living pancreas donors have a 13% risk of minor postoperative complications, such as peripancreatic fluid accumulation.[85] Surgical mortality in live kidney donors is extremely low at 3.1 per 10,000 donors, which has not change during the last 15 years, despite differences in practice and selection.[86] Although the immediate recovery is usually uneventful, the long-term health consequences of organ donation are not yet fully understood: 10.8% of living liver donors have delayed recovery of their liver function (defined as increases in international normalized ratio of prothrombin time and concomitant hyperbilirubinemia on or after postoperative day 5).[87] In the long-term, kidney donors seem to be at greater risk of developing ESRD than the general population.[88] Pancreatic donors have a 10% to 25% risk of developing insulin-dependent diabetes after donation.[89]

Predonation psychiatric problems are considered to be a risk factor for perioperative surgical complications among living kidney donors.[83] Psychiatric complications are usually associated with a longer length of hospital stay.[81] Depression before surgery is often associated with worse postsurgical donation pain.[90] Preoperative motivational interviewing centered on the ambivalence about donation has been associated with fewer physical symptoms, lower rates of pain, and shorter recovery times among liver donors.[91] Immediately postoperatively, the psychiatrist may be asked to address new-onset psychiatric problems, such as anxiety and CI, or to assist in pain management. Given the excellent health usually associated with the living donor status, patients are usually fully alert in the ICU; therefore, they are often quite aware of the ICU environment, which many may find stressful. During the posttransplant period, donors should be monitored for the development of emotional distress in the critical care environment.[1] Donation-related psychological issues may increase in the immediate perioperative period, such as feelings of vulnerability, a need to follow the recipient's progress, or feeling a closer relationship with the donor.[92] Mild frontal lobe impairment and attention deficits have been found 1 week after living liver donation surgery.[93] Contrary to earlier reports, recent studies have shown that organ donors report less intense postoperative pain than anticipated.[94] Studies have found that smoking in living kidney donors is associated with worse outcomes for both donors and recipients; some kidney transplant programs may require help with smoking cessation or maintaining abstinence in the preoperative or postoperative setting.[95] Psychiatric complications, such depression, tend to develop later after donation: cumulative frequency of depression diagnosis was 4.2% at 1 year and 11.5% at 5 years.[96] Nonspousal, unrelated donors seem to have the highest risk for developing depression, whereas loss of the graft or death of the recipient may also play a role,[96,97] as did the recipient's hospitalization.[98] New-onset psychiatric problems after living liver donation occurs in 4% of donors, with depression and anxiety being the most common problems, followed by substance misuse and conversion disorder.[99] Predonation characteristics associated with more psychological distress after donation include not having a partner, younger age, lack of social support, and an avoidant coping style.[100] Little is known about the psychological risks of emergency organ donation, defined by performing liver transplantation within 10 days from diagnosis of liver failure that occurs sporadically.[101]

Despite the aforementioned risks, it is important to remember that more than 85% of the donors do not regret having donated.[102] In fact, organ donation was associated with psychological benefits, such as with moderate increase in self-esteem and psychological growth.[97]

CAREGIVERS
Patient Caregivers

Patient caregivers constitute an integral part of the transplant recipient's recovery and posttransplant functioning. In fact, most programs consider the lack of an adequate psychosocial support network to be an absolute contraindication to transplantation. Caregivers sacrifice their time, take time off work, relocate, and frequently put their lives on hold while taking care of transplant recipients. While attempting to be a cheerleader for patients, they face their own fears about losing their loved one and witnessing the recipient's health decline and suffering. At times, they have to make difficult decisions on behalf of transplant patients', especially when patients are unable to make their own medical decisions. They continue to support patients long after their ICU stay: nursing them to health, assisting with their medication and appointment needs, and serving as their advocates.

This experience can take a significant toll on caregivers. In fact, patient caregivers are at increased risk for post-ICU PTSD. In one study, 15% of family caregivers of patients with critical illness requiring ICU hospitalization showed clinical relevant scores of posttraumatic stress 3 to 6 months after the hospital stay.[103] Patients' diagnosis of PTSD was a risk factor for the caregiver PTSD, whereas a good relationship with patients was protective. In another study of heart transplant recipient caregivers (n = 190) followed up to 3 years, 56.3% of caregivers had any psychiatric disorder, 31.6% had MDD, 35% had adjustment disorder, and 22.5% had PTSD-T.[104] Risk factors included increasing burden of caregiving and poorer relationship with patients.[104]

Critical care staff are able to observe the availability of the caregivers and their relationships with the recipients and advise the transplant teams of a particular need for further evaluation and intervention. They can also provide invaluable support to the caregivers. Interventions that have been found to be helpful for transplant patients' caregivers' well-being include Internet-based intervention based on coping skills building, support, and education[105] and interventions directed at teaching mindfulness meditation.[106]

Health Care Provider Caregivers

The health care caregivers are the fundamental part of patients' journey, recovery, and dying. The ICU providers interact with patients and their families amid the most acute medical and psychological crises, and this can have a profound effect on the well-being of providers. Daily traumatic and ethical challenges faced by ICU personnel can overwhelm anyone's coping mechanisms and defenses. A burnout syndrome can develop among providers resulting in feelings of frustration, anger, fear, hopelessness, disillusionment, lack of empathy, and dissatisfaction and may be accompanied by somatic symptoms.[107] This syndrome in turn has negative effects on patients' care and outcomes.[107] Based on multiple studies, up to 33% of critical care nurses and up to 45% of critical care physicians manifest symptoms of severe burnout syndrome.[107]

Moreover, providers can experience full-blown PTSD as a result of their work. In one study, 24% of the ICU nurses tested positive for symptoms of PTSD related to their work environment, as compared with 14% of general floor nurses.[108] PTSD among ICU nurses is usually associated with the following factors: a poor social network, lack of identification with a role model, disruptive thoughts, regret, and lost optimism as compared with ICU nurses without PTSD.[109]

It is important for ICU staff to be vigilant about their own and their colleagues' psychological well-being. In fact, the Critical Care Societies Collaborative recently developed the Call to Action campaign to increase awareness about burnout syndrome in critical care staff and to work on potential solutions.[107] An important strategy is to establish and sustain a healthy work environment fostering respect, develop awareness to recognize burnout symptoms in self and others, and ask for appropriate assistance, when needed.[107] Avoiding burnout syndrome requires sensitivity regarding the impact that end-of-life issues and patients' deaths have on the critical care staff, the management of the clinical workload, appropriate support after the loss of a patient, and added support from colleagues.[1]

SUMMARY

Transplant patients face challenging medical journeys, with many detours to the ICU. Before and after transplantation they have significant psychological and cognitive comorbidities, which decrease their QoL and potentially compromise their medical outcomes. Critical care staff are essential in these journeys. Being cognizant of relevant psychosocial and mental health aspects of transplant patients' experiences can help critical care personnel take comprehensive care of these patients. This knowledge can empower them to understand their patients' psychological journeys, recognize patients' mental health needs, provide initial interventions, and recognize need for expert consultations.

REFERENCES

1. DiMartini A, Crone C, Fireman M, et al. Psychiatric aspects of organ transplantation in critical care. Crit Care Clin 2008;24(4):949–81, x.
2. Organ Procurement and Transplantation Network. 2016. Available at: https://optn.transplant.hrsa.gov/. Accessed November 29, 2016.
3. Owen JE, Bonds CL, Wellisch DK. Psychiatric evaluations of heart transplant candidates: predicting post-transplant hospitalizations, rejection episodes, and survival. Psychosomatics 2006;47(3):213–22.
4. Maldonado JR, Sher Y, Lolak S, et al. The Stanford integrated psychosocial assessment for transplantation: a prospective study of medical and psychosocial outcomes. Psychosom Med 2015;77(9):1018–30.
5. Maldonado JR, Dubois HC, David EE, et al. The Stanford integrated psychosocial assessment for transplantation (SIPAT): a new tool for the psychosocial evaluation of pre-transplant candidates. Psychosomatics 2012;53(2):123–32.
6. Hitschfeld MJ, Schneekloth TD, Kennedy CC, et al. The psychosocial assessment of candidates for transplantation: a cohort study of its association with survival among lung transplant recipients. Psychosomatics 2016;57(5):489–97.
7. Twillman RK, Manetto C, Wellisch DK, et al. The transplant evaluation rating scale. A revision of the psychosocial levels system for evaluating organ transplant candidates. Psychosomatics 1993;34(2):144–53.
8. Presberg BA, Levenson JL, Olbrisch ME, et al. Rating scales for the psychosocial evaluation of organ transplant candidates. Comparison of the PACT and

TERS with bone marrow transplant patients. Psychosomatics 1995;36(5): 458–61.

9. Flynn K, Daiches A, Malpus Z, et al. 'A post-transplant person': narratives of heart or lung transplantation and intensive care unit delirium. Health (London) 2014;18(4):352–68.

10. Caro MA, Rosenthal JL, Kendall K, et al. What the psychiatrist needs to know about ventricular assist devices: a comprehensive review. Psychosomatics 2016;57(3):229–37.

11. Kirklin JK, Naftel DC, Pagani FD, et al. Seventh INTERMACS annual report: 15,000 patients and counting. J Heart Lung Transplant 2015;34(12):1495–504.

12. Yost GL, Bhat G, Ibrahim KN, et al. Psychosocial evaluation in patients undergoing left ventricular assist device implantation using the transplant evaluation rating scale. Psychosomatics 2016;57(1):41–6.

13. Gordon RJ, Weinberg AD, Pagani FD, et al. Prospective, multicenter study of ventricular assist device infections. Circulation 2013;127(6):691–702.

14. Snipelisky D, Stulak JM, Schettle SD, et al. Psychosocial characteristics and outcomes in patients with left ventricular assist device implanted as destination therapy. Am Heart J 2015;170(5):887–94.

15. Petrucci RJ, Rogers JG, Blue L, et al. Neurocognitive function in destination therapy patients receiving continuous-flow vs pulsatile-flow left ventricular assist device support. J Heart Lung Transplant 2012;31(1):27–36.

16. Dew MA, Kormos RL, Winowich S, et al. Quality of life outcomes after heart transplantation in individuals bridged to transplant with ventricular assist devices. J Heart Lung Transplant 2001;20(11):1199–212.

17. Abshire M, Prichard R, Cajita M, et al. Adaptation and coping in patients living with an LVAD: a meta-synthesis. Heart Lung 2016;45(5):397–405.

18. Tigges-Limmer K, Schonbrodt M, Roefe D, et al. Suicide after ventricular assist device implantation. J Heart Lung Transplant 2010;29(6):692–4.

19. Baba A, Hirata G, Yokoyama F, et al. Psychiatric problems of heart transplant candidates with left ventricular assist devices. J Artif Organs 2006;9(4):203–8.

20. Tramm R, Ilic D, Davies AR, et al. Extracorporeal membrane oxygenation for critically ill adults. Cochrane Database Syst Rev 2015;(1):CD010381.

21. Biscotti M, Sonett J, Bacchetta M. ECMO as bridge to lung transplant. Thorac Surg Clin 2015;25(1):17–25.

22. Tramm R, Ilic D, Murphy K, et al. A qualitative exploration of acute care and psychological distress experiences of ECMO survivors. Heart Lung 2016;45(3): 220–6.

23. Sher Y, Lolak S, Maldonado JR. The impact of depression in heart disease. Curr Psychiatry Rep 2010;12(3):255–64.

24. Quittner AL, Goldbeck L, Abbott J, et al. Prevalence of depression and anxiety in patients with cystic fibrosis and parent caregivers: results of the International Depression Epidemiological Study across nine countries. Thorax 2014;69(12): 1090–7.

25. Matte DL, Pizzichini MM, Hoepers AT, et al. Prevalence of depression in COPD: a systematic review and meta-analysis of controlled studies. Respir Med 2016; 117:154–61.

26. Soyseth TS, Lund MB, Bjortuft O, et al. Psychiatric disorders and psychological distress in patients undergoing evaluation for lung transplantation: a national cohort study. Gen Hosp Psychiatry 2016;42:67–73.

27. Cron DC, Friedman JF, Winder GS, et al. Depression and frailty in patients with end-stage liver disease referred for transplant evaluation. Am J Transplant 2016; 16(6):1805–11.
28. Dew MA, DiMartini AF, DeVito Dabbs AJ, et al. Onset and risk factors for anxiety and depression during the first 2 years after lung transplantation. Gen Hosp Psychiatry 2012;34(2):127–38.
29. Davydow DS, Lease ED, Reyes JD. Posttraumatic stress disorder in organ transplant recipients: a systematic review. Gen Hosp Psychiatry 2015;37(5):387–98.
30. Davydow DS, Gifford JM, Desai SV, et al. Posttraumatic stress disorder in general intensive care unit survivors: a systematic review. Gen Hosp Psychiatry 2008;30(5):421–34.
31. Parker AM, Sricharoenchai T, Raparla S, et al. Posttraumatic stress disorder in critical illness survivors: a meta-analysis. Crit Care Med 2015;43(5):1121–9.
32. Beg M, Scruth E, Liu V. Developing a framework for implementing intensive care unit diaries: a focused review of the literature. Aust Crit Care 2016;29(4):224–34.
33. Dew MA, Rosenberger EM, Myaskovsky L, et al. Depression and anxiety as risk factors for morbidity and mortality after organ transplantation: a systematic review and meta-analysis. Transplantation 2015;100(5):988–1003.
34. Rosenberger EM, DiMartini AF, DeVito Dabbs AJ, et al. Psychiatric predictors of long-term transplant-related outcomes in lung transplant recipients. Transplantation 2016;100(1):239–47.
35. Crone C, DiMartini A. Liver transplant for intentional acetaminophen overdose: a survey of transplant clinicians experiences with recommendations. Psychosomatics 2014;55(6):602–12.
36. Karvellas CJ, Safinia N, Auzinger G, et al. Medical and psychiatric outcomes for patients transplanted for acetaminophen-induced acute liver failure: a case-control study. Liver Int 2010;30(6):826–33.
37. Levenson JL, Olbrisch ME. Psychosocial evaluation of organ transplant candidates. A comparative survey of process, criteria, and outcomes in heart, liver, and kidney transplantation. Psychosomatics 1993;34(4):314–23.
38. Zimbrean P, Emre S. Patients with psychotic disorders in solid-organ transplant. Prog Transplant 2015;25(4):289–96.
39. Okayasu H, Ozeki Y, Chida M, et al. Lung transplantation in a Japanese patient with schizophrenia from brain-dead donor. Gen Hosp Psychiatry 2013;35(1): 102.e11-3.
40. Murray AM, Tupper DE, Knopman DS, et al. Cognitive impairment in hemodialysis patients is common. Neurology 2006;67(2):216–23.
41. Lee Y, Kim C, Suk KT, et al. Differences in cognitive function between patients with viral and alcoholic compensated liver cirrhosis. Metab Brain Dis 2016; 31(2):369–76.
42. Ahluwalia V, Wade JB, White MB, et al. Liver transplantation significantly improves global functioning and cerebral processing. Liver Transpl 2016;22(10): 1379–90.
43. Smith PJ, Rivelli S, Waters A, et al. Neurocognitive changes after lung transplantation. Ann Am Thorac Soc 2014;11(10):1520–7.
44. Lescot T, Karvellas CJ, Chaudhury P, et al. Postoperative delirium in the intensive care unit predicts worse outcomes in liver transplant recipients. Can J Gastroenterol 2013;27(4):207–12.
45. Choi JY, Kim JM, Kwon CH, et al. Use of dexmedetomidine in liver transplant recipients with postoperative agitated delirium. Transplant Proc 2016;48(4): 1063–6.

46. Smith PJ, Rivelli SK, Waters AM, et al. Delirium affects length of hospital stay after lung transplantation. J Crit Care 2015;30(1):126–9.

47. Smith PJ, Blumenthal JA, Hoffman BM, et al. Reduced cerebral perfusion pressure during lung transplant surgery is associated with risk, duration, and severity of postoperative delirium. Ann Am Thorac Soc 2016;13(2):180–7.

48. Santacruz J, Mireles-Cabodevila E, Guzman Zavala E, et al. Post-operative delirium in lung transplant recipients: incidence and associated risk factors and morbidity Paper presented at: Chest. San Diego (CA), November 3, 2009.

49. Barr J, Fraser GL, Puntillo K, et al. Clinical practice guidelines for the management of pain, agitation, and delirium in adult patients in the intensive care unit. Crit Care Med 2013;41(1):263–306.

50. Siddiqi N, Harrison JK, Clegg A, et al. Interventions for preventing delirium in hospitalised non-ICU patients. Cochrane Database Syst Rev 2016;(3):CD005563.

51. DiMartini A, Crone C, Dew MA. Alcohol and substance use in liver transplant patients. Clin Liver Dis 2011;15(4):727–51.

52. Dew MA, DiMartini AF, Steel J, et al. Meta-analysis of risk for relapse to substance use after transplantation of the liver or other solid organs. Liver Transpl 2008;14(2):159–72.

53. Mathurin P, Moreno C, Samuel D, et al. Early liver transplantation for severe alcoholic hepatitis. N Engl J Med 2011;365(19):1790–800.

54. Lee BP, Chen PH, Haugen C, et al. Three-year results of a pilot program in early liver transplantation for severe alcoholic hepatitis. Ann Surg 2016;265(1):20–9.

55. Mueller SW, Preslaski CR, Kiser TH, et al. A randomized, double-blind, placebo-controlled dose range study of dexmedetomidine as adjunctive therapy for alcohol withdrawal. Crit Care Med 2014;42(5):1131–9.

56. Bielka K, Kuchyn I, Glumcher F. Addition of dexmedetomidine to benzodiazepines for patients with alcohol withdrawal syndrome in the intensive care unit: a randomized controlled study. Ann Intensive Care 2015;5(1):33.

57. Weinrieb RM, Barnett R, Lynch KG, et al. A matched comparison study of medical and psychiatric complications and anesthesia and analgesia requirements in methadone-maintained liver transplant recipients. Liver Transpl 2004;10(1):97–106.

58. Liu LU, Schiano TD, Lau N, et al. Survival and risk of recidivism in methadone-dependent patients undergoing liver transplantation. Am J Transplant 2003;3(10):1273–7.

59. Acute adverse reactions to prednisone in relation to dosage. Clin Pharmacol Ther 1972;13(5):694–8.

60. Fardet L, Petersen I, Nazareth I. Suicidal behavior and severe neuropsychiatric disorders following glucocorticoid therapy in primary care. Am J Psychiatry 2012;169(5):491–7.

61. Dubovsky AN, Arvikar S, Stern TA, et al. The neuropsychiatric complications of glucocorticoid use: steroid psychosis revisited. Psychosomatics 2012;53(2):103–15.

62. Judd LL, Schettler PJ, Brown ES, et al. Adverse consequences of glucocorticoid medication: psychological, cognitive, and behavioral effects. Am J Psychiatry 2014;171(10):1045–51.

63. West S, Kenedi C. Strategies to prevent the neuropsychiatric side-effects of corticosteroids: a case report and review of the literature. Curr Opin Organ Transplant 2014;19(2):201–8.

64. Fardet L, Nazareth I, Whitaker HJ, et al. Severe neuropsychiatric outcomes following discontinuation of long-term glucocorticoid therapy: a cohort study. J Clin Psychiatry 2013;74(4):e281–286.

65. DiMartini AF, Crone CC, Fireman M. Organ transplantation. In: Ferrando S, Levenson J, Owen JA, editors. Clinical manual psychopharmacology in the medically Ill. Washington, DC: American Psychiatric Publishing, Inc; 2010. p. 469–99.

66. Falk WE, Mahnke MW, Poskanzer DC. Lithium prophylaxis of corticotropin-induced psychosis. JAMA 1979;241(10):1011–2.

67. Roxanas MG, Hunt GE. Rapid reversal of corticosteroid-induced mania with sodium valproate: a case series of 20 patients. Psychosomatics 2012;53(6): 575–81.

68. Fireman M, DiMartini AF, Armstrong SC, et al. Immunosuppressants. Psychosomatics 2004;45(4):354–60.

69. Bechstein WO. Neurotoxicity of calcineurin inhibitors: impact and clinical management. Transpl Int 2000;13(5):313–26.

70. Barr J, Kishman CP Jr, Jaeschke R. The methodological approach used to develop the 2013 pain, agitation, and delirium clinical practice guidelines for adult ICU patients. Crit Care Med 2013;41(9 Suppl 1):S1–15.

71. Caroff DA, Szumita PM, Klompas M. The relationship between sedatives, sedative strategy, and healthcare-associated infection: a systematic review. Infect Control Hosp Epidemiol 2016;37(10):1234–42.

72. Beach SR, Celano CM, Noseworthy PA, et al. QTc prolongation, torsades de pointes, and psychotropic medications. Psychosomatics 2013;54(1):1–13.

73. Watanabe N, Omori IM, Nakagawa A, et al. Mirtazapine versus other antidepressants in the acute-phase treatment of adults with major depression: systematic review and meta-analysis. J Clin Psychiatry 2008;69(9):1404–15.

74. Rastogi R, Swarm RA, Patel TA. Case scenario: opioid association with serotonin syndrome: implications to the practitioners. Anesthesiology 2011;115(6): 1291–8.

75. Gillman PK. A review of serotonin toxicity data: implications for the mechanisms of antidepressant drug action. Biol Psychiatry 2006;59(11):1046–51.

76. Levenson JL. High-dose intravenous haloperidol for agitated delirium following lung transplantation. Psychosomatics 1995;36(1):66–8.

77. Devlin JW, Roberts RJ, Fong JJ, et al. Efficacy and safety of quetiapine in critically ill patients with delirium: a prospective, multicenter, randomized, double-blind, placebo-controlled pilot study. Crit Care Med 2010;38(2):419–27.

78. Living Kidneys Donors Network. 2016. Available at: http://lkdn.org/paired_kidney_exchange.html. Accessed November 29, 2016.

79. Iacoviello BM, Shenoy A, Braoude J, et al. The live donor assessment tool: a psychosocial assessment tool for live organ donors. Psychosomatics 2015; 56(3):254–61.

80. Janki S, Dor FJ, IJzermans JN. Surgical aspects of live kidney donation: an updated review. Front Biosci (Elite Ed) 2015;7:346–65.

81. Schold JD, Goldfarb DA, Buccini LD, et al. Comorbidity burden and perioperative complications for living kidney donors in the United States. Clin J Am Soc Nephrol 2013;8(10):1773–82.

82. Date H, Sato M, Aoyama A, et al. Living-donor lobar lung transplantation provides similar survival to cadaveric lung transplantation even for very ill patients dagger. Eur J Cardiothorac Surg 2015;47(6):967–72 [discussion: 972–3].

83. Lentine KL, Lam NN, Axelrod D, et al. Perioperative complications after living kidney donation: a national study. Am J Transplant 2016;16(6):1848–57.
84. Ran S, Wen TF, Yan LN, et al. Risks faced by donors of right lobe for living donor liver transplantation. Hepatobiliary Pancreat Dis Int 2009;8(6):581–5.
85. Kirchner VA, Finger EB, Bellin MD, et al. Long-term outcomes for living pancreas donors in the modern era. Transplantation 2016;100(6):1322–8.
86. Segev DL, Muzaale AD, Caffo BS, et al. Perioperative mortality and long-term survival following live kidney donation. JAMA 2010;303(10):959–66.
87. Choi SS, Cho SS, Ha TY, et al. Intraoperative factors associated with delayed recovery of liver function after hepatectomy: analysis of 1969 living donors. Acta Anaesthesiol Scand 2016;60(2):193–202.
88. Gibney EM, Parikh CR, Garg AX. Age, gender, race, and associations with kidney failure following living kidney donation. Transplant Proc 2008;40(5): 1337–40.
89. Lam NN, Schnitzler MA, Segev DL, et al. Diabetes mellitus in living pancreas donors: use of integrated national registry and pharmacy claims data to characterize donation-related health outcomes. Transplantation 2016. [Epub ahead of print].
90. Mandell MS, Smith AR, Dew MA, et al. Early postoperative pain and its predictors in the adult to adult living donor liver transplantation cohort study. Transplantation 2016;100(11):2362–71.
91. Dew MA, DiMartini AF, DeVito Dabbs AJ, et al. Preventive intervention for living donor psychosocial outcomes: feasibility and efficacy in a randomized controlled trial. Am J Transplant 2013;13(10):2672–84.
92. Agerskov H, Ludvigsen MS, Bistrup C, et al. From donation to everyday life: living kidney donors' experiences three months after donation. J Ren Care 2016;42(1):43–52.
93. Bucak N, Begec Z, Erdil F, et al. Postoperative cognitive dysfunction in living liver transplant donors. Exp Clin Transpl 2014;12(Suppl 1):81–5.
94. Holtzman S, Clarke HA, McCluskey SA, et al. Acute and chronic postsurgical pain after living liver donation: incidence and predictors. Liver Transpl 2014; 20(11):1336–46.
95. Heldt J, Torrey R, Han D, et al. Donor smoking negatively affects donor and recipient renal function following living donor nephrectomy. Adv Urol 2011; 2011:929263.
96. Lentine KL, Schnitzler MA, Xiao H, et al. Depression diagnoses after living kidney donation: linking U.S. Registry data and administrative claims. Transplantation 2012;94(1):77–83.
97. Butt Z, Dew MA, Liu Q, et al. Psychological outcomes of living liver donors from a multi-center, prospective study: results from the adult to adult living donor liver transplantation cohort study (A2ALL). Am J Transplant 2016. [Epub ahead of print].
98. Timmerman L, Laging M, Timman R, et al. The impact of the donors' and recipients' medical complications on living kidney donors' mental health. Transpl Int 2016;29(5):589–602.
99. Kimura H, Onishi Y, Sunada S, et al. Postoperative psychiatric complications in living liver donors. Transplant Proc 2015;47(6):1860–5.
100. Timmerman L, Timman R, Laging M, et al. Predicting mental health after living kidney donation: the importance of psychological factors. Br J Health Psychol 2016;21(3):533–54.

101. Takeda K, Tanaka K, Kumamoto T, et al. Emergency versus elective living-donor liver transplantation: a comparison of a single center analysis. Surg Today 2012; 42(5):453–9.
102. Parikh ND, Ladner D, Abecassis M, et al. Quality of life for donors after living donor liver transplantation: a review of the literature. Liver Transpl 2010; 16(12):1352–8.
103. Wintermann GB, Weidner K, Strauss B, et al. Predictors of posttraumatic stress and quality of life in family members of chronically critically ill patients after intensive care. Ann Intensive Care 2016;6(1):69.
104. Dew MA, Myaskovsky L, DiMartini AF, et al. Onset, timing and risk for depression and anxiety in family caregivers to heart transplant recipients. Psychol Med 2004;34(6):1065–82.
105. Dew MA, Goycoolea JM, Harris RC, et al. An internet-based intervention to improve psychosocial outcomes in heart transplant recipients and family caregivers: development and evaluation. J Heart Lung Transplant 2004;23(6): 745–58.
106. Haines J, Spadaro KC, Choi J, et al. Reducing stress and anxiety in caregivers of lung transplant patients: benefits of mindfulness meditation. Int J Organ Transplant Med 2014;5(2):50–6.
107. Moss M, Good VS, Gozal D, et al. An official critical care societies collaborative statement: burnout syndrome in critical care healthcare professionals: a call for action. Crit Care Med 2016;44(7):1414–21.
108. Mealer ML, Shelton A, Berg B, et al. Increased prevalence of post-traumatic stress disorder symptoms in critical care nurses. Am J Respir Crit Care Med 2007;175(7):693–7.
109. Mealer M, Jones J, Moss M. A qualitative study of resilience and posttraumatic stress disorder in United States ICU nurses. Intensive Care Med 2012;38(9): 1445–51.

Neuropsychiatric Aspects of Infectious Diseases
An Update

Sahil Munjal, MD[a], Stephen J. Ferrando, MD[a],*,
Zachary Freyberg, MD, PhD[b,c]

KEYWORDS

- Neuropsychiatric disturbances • Infectious diseases • Delirium • HIV-AIDS
- Pediatric autoimmune neuropsychiatric disorders associated with streptococcal infections • Herpes simplex encephalitis • Neurocysticercosis • Neurosyphilis
- Creutzfeldt-Jakob disease • Neuroborreliosis

KEY POINTS

- Among the critically ill, infectious diseases can play a significant role in the etiology of neuropsychiatric disturbances.
- All critical care physicians are familiar with delirium as a secondary complication of systemic infection.
- This article focuses on key infectious diseases that commonly and directly produce neuropsychiatric symptoms, including direct infection of the central nervous system, human immunodeficiency virus infection, and AIDS.

INTRODUCTION

Among the critically ill, infectious diseases can play a significant role in the etiology of neuropsychiatric disturbances. All critical care physicians are familiar with delirium as a secondary complication of systemic infection. This article focuses on key infectious diseases that commonly and directly produce neuropsychiatric symptoms, including direct infection of the central nervous system (CNS), human immunodeficiency virus (HIV) infection, and AIDS.

HIV-AIDS is often seen as the modern "great imitator," a complex infectious disease with multiple manifestations and interplay of myriad biopsychosocial factors, including

This article is an update of an article previously published in *Critical Care Clinics*, Volume 24, Issue 4, October 2008.
[a] Department of Psychiatry, Westchester Medical Center, New York Medical College, 100 Woods Road, Valhalla, NY 10595, USA; [b] Department of Psychiatry, University of Pittsburgh, 3811 O'Hara Street, Pittsburgh, PA 15213, USA; [c] Department of Cell Biology, University of Pittsburgh, 3811 O'Hara Street, Pittsburgh, PA 15213, USA
* Corresponding author.
E-mail address: Stephen.Ferrando@wmchealth.org

neuropsychiatric disorders related to direct HIV-1 brain invasion, CNS opportunistic infections, manifestations of concurrent drug abuse, hepatitis C coinfection, and iatrogenic complications. Differential diagnosis and management of HIV-AIDS–related neuropsychiatric disturbances can serve as a paradigm for other infectious diseases that have neuropsychiatric manifestations.

MEDICAL HOSPITALIZATION IN HUMAN IMMUNODEFICIENCY VIRUS–AIDS

With the widespread availability of highly active antiretroviral therapy (HAART) for HIV infection in developed countries, there have been dramatic declines in HIV-related hospital admissions. Between 1995 and 1997, admissions dropped 33% to 75%.[1–4] Since that time, rates have stabilized or rebounded slightly. The reasons for medical hospital admission have also shifted. In 2 urban hospital studies,[3,4] a drop in hospitalization caused by opportunistic infections and cancers was observed, contrasting with a rise in nonopportunistic complications, such as hepatitis C and cardiovascular disease. Mean CD4 counts of HIV inpatients were seen to increase by more than 100 cells/mm^3 from 1995 to 2001.[3] During 1990 to 2011, among persons with AIDS, the annual rate of death due to HIV-attributable causes has also decreased by 89%.[5]

Factors that seem to confer risk for medical hospitalization in the HAART era include low CD4 count, female gender, lack of antiretroviral treatment, and injection drug use.[3,4] The sociodemographic characteristics of those at risk reflect the shifting demographics of the HIV epidemic, limitations in access to care, and poor adherence to antiretroviral treatment.

EPIDEMIOLOGY OF PSYCHIATRIC DISORDERS IN MEDICAL INPATIENTS WITH HUMAN IMMUNODEFICIENCY VIRUS–AIDS

There are extensive epidemiologic data regarding psychiatric disorders in ambulatory patients with HIV-AIDS. Overall, studies reveal high rates of lifetime and current substance abuse and depressive and anxiety disorders (see Ferrando and Tiamson[6] for a review of this literature). As seen in **Table 1**, among medially hospitalized patients with HIV, studies indicate a similar profile; however, delirium, dementia, and manic-spectrum disorders seem to be more common.[7–11] The most frequently diagnosed disorders are in the depressive spectrum (range, 27%–83%), including depression secondary to medical condition (or organic mood disorder), adjustment disorder with depressed mood, major depressive disorder, or dysthymic disorder. Delirium is diagnosed in 8% to 29% of patients, regardless of HIV stage, and is often reported to be concurrent with HIV-associated dementia, diagnosed in 8% to 22% of cases. Substance use disorders are diagnosed in 11% to 36% of inpatients with AIDS and up to 63% in patients who are HIV-positive without AIDS. One study found that bipolar disorder and HIV-associated mania occurred in 11% of medical inpatients.[11]

HUMAN IMMUNODEFICIENCY VIRUS AND THE BRAIN

Since the beginning of the HIV epidemic, it has been recognized that HIV can infect the CNS and produce a range of cognitive and behavioral symptoms that become more frequent and severe as the immune system declines and symptomatic illness and AIDS ensue. In 1991, the American Academy of Neurology published research diagnostic criteria for HIV-associated cognitive, motor, and behavior disorders,[12] which remained in widespread use until the diagnostic criteria were recently updated by a work group convened at the National Institute of Mental Health.[13] Based on cumulative research and clinical evidence, this group described 3 HIV-associated

Table 1
Frequency of psychiatric disorders reported in the inpatient medical setting

Authors	n	% Male	HIV Risk	Medical Illnesses	Depressive Disorders	% Dementia	% Delirium	% Substance Use Disorder	% Other Psychiatric Disorders
Perry & Tross,[7] 1984	52 AIDS	98	Homosexual 79% Homosexual + IVDU 12% Other 9%	OI 71% KS 17% OI + KS 12%	Any 83%	11	29	11	Schizophrenia 2
Dilley et al,[8] 1985	13 AIDS	100	Homosexual 100%	OI 70% OI + KS 15% Other 15%	Adjustment disorder 54% MDD 15%	8	8	31	Panic 8
O'Dowd & Mc Kegney,[9] 1990	67 AIDS	69	Not reported	Not reported	Adjustment disorder 42% MDD 3%	22	27	20	Axis II 6
Bialer et al,[10] 1996	433 AIDS 116 HIV+	79	Not reported	Not reported	Organic mood 13%	22	29	36	Axis II 9
Ferrando et al,[48] 1997	36 AIDS 4 HIV+	60	Homosexual 34% IVDU 31% Heterosexual 31%	OI 89%	Adjustment disorder 13% MDD 1% MDD or 31% dysthymic disorder	19	19	19	Mania/hypomania 11 Anxiety 8

Abbreviations: HIV, human immunodeficiency virus; IVDU, intravenous drug user; KS, Kaposi sarcoma; MDD, major depressive disorder; OI, opportunistic illnesses.

neurocognitive disorders (HANDs): (1) asymptomatic neurocognitive impairment, (2) mild neurocognitive disorder, and (3) HIV-associated dementia. The asymptomatic neurocognitive impairment category recognizes that a substantial percentage of patients who infected with HIV have demonstrable impairment on neuropsychologic testing but little or no perceptible functional impairment. The latter 2 disorders (mild neurocognitive disorder and HIV-associated dementia) present with cognitive and behavioral symptoms associated with functional impairment (mild in mild neurocognitive disorder, moderate to severe in HIV-associated dementia). HANDs have been found to predict shorter survival,[14,15] especially in the setting of virologic failure on HAART.[16] The cognitive symptoms of HANDs are characteristic of subcortical-frontal pathology and include impairment in psychomotor processing speed, executive function, and verbal memory. The potential behavioral manifestations are broad and include apathy, depression, anxiety, mania, and psychosis.

Neuropathologically, HIV traverses the blood-brain barrier primarily by infected blood mononuclear cells, becoming activated macrophages once they enter the brain. Onset of neural injury may date to initial viral invasion and the transient early period of unchecked viremia and marked immunosuppression of the seroconversion period.[17] Neuropathologic changes seem to be a result of CNS immune activation with release of neurotoxic cytokines and metabolites. Substance abuse is an important cofactor for HIV neuropathology.[18] Subcortical brain structures, such as the basal ganglia and periventricular white matter, are most affected. If unchecked, this immune cascade leads to neuronal cell apoptosis. Effective suppression of CNS viral replication and the resulting immune activation has the potential, however, to reverse at least some of the neuropathologic changes.

HIV-associated neuropathology has received heightened attention in recent years because of 2 associated developments. First, HIV-1 viral load monitoring has demonstrated that the CNS is an independent sanctuary site of viral replication.[19] The level and genetic profile of HIV in the peripheral circulation may not correlate with that in the CNS. The second development relates to the recognition that antiretroviral medications have differing levels of penetration into the CNS. It is hypothesized that poorly penetrating antiretrovirals might inadequately treat CNS infection despite being effective peripherally. This has led to concerns that actively replicating virus in the CNS could cause progressive cognitive decline in otherwise healthy HIV-positive individuals and could also lead to a reseeding of the virus into the peripheral circulation. Indeed, better CNS antiretroviral penetrance has been found to correlate with better suppression of HIV in the cerebrospinal fluid (CSF).[20] However, this approach is controversial, as higher CSF Penetration Effectiveness scores correlate with lower HIV RNA load in the CSF but do not necessarily correlate with better cognition.[21] HAND is common in patients with HIV on combination treatment with a reported frequency of 25% to 47%.[22] There has been a reduction in the incidence of HIV-associated dementia from 7% per year in the pre-HAART era to approximately 2% to 3%.[23] However, cases still occur in patients with HIV who are untreated, inadequately treated, or in persons who have "CNS escape" (a phenomenon in which antiretroviral therapy [ART] controls HIV in the periphery but not in the CNS).[24] HAART regimens have been shown to reduce CSF viral load to undetectable levels,[19] to reverse white matter lesions on MRI,[25] to reverse brain metabolic abnormalities detected by proton magnetic resonance spectroscopy,[26] and also to improve neuropsychologic test performance.[27–29] Despite these hopeful findings, however, functionally significant cognitive and behavioral disturbances, without frank dementia, may persist in approximately one-fourth of patients treated with HAART,[30,31] impeding adherence to treatment[32] and ability to work.[33]

DIFFERENTIAL DIAGNOSIS

Differential diagnosis is paramount when investigating for medical and neuropsychiatric etiologic factors related to HIV illness and its treatment (**Box 1**).

First, in assessing the hospitalized patient with HIV-AIDS, it is important to query for personal and family psychiatric history because neuropsychiatric complications may be a manifestation of preexisting psychopathology.[34,35] Even in the presence of a prior psychiatric history, however, it is imperative to rule out potentially exacerbating, if not etiologic, medical factors. HANDs are associated with a range of cognitive or behavioral symptoms, including apathy, depression, sleep disturbances, mania, and psychosis. CNS opportunistic illnesses and cancers also can present with a wide range of neuropsychiatric symptoms as a result of both focal and generalized neuropathologic processes (**Table 2**).

Substance intoxication and withdrawal also are common in the medical inpatient setting. HIV-infected substance users have high rates of preexisting comorbid psychopathology that may be exacerbated by ongoing substance use. Further, abuse of multiple substances concurrently (eg, opioids, cocaine, benzodiazepines, alcohol) can result in complex intoxication and withdrawal states that may be very difficult to treat.

Hepatitis C coinfection is associated with multiple neuropsychiatric complaints, most frequently fatigue, depression, and cognitive dysfunction. The pattern of cognitive impairment is similar to that of HIV, with impairment in attention, concentration, psychomotor processing speed, verbal memory, and executive dysfunction. Patients with end-stage liver disease and cirrhosis experience superimposed delirium (hepatic encephalopathy). Combination pegylated interferon alpha-2a treatment for hepatitis C has been extensively documented to cause neuropsychiatric side effects, including depression, suicidal ideation, anxiety, sleep disturbance, fatigue, mania, psychosis, delirium, and cognitive dysfunction.[36]

Multiple antiretroviral and other medications used in the context of HIV have been reported to have neuropsychiatric side effects. These include zidovudine, didanosine, abacavir, nevirapine, efavirenz, and interferon alpha-2a.[37] Most of these are uncommon or rare and causal relationships are often difficult to determine. The most widespread clinical concern has been generated by reports of sudden-onset depression and suicidal ideation associated with interferon alpha-2a and efavirenz. Early reports suggested that efavirenz may be associated with at least transient neuropsychiatric

---

Box 1
Differential diagnosis of psychiatric disorders and symptoms in medical inpatients with HIV-AIDS

- Primary psychiatric disorder
- CNS HIV infection (minor neurocognitive disorder and HIV-associated dementia)
- CNS opportunistic illnesses and cancers (see **Table 2**)
- Substance intoxication and withdrawal
- Neuropsychiatric complications of hepatitis C and its treatments
- Neuropsychiatric side effects of HIV medications
- Drug-drug interactions
- Endocrine abnormalities (eg, hypogonadism, adrenal insufficiency, thyroid disease)

Abbreviations: CNS, central nervous system; HIV, human immunodeficiency virus.

Table 2
Opportunistic illnesses of the central nervous system in AIDS

OI	CD4	Signs	Focal	CT/MRI	Lumbar Puncture
Toxoplasmosis	<100	Fever Delirium Headache Seizures	Y	Ring-enhancing lesions Basal ganglia Gray-white junction	*Toxoplasma gondii* antibody or PCR High specificity/low sensitivity Other routine CSF studies not generally diagnostic
Cytomegalovirus	<50	Delirium Infections found at diagnosis Retina Blood Adrenal gland Gastrointestinal tract	Y/N	Ventricular enlargement Increased periventricular signal (T2 image)	CMV PCR Variable specificity/variable sensitivity Elevated protein level, pleocytosis, hypoglycorrhachia
Cryptococcal meningitis	<100	Fever Delirium Not universally seen Increased intracranial pressure (50%) Seizures	N	Nonspecific	*Cryptococcus neoformans*, India ink, latex agglutination or PCR High specificity/high sensitivity Other routine CSF studies not generally diagnostic
Progressive multifocal leukoencephalopathy (JCV)	<100	Mono/hemiparesis Dysarthria Gait disturbance Sensory deficit Progressive dementia Occasional Visual loss Seizures	Y	Attenuated signal/(T2 images) Periventricular White matter Other areas: Gray matter Brainstem Cerebellum Spinal cord	JCV PCR High specificity/high sensitivity Other routine CSF studies not generally diagnostic
Central nervous system neoplasm/lymphoma	<100	Afebrile delirium Seizures (10%) Increased intracranial pressure	Y	Lesions Hypodense/patchy Nodular Enhancing SPECT thallium differentiates from toxoplasmosis	EBV PCR High specificity/high sensitivity Other routine CSF studies not generally diagnostic

Abbreviations: CMV, cytomegalovirus; CSF, cerebrospinal fluid; CT, computed tomography; EBV, Epstein-Barr virus; JCV, JC virus; N, no; OI, opportunistic illnesses; PCR, polymerase chain reaction; SPECT, single-photon emission computed tomography; Y, yes.

side effects in excess of 50% of patients.[38] Reported effects are protean and include depression, suicidal ideation, vivid nightmares, anxiety, insomnia, psychosis, cognitive dysfunction, and antisocial behavior. Drug interactions between antiretroviral and psychotropic medications are important aspects of differential diagnosis in the hospital setting. In one study, HIV-AIDS medical inpatients were prescribed an average of 7 medications during their admission.[11] Factors influencing drug-drug interactions include medical illness severity, prior substance abuse, the likelihood of multiple medications being initiated simultaneously, changes in volume of distribution and protein binding, and hepatic and renal impairment.

Inpatients with HIV-AIDS often experience endocrinologic derangements that may produce behavioral symptoms. These include clinical and subclinical hypothyroidism,[39] hypogonadism,[40] adrenal insufficiency,[41] and Graves disease (autoimmune thyroiditis).[39] Thyroid deficiency, including its subclinical forms, is present in approximately 36% of HIV- infected patients.[39] Testosterone deficiency, with clinical symptoms of hypogonadism, is present in up to 50% of men with symptomatic HIV or AIDS and is likely to be present with concurrent acute medical illness.[40] Deficiency of adrenal glucocorticoid production is present in up to 50% of severely ill patients with HIV.[41] These endocrine deficiency states have been associated with fatigue, low mood, low libido, and loss of lean body mass and may be ameliorated by correction of the deficiency. Graves disease presents in the acute stages with activation symptoms including anxiety, irritability, insomnia, weight loss, mania, and agitation.

DIAGNOSTIC EVALUATION

The psychiatric evaluation of the inpatient with HIV-AIDS is consistent with the broad differential diagnosis and is focused on identifying potentially reversible underlying etiologies. A thorough psychiatric evaluation, including presenting symptoms, personal and family history of psychiatric illness and substance abuse, and a cognitive functioning examination are essential. **Box 2** contains a listing of such diagnostic tests.

Box 2
Diagnostic evaluation of the medical inpatient with HIV-AIDS and neuropsychiatric disturbances

- Medical evaluation with screening laboratories: complete blood count, chemistry screen (including liver and renal function tests), urinalysis, chest radiograph, electrocardiogram, blood and urine cultures (when applicable)

- Psychiatric diagnostic interview including personal and family history

- Cognitive screen (HIV Dementia Scale)

- Additional laboratories when applicable: illicit drug toxicology screen, serum psychotropic drug levels, thyroid function tests, antithyroid antibodies, vitamin B12 and B6 levels, total or bioavailable testosterone, dehydroepiandrosterone sulfate, adrenocorticotropic stimulation test, 24-hour urine cortisol

- Evaluation for hepatitis C (including viral load)

- Review of antiretroviral regimen for neuropsychiatric side effects

- Review of psychotropic mediations for efficacy, neuropsychiatric side effects, drug interactions

- Neuroimaging (MRI, magnetic resonance spectroscopy)

- Lumbar puncture

In general, the diagnostic workup should include complete blood count with differential, serum chemistries (including liver and renal function tests, fasting glucose, and creatine phosphokinase), chest radiograph, electrocardiogram, blood and urine cultures (if indicated), toxicology screen, and psychotropic medication serum levels (when available). Depending on the clinical presentation, assays of thyroid function; vitamins B6 and B12; Venereal Disease Research Laboratory; serum total, free, or bioavailable testosterone; adrenocorticotropic hormone stimulation; and 24-hour urinary cortisol may be obtained. If brain imaging is required, MRI of the brain with gadolinium contrast is preferred over computed tomography (CT) because it produces better visualization of brain tissue and of subcortical and posterior fossa structures and focal lesions. A lumbar puncture also may be obtained if necessary under sedation with fluoroscopic guidance. Results are often nonspecific, but important studies include opening pressure; culture (viral, fungal, mycobacterial); cell count; protein; neopterin; b2-microglobulin; and polymerase chain reaction testing for cytomegalovirus, Epstein-Barr virus, John Cunningham (JC) virus, herpes simplex virus (HSV), and HIV-1.

PSYCHIATRIC DISORDERS IN HUMAN IMMUNODEFICIENCY VIRUS–AIDS AND THEIR TREATMENT
Depression

Depression is the most common psychiatric symptom and diagnosis among medical inpatients with HIV-AIDS. Symptoms are often attributed to adjustment disorder or to medically related (organic) factors that may be transient, related to improvement in physical symptoms. Major depressive disorder (MDD) may be a reaction to an HIV diagnosis, medical illness, HIV stigma, or the direct CNS effects of HIV as mediated by altered cytokine and neurotransmitter metabolism.[42] Identifying and treating MDD is important to long-term management because prolonged MDD is associated with decreased adherence to ART.[43,44] In one prospective study assessing depressive symptoms at admission and discharge, however, 28% of medical inpatients with HIV-AIDS had severe depression that persisted at discharge.[45] In another study, 76% of patients who had a depressive disorder during their admission continued to have significant depressive symptoms 3 to 6 weeks after discharge, with significant predictors of depression during and after medical hospitalization including being a woman, having an AIDS diagnosis, and having poor social support.[11]

In the medical inpatient setting in particular, the diagnosis of depressive disorder in HIV-infected patients may be confounded by somatic symptoms common to depression, HIV illness, and its complications. HIV infection stimulates rising levels of proinflammatory cytokines, such as interleukin-6, interleukin-1 beta, tumor necrosis factor-alpha and interferon-gamma, that are associated with "sickness behavior" (fever, hypersomnia, anorexia, decreased motor activity, and loss of interest in the environment).[46] These include fatigue, appetite loss, sleep disturbance, and cognitive disturbances. Generally, in the presence of persistent depressed mood or loss of interest, an inclusive approach toward somatic symptoms is preferred. This is because affective and somatic subscales of depression screening instruments (eg, the Beck Depression Inventory) are highly intercorrelated, that these symptoms are more closely linked to measures of depression than to measures of HIV disease severity, and that both affective and somatic symptoms improve with antidepressant treatment.[47,48] However, persons with HIV may be screened using the Beck Depression Inventory for Primary Care, a tool that focuses on nonphysical symptoms as well.[49]

In the medical inpatient setting, when antidepressant medication treatment is considered, particular attention must be paid to side-effect profile, hepatic and renal function, and the potential for drug interactions. In addition to standard antidepressants, such as serotonin and serotonin-norepinephrine reuptake inhibitors, the initiation of psychostimulants and anabolic steroids, particularly testosterone, is frequently used in the inpatient setting and is given particular attention here.

Psychostimulants have been studied for the treatment of depressed mood, fatigue, and cognitive impairment in the context of HIV infection, particularly in advanced illness and where rapid onset of action is desirable. Agents studied include methylphenidate (5–90 mg/d), dextroamphetamine (5–20 mg/d), pemoline (35–150 mg/d), and the wakefulness agent modafinil (50–200 mg/d).[50–53] These agents are efficacious in treating depressive symptoms in patients with advanced HIV. The primary side effect is overstimulation.

Testosterone deficiency, with clinical symptoms of hypogonadism (depressed mood, fatigue, diminished libido, decreased appetite, and loss of lean body mass) is present in up to 50% of men and women with symptomatic HIV or AIDS.[40] The most common screening test for testosterone deficiency is total serum testosterone (deficiency is defined as <300–400 ng/dL in men); however, serum-free (deficiency: <5–7 pg/mL in men; <3 pg/mL in women) and bioavailable testosterone may be more accurate measures. For testosterone replacement in men, commonly used testosterone preparations include esterified depot testosterone (propionate, enanthate, cypionate, initiated at 100–200 mg intramuscularly every 2 weeks, maximum 400 mg intramuscularly weekly), transdermal skin patches (1 to 2 patches, 5–10 mg, to clean, dry skin daily), and transdermal testosterone gel (1 to 4 packets, 25–100 mg, to clean, dry skin daily), with the depot preparations being the least expensive and most studied. Patch and gel formulations may produce less variability in serum testosterone levels and in target symptoms. In women, transdermal testosterone, 150 mg per day or equivalent, may be used to improve energy, well-being, muscle mass, and restore normal menstrual functioning.[40] Reported side effects for men include irritability, tension, reduced energy, hair loss, testicular atrophy, reduced ejaculate volume, and acne. For women, there is particular concern for virilizing side effects; however, clinically these have been minimal in the setting of physiologic replacement dosing in the range described.

Delirium

The most common neuropsychiatric complication in hospitalized patients with AIDS is delirium.[54] Delirium is diagnosed in 11% to 29% of hospitalized patients with HIV-AIDS.[11] There are no data regarding specific or distinguishing symptom characteristics for the delirium seen in patients with HIV. Both the hypoactive and hyperactive variants of delirium are seen, and in addition to cognitive disturbance, symptom manifestations include apathy, dysphoria, agitation, fearfulness, delusions, and hallucinations.[55]

Delirium in the patient with HIV-AIDS is often superimposed on HANDs, particularly dementia, and patients with these disorders are at increased risk for the development of delirium when medically hospitalized. The etiology of delirium in patients with HIV-AIDS is generally multifactorial. Breitbart and colleagues[55] reported a mean of 12.6 medical complications in 30 delirious patients with AIDS, with the most common being hematologic (anemia, leukopenia, thrombocytopenia, hypoalbuminemia) and infectious diseases (eg, septicemia, systemic fungal infections, *Pneumocystis carinii* pneumonia, tuberculosis, and disseminated viral infections). Other potential etiologies were discussed previously in the differential diagnosis section.

Central to the treatment of delirium is treatment of its underlying medical causes. Symptomatic treatment includes educational, environmental, and psychopharmacologic interventions. Education regarding the risk and nature of delirium delivered to patients, their families, and the treatment team can be preventive and can result in earlier treatment and improved outcomes. Environmental interventions include titrating the level of stimulation, sitting the patient up, placing patients next to a window, frequent orientation, stabilizing sleep-wake cycles, and placing familiar people and orienting objects in the room.

In terms of pharmacologic treatment, most practitioners treat delirium with atypical antipsychotics, including olanzapine (available with dissolving oral preparation and intramuscularly), risperidone (available in dissolving oral preparation), quetiapine, aripiprazole (available intramuscularly), and ziprasidone (available intramuscularly). The only double-blind clinical trial of delirium treatment in AIDS, however, compared haloperidol, chlorpromazine, and lorazepam.[55] In that study, Breitbart and colleagues[55] screened medical inpatients with HIV for delirium. Treatment was initiated early, and when symptoms were mild to moderate in degree. Patients were severely medically ill, because 9 (30%) of the 30 patients died within 1 week after completing the protocol. There were 3 important findings. First, haloperidol (mean dose, 2.8 mg/d acutely and 1.4 mg/d maintenance) and chlorpromazine (mean dose, 50 mg/d acutely and 36 mg/d maintenance) were equally efficacious. Second, the lorazepam arm (mean dose, 3 mg acutely) was stopped early because of worsening of delirium symptoms, including oversedation, disinhibition, ataxia, and increased confusion. Third, adverse effects in the antipsychotic arms were limited and included mild extrapyramidal symptoms (EPS), such as decreased expressiveness, rigidity, tremor, and mild akathisia. Open-label studies and case reports suggest that the atypical antipsychotics clozapine, risperidone, and ziprasidone benefit patients with AIDS with psychosis and/or delirium.[56]

Delirium is common in hospitalized patients with HIV-AIDS, who should be assessed frequently for early detection and treatment. A combination of psychoeducational, environmental, and pharmacologic interventions, primarily with neuroleptic medications, is recommended. Benzodiazepines should be avoided, except in cases of severe agitation that fails to respond to antipsychotic agents or patients experiencing delirium secondary to alcohol or other CNS-depressant agent withdrawal, and patients should be monitored closely for the emergence of EPS. There is a higher susceptibility of patients with HIV to EPS, even with exposure to drugs with low potential for inducing EPS.[57] Extreme sensitivity to EPS is encountered in patients with HIV-dementia.[58] Marked neuronal degeneration in the basal ganglia of patients with HIV may contribute to these findings because of the accompanying dopaminergic neuron destruction and/or alteration.[59]

Mania

Manic symptomatology has been reported in 11% of all medically hospitalized patients with HIV-AIDS[11] and may be seen in conjunction with primary bipolar illness or with CNS HIV infection (HIV-associated mania). Descriptively, HIV-associated mania is found to be a late-onset, secondary affective illness associated with HIV infection of the brain, being less associated with a personal or family history of mood disorder. In addition, the symptomatology of HIV-associated mania may include more irritability, less hypertalkativeness, and more psychomotor slowing and cognitive impairment compared with primary bipolar mania.[60] Given that HIV-associated mania is directly related to HIV brain infection, antiretroviral agents that penetrate the blood-brain barrier may offer some protection from incident mania.[61] The mechanisms are poorly understood; however, the HIV nef protein is reported to alter CNS dopamine metabolism leading to hyperactive, "maniclike" behaviors in animal models.[62]

The choice of psychotropic drugs to treat HIV mania is based on case reports, and open-label studies, rather than randomized controlled trials, as well as the desire to avoid adverse drug interactions, and the avoidance of HIV-specific side effects. HIV mania may improve with an approach that combines resolution of the underlying CNS process, use of a mood-stabilizing drug, and/or addition of an antipsychotic drug.[63] Valproic acid is metabolized in the liver, and liver disease is common in HIV-positive persons; further, valproic acid has interactions with many ART drugs.[64,65] This must be weighed against the potential disadvantages of other mood stabilizers, such as lithium, which can exacerbate renal disease, or carbamazepine, which can induce bone marrow suppression, hepatotoxicity, and induce the metabolism of ART (particularly protease inhibitors).[64,66] Lamotrigine has been tested for HIV-associated peripheral neuropathy and may be useful for treating mixed mania or bipolar depression in HIV; however, patients with overt manic symptomatology generally require a traditional mood stabilizer. This anticonvulsant requires careful upward dose titration because of risk of severe hypersensitivity (Stevens-Johnson syndrome).

Given the limitations of mood stabilizers in HIV, there is widespread clinical use of atypical antipsychotics for acute and maintenance treatment of HIV-associated mania; however, there are no clinical trial data. Clinicians generally choose olanzapine, risperidone, ziprasidone, or quetiapine as alternatives to traditional mood stabilizers[58,67]; however, these agents may exacerbate metabolic syndrome or cause EPS in patients with extensive basal ganglia HIV involvement. Benzodiazepines may be useful for adjunctive treatment, but acute and maintenance therapy may be complicated by tolerance, dependence, and cognitive impairment, including the possibility of causing delirium and disinhibition.

Psychosis

HIV infection may be directly linked to the onset of psychosis, which is defined by the presence of thought disorder, hallucinations, or delusions. Psychosis in HIV is most often a manifestation of substance intoxication or withdrawal, delirium, HANDs, mood disorders with psychotic features, or schizophrenia. Estimates of the prevalence of new-onset psychosis in patients with HIV range from 0.5% to 15.0%.[68] One study compared 20 HIV-infected patients with new-onset psychosis (and no prior psychotic episodes or current substance abuse) with 20 nonpsychotic patients matched for demographics and HIV illness. The former group tended to have worse global neuropsychologic impairment, was more likely to have a prior history of substance abuse, and had significantly higher mortality at follow-up, suggesting that psychotic patients with HIV-AIDS had an increased CNS vulnerability.[69]

Persons with HIV-associated secondary psychosis are reported to show more disorders of consciousness, orientation, attention, and memory than patients with primary serious mental illness.[70] They also tend to report less bizarre delusions, have a more variable course, and are more likely to have eventual remission of their psychosis.[71]

Patients infected with HIV with primary psychotic disorders, such as schizophrenia and schizoaffective disorder, may have poor access to HIV care, may present to the emergency and medical inpatient setting with untreated advanced HIV illness, and may be at risk for poor adherence to care, unless provided with comprehensive supportive services, including psychiatric treatment, housing, and community case management.

In general, treatment with antipsychotic medication requires awareness of HIV-infected patients' susceptibility to neuroleptic-induced EPS as a result of HIV-induced neuronal damage to the basal ganglia. Movement disorders (acute dystonia, parkinsonism, ataxia) can be seen in advanced HIV disease in the absence of antipsychotic exposure. General recommendations include avoidance of high-potency D2 blocking agents (eg, haloperidol), avoidance of depot neuroleptics, and the consideration that maintenance antipsychotic medication may not be necessary for the complete remission of new-onset or transient psychotic symptoms. Most clinicians prefer the use of atypical antipsychotics in this population; however, they are associated with development of metabolic syndrome, cardiac problems, and obesity.[72]

A literature search on the use of antipsychotic medication in HIV-AIDS revealed 6 studies published since 1993; these studies described treatment of psychosis occurring in delirious, schizophrenic, and manic patients. Agents reported in the literature include haloperidol (mean dose, 3 mg),[73] clozapine (mean dose, 27 mg/d),[74] risperidone (mean dose, 3.3 mg/d),[75] and olanzapine (10–15 mg/d).[76] Haloperidol was reported to have a high incidence of EPS and caution is encouraged with clozapine because of the risk for agranulocytosis and interaction with ritonavir.

Anxiety

Anxiety is common in patients who are HIV-positive, estimated to occur in 22% to 47%. Generalized anxiety disorder has been found to range between 6.5% and 20.0% in HIV samples.[77,78] Posttraumatic stress disorder is a common anxiety disorder in persons with HIV, estimated at 10% to 54% among populations such as men who have sex with men, minority women, and those with persistent pain.[79,80] Patients who are HIV positive with subclinical or overt neurocognitive impairment are more sensitive to the side effects of anxiolytic medications and should start at low doses. Drug-drug interactions have been reported with anxiolytics and AIDS medications; for example, there are case reports of patients who are HIV-positive on protease inhibitors who experienced prolonged sedation when given midazolam.[81] Buspirone, a popular antianxiety agent and 5HT1A agonist, has been reported to cause extrapyramidal signs when given with protease inhibitors such as ritonavir.[82] Anxiety also interferes with ART adherence.[83]

Members of the Organization of AIDS Psychiatry participated in a Web-based survey. Consensus emerged regarding first-line treatment for depression (escitalopram/citalopram), for psychosis and secondary mania (quetiapine), and for anxiety (clonazepam).[84]

Herpes Simplex Encephalitis

Several viruses can cause viral encephalitis including HSV.[85] HSV is the etiologic agent for herpes simplex encephalitis (HSE), the most common source of acute viral encephalitis in the United States, with an annual incidence of 2000 cases yearly.[85,86] Two principal forms of HSV exist: HSV-1, which typically leads to orolabial lesions; and HSV-2, which is responsible for genital herpes lesions. HSV-2 infections more typically result in aseptic meningitis, whereas HSV-1 causes HSE. HSE is a potentially lethal infection with a mortality rate of up to 70% if left untreated and 14% to 20% with treatment.[85,87] Half of HSE cases occur in people older than 50, whereas a third of cases are in people younger than 20.[88]

Clinically, HSE often presents with acute onset of symptoms, such as fever, altered mental status, seizures, and focal neurologic signs, such as aphasia and hemiparesis. Without treatment, patients may progress to coma.[86] Before the acute presentation, there may be a prodrome characterized by headache, fatigue, mild fever, and irritability. It is hypothesized that HSV-1 enters the brain via the olfactory nerves and spreads into the limbic system, frontal, and temporal lobes. Infected neurons and other cells can undergo cytolysis, causing hemorrhagic destruction of brain tissue. Particularly vulnerable areas include the fronto-orbital region, temporal lobes, hippocampus, cingulate gyrus, and insular cortex.[89]

HSE leaves up to 80% of people who survive infection with a number of residual cognitive and neuropsychiatric sequelae.[85] Cognitively, patients may experience significant limitations in anterograde memory formation with additional impairment in retrograde memory. The cognitive effects of HSE are dependent on the sites of the brain involved. Although HSV-1 infection is often bilateral, impairments seen clinically may be dependent on lateralization of HSV-1–related brain injuries. In particular, right hemispheric involvement often leads to subtle deficits with less functional impairment. Left hemispheric neuronal damage, however, creates difficulties in language function and verbal memory.[85] Additional impairments, such as semantic aphasia or mutism, are found in up to 46% of patients with HSE and, more rarely, auditory agnosia also has been documented.[85,86] Long-term consequences of HSE include memory impairment and behavioral and personality changes.[85] Neuropsychiatrically, patients may exhibit symptoms of aggression and disinhibition consistent with a Klüver-Bucy syndrome. Early treatment may ameliorate some of these symptoms; however, particularly in the young and old, cognitive impairments secondary to HSE may lead to postencephalitic dementia.[85,90]

HSE is diagnosed by using a combination of clinical features and laboratory and imaging findings (**Table 3**). Noncontrast CT imaging demonstrates abnormalities in up to 50% of scans, including a midline shift. MRI, however, remains the most sensitive imaging tool in diagnosing HSE and is recommended as the first diagnostic step after the clinical examination.[86] MRI findings include focal hyperintensities on T2-weighted imaging. Electroencephalography (EEG) also may be used and initially may show some generalized or focal slowing over the temporal lobes (sites that are commonly a focus for HSV-1 infection), but may change to lateralized, epileptiform activity.[85] Lumbar puncture may demonstrate an elevated opening pressure, CSF leukocytosis, and xanthochromia in addition to a normal CSF glucose level. Polymerase chain reaction demonstrates the presence of HSV-1 infection in the CSF.

HSE is treated with intravenous acyclovir (60 mg/kg per day, given in 3 divided doses) for 21 days.[91] A repeat CSF examination should be performed at the end of therapy to ensure that the virus has cleared. The use of continued outpatient treatment with oral valacyclovir is common but has not been shown to improve outcomes.[92] Recovery is determined in part by how quickly treatment is begun, with increased morbidity and mortality associated with delays in treatment.[88] Although acyclovir treatment of HSV infection in HSE is widely accepted, there is no well-defined treatment specific for the cognitive and neuropsychiatric symptoms associated with HSE. It has been proposed that using dopamine antagonists in a carefully monitored manner may be useful in treating the behavioral disturbances associated with HSE in the acute period. This is based on evidence from an animal study suggesting activation of the mesostriatal dopamine system in HSE. Other treatments used in clinical practice for the neurobehavioral sequelae of HSE include anticonvulsants, benzodiazepines, antipsychotics, stimulants, mood stabilizers, and cholinesterase inhibitors.[85,93]

PEDIATRIC AUTOIMMUNE NEUROPSYCHIATRIC DISORDERS ASSOCIATED WITH STREPTOCOCCAL INFECTIONS

Over the past 25 years, there has been mounting evidence for connections between group A b-hemolytic streptococcal (GAS) infections and the development

Table 3
Clinical features and diagnosis of non-HIV infectious diseases with neuropsychiatric manifestations

Disease	Signs	Focal	CT/MRI	Laboratory Tests	Neuropsychiatric Sequelae	Treatment
Herpes encephalitis	Fever Altered mental Status Focal neurologic Signs Seizures Aggression/ disinhibition Language impairments	Yes	Midline shift T2 focal hyperintensities	EEG Lumbar puncture PCR	Difficulties in language function and verbal memory Semantic aphasia or autism Behavioral and personality changes Klüver-Bucy syndrome	Intravenous acyclovir
Pediatric autoimmune neuropsychiatric disorders associated with streptococcal infections	Age of onset between ages 3 and 11 y OCD or tic disorder symptoms Temporal association between symptoms and group A-hemolytic streptococcal infection	No	Basal ganglia enlargement	Antistreptococcal antibody titers ESR, CRP D8/17 B-lymphocyte marker ↑antibasal ganglia Ab's	OCD or tic disorder symptoms Other movement disorders	Plasma exchange intravenous immunoglobulin ±PCN or azithromycin
Neurocysticercosis	Seizures Agitation Psychosis Focal neurologic signs Depression Dementia	Yes	Ring-enhancing lesions Visualization of scolex in cystic structure	ELISA EITB	Seizures Psychosislike states Dementia	Antihelminthic agents: praziquantel, albendazole Steroids Anticonvulsants

Disease	Symptoms	Lesions correlate to specific deficits	Imaging	Diagnostic tests	Psychiatric features	Treatment
Neurosyphilis	General paresis Psychosis Emotional lability Anhedonia Social withdrawal Dementia	No	Lesions correlate to specific deficits	VDRL Rapid plasma regain Fluorescent treponemal antibody-absorption assay Lumbar puncture	Mood disorders Psychosislike states Behavioral changes: disinhibition Dementia	PCN Ceftriaxone
Creutzfeldt-Jakob disease	Rapidly progressive cognitive decline Extrapyramidal signs, ataxia, myoclonus, dysphagia Akinetic mutism Agitation Psychosis Depression	No	Cortical ribboning Basal ganglia and cortical abnormalities Variant Creutzfeldt-Jakob disease: hyperintensity in pulvinar thalami	EEG: periodic sharp wave complexes Tonsil biopsy for variant Creutzfeldt-Jakob disease 14-3-3 assay	Rapidly progressive dementia Cerebellar signs Visual signs Myoclonus Pyramidal symptoms Extrapyramidal symptoms Akinetic mutism Mood disorders Psychosislike states	No effective treatment has been identified

Abbreviations: ↑, increasing; Ab, antibody; CRP, C-reactive protein; CT, computed tomography; EEG, electroencephalogram; EITB, enzyme-linked immunoelectrotransfer; ELISA, enzyme-linked immunosorbent assay; ESR, erythrocytic sedimentation rate; HIV, human immunodeficiency virus; OCD, obsessive-compulsive disorder; PCN, penicillin; PCR, polymerase chain reaction; VDRL, Venereal Disease Research Laboratory.

of neuropsychiatric symptoms. Sir William Osler made the original observation that patients with Sydenham chorea, a complication of GAS infection, also exhibited behaviors consistent with tics and obsessive-compulsive disorder (OCD). Later work demonstrated that as many as 70% to 80% of patients with Sydenham chorea also have clinical features meeting diagnostic criteria for OCD, particularly in children.[94,95] Based on work with children who exhibited abrupt onset of OCD symptoms or tics following GAS infection, the development of these symptoms was linked to an immune system–mediated response to the original infection, termed "pediatric autoimmune neuropsychiatric disorders associated with streptococcal infections" (PANDAS).[94,96] Age of symptom onset is approximately 3 years younger in PANDAS than childhood-onset OCD. Additionally, the abrupt onset and relapsing-remitting pattern of symptoms in PANDAS differs from the more gradual onset and chronic pattern in childhood OCD.[95,97] There may be a heritable component to PANDAS, because children with PANDAS have parents and grandparents with significantly higher rates of streptococcal infection complications, such as rheumatic fever, compared with controls.[96]

Diagnostic criteria for PANDAS include (1) age of onset between the ages of 3 and 11 years; (2) meeting criteria for OCD or a tic disorder; (3) episodic severity of symptoms; (4) association with GAS infection; and (5) association with neurologic abnormalities, including hyperactivity, tic, or choreoform movements.[94,95] Although resembling childhood-onset OCD, PANDAS is distinguished clinically by a distinct temporal relationship between a GAS infection and onset of OCD or tics.

Experts convened at the National Institutes of Health in July 2010, given the agreement that a subgroup of children with OCD have an abrupt onset of symptoms accompanied by a variety of severe and acute neuropsychiatric symptoms. Given the ongoing controversy about the etiology of the symptoms, experts proposed an expanded clinical syndrome, pediatric acute-onset neuropsychiatric syndrome (PANS) or childhood acute neuropsychiatric symptoms (CANS), which may be caused by noninfectious (eg, drugs, metabolic abnormalities) or infectious (eg, group A streptococci) triggers. Proposed diagnostic criteria for PANS/CANS include the following:

- Abrupt, dramatic onset of OCD or severely restricted food intake
- At least 2 concurrent severe neuropsychiatric symptoms (eg, anxiety, depression, emotional lability), also with acute onset
- Symptoms not better explained by a known neurologic or medical disorder (for example, Sydenham chorea, systemic lupus erythematosus, Tourette disorder)[98,99]

To make a more definitive diagnosis (see **Table 3**), obtaining antistreptococcal antibody titers (including antistreptolysin O [ASO] and antideoxyribonuclease B [ADB] antibodies) that rise during a symptomatic exacerbation and fall with symptomatic improvement is often needed. Serologic diagnosis of recent GAS infection can be made by demonstrating a 0.2 log10 rise (a 58% increase) in either ASO or ADB, ordinarily obtained 4 to 8 weeks apart, although only 62% of new GAS acquisitions were followed by such a rise. A single high titer, rather than serial acute and convalescent titers, is not diagnostically reliable, but may be considered contributory if levels exceed twofold (0.3 log10) above the laboratory's stated upper limit of normal, because these higher levels are uncommon in children without recent streptococcal infection.[100] Use of these antistreptococcal antibody titers, however, is complicated because titers may remain high for months after infection.[95] There is also evidence that antibodies directed against the basal ganglia are found more commonly in patients with PANDAS relative to people with uncomplicated streptococcal infections.[101]

This finding may shed further light on the pathophysiology of PANDAS, given that preliminary MRI suggests basal ganglia enlargement in patients with PANDAS.[102] In determining susceptibility to PANDAS, studies have indicated that patients with PANDAS are more likely to also have lymphocytes that are positive for the D8/17 marker. This B-lymphocyte alloantigen marker is also associated with other streptococcal-related conditions, such as rheumatic fever and Sydenham chorea, further suggesting an immune basis.[94,95]

Ultimately, based on the clinical and diagnostic features of PANDAS, it has been suggested that the pathophysiology of PANDAS is based on the development of an autoimmune reaction in patients who are susceptible (ie, based on family history, immunologic markers). This reaction occurs in response to infection with GAS in which the immune system inappropriately generates antibodies against epitopes on the basal ganglia that resemble streptococcal antigens through the process of molecular mimicry.[95] The resulting immune-mediated inflammatory process in the basal ganglia then may lead to the clinical features of PANDAS.[96]

Most instances of PANS are suspected to be postinfectious in origin, although no single microbe other than GAS has yet been consistently associated with the onset of PANS. Therefore, a detailed review and documentation of associated febrile and nonfebrile infectious illnesses, including signs and symptoms and diagnostic testing, is advised. The most commonly observed antecedent infection seems to be upper respiratory infection, including rhinosinusitis, pharyngitis, or bronchitis. It is not yet clear if any 1 of those 3 presentations is more likely than the others to be associated with the initiation of PANS. *Mycoplasma pneumoniae*, influenza, Epstein-Barr virus, and Lyme disease have been implicated to PANS onset or flares.[103]

Treatment of PANDAS has been largely based on immunomodulatory therapies. Notably, significant symptomatic improvements have been demonstrated in patients following use of plasma exchange and intravenous immunoglobulin (IVIG). In one study, severity of OCD symptoms diminished by 45% to 58% following treatment with either plasma exchange or IVIG.[96,104] Despite this, immunomodulatory therapies have not been recommended as the routine treatment of PANDAS.[95] IVIG and plasma exchange both carry a substantial risk of adverse effects, and use of these modalities should be reserved for children with particularly severe symptoms and a clear-cut PANDAS presentation.[105] The US National Institutes of Health and American Academy of Neurology 2011 guidelines state there are inadequate data to determine the efficacy of plasmapheresis in the treatment of acute OCD and tic symptoms in the setting of PANDAS and insufficient evidence to support or refute the use of plasmapheresis in the treatment of acute OCD and tic symptoms in the setting of PANDAS.[106] Use of antibiotic prophylaxis to prevent neuropsychiatric exacerbations following recurrent streptococcal infections has yielded mixed results. Although one double-blind, placebo-controlled trial found no benefit over placebo in preventing PANDAS exacerbations, another trial found that either penicillin or azithromycin were able not only to lower rates of streptococcal infections but also to decrease symptom exacerbations in patients with PANDAS.[107,108] Evidence is insufficient to determine if tonsillectomy is effective.[109]

Children with OCD and/or tic disorders should receive standard neuropsychiatric treatment for these disorders (whether or not the children have evidence of recent GAS infection).[110,111] Treatment of neuropsychiatric symptoms should not be delayed pending confirmation of PANDAS (eg, documenting rise in antistreptococcal antibodies or while monitoring for a second episode).

The neuropsychiatric manifestations of children in the PANDAS subgroup respond to treatment with standard pharmacologic and behavior therapies.[110] OCD symptoms generally respond to a combination of pharmacotherapy (typically a selective seroto-nin reuptake inhibitor) and cognitive behavior therapy. Motor and vocal tics can be treated with a variety of medications.

NEUROCYSTICERCOSIS

Neurocysticercosis (NCC) is the most common parasitic disease of the nervous sys-tem, particularly in developing countries in Asia, Latin America, and Africa. Because of rising rates of immigration from areas in which it is more prevalent, however, NCC is appearing more frequently in North America and Europe. Annually, more than 50,000 deaths worldwide are attributable to NCC. Even more patients are left alive with chronic, irreversible brain damage. Moreover, NCC is the major etiology for acquired epilepsy in endemic areas.[112] NCC is caused by infection with the tape-worm *Taenia solium*. Humans are the definitive host for *T solium*, whereas pigs serve as the intermediate host. NCC results generally from fecal-oral transmission in which people ingest the eggs of the tapeworm from contaminated food or water. Commonly, this route of transmission occurs through handling of food by others already infected or from improperly cleaned food. Autoinfection also occurs, albeit less frequently.[95] Once in the intestine, the eggs hatch and migrate throughout the body by way of the bloodstream, ultimately depositing into various tissues where they develop into the larval cysticercus form. When the site of larval deposition is in the CNS, NCC de-velops. Symptoms of NCC are dependent on the area and extent of nervous system involvement. The 4 main types of NCC are (1) parenchymal, (2) subarachnoid, (3) ven-tricular, and (4) spinal.[95]

Neurologically, seizures are the most common manifestation of NCC, occurring in 80% of infected patients, especially in the parenchymal form of the disease.[113] The seizures are typically simple partial or generalized tonic-clonic, although patients also may present with focal neurologic deficits based on the sites of infection. Stroke, intracranial hypertension, hydrocephalus, meningeal inflammation, fibrosis, or cyst formation also may occur.[112] As a result, NCC is on the differential diagnosis of most neurologic disorders in endemic regions.[114]

Given the varied neurologic presentations of NCC, it is not surprising that NCC also has many different psychiatric manifestations. Up to 15% of people infected with NCC exhibit only psychiatric sequelae.[115] In a study examining rates of *T solium* infection among chronic psychiatric inpatients in a community in Venezuela, 18.5% of the inpa-tients were infected versus 1.6% of controls.[116] Commonly, patients present with acute psychiatric decompensation,[95] mimicking psychotic states, such as schizo-phrenia. In one case report, NCC was marked by acute psychosis characterized by agitation, thought disorganization, paranoia, and auditory-visual hallucinations.[112,117] Other psychiatric manifestations of NCC include depression or dementia; suspicion for NCC-related dementia ought to be high if it occurs in patients who are younger, also have a history of seizures, have acute onset of symptoms, and are from an area in which NCC is endemic.[95] In a recent study from Brazil, more than 80% of the patients with NCC reported depressive symptoms.[118]

The diagnosis of NCC is often difficult because the symptoms often resemble those from a broad differential of other disorders (see **Table 3**). NCC most commonly is diag-nosed, however, from clinical history, imaging, and laboratory techniques. Besides bi-opsies that often prove difficult to do, brain imaging using CT and MRI scans allows for visualization of lesions from *Taenia* infection. In active disease, ring-enhancing lesions are most typically seen; visualization of the parasite's scolex within a cystic structure is pathognomonic for NCC.[112] Infection outside the brain parenchyma makes visualization more difficult.[95] Laboratory studies are often used to confirm the diagnosis by investigating patient serology for antibodies related to *Taenia* infection. Enzyme-linked immunosorbent assay and enzyme-linked immunoelectrotransfer are often used for antibody detection.[95] However, a weakness of the test is that it may be false negative in approximately 50% of patients with a single cerebral cyst or in those with calcifications alone. Another weakness is that it may be false positive in persons who had been exposed to the adult parasite without developing the disease.[119]

NCC treatment has been controversial, with few rigorous, large-scale studies conducted examining the various treatment options. The location of cysts; degree, size, and severity of local inflammation around lesions; and symptom severity all affect the treatment choice. This is complicated by findings that the treatments themselves may exacerbate the already present inflammatory response leading to symptomatic worsening.[120] Nevertheless, NCC has been treated for more than 20 years using antihelminthic agents, such as praziquantel and albendazole.[95,112,120] Other agents may be given in concert with these drugs, including steroids (to treat pericystic inflammation and NCC-related encephalitis) and anticonvulsants (because of NCC-related seizures). The American Academy of Neurology issued a guideline document and concluded that albendazole plus corticosteroids should be considered for patients with neurocysticercosis, as the use of these drugs reduces the number of viable cysts on control neuroimaging studies (level B of evidence) and the long-term risk of seizure recurrence (level B evidence).[121] In some instances, surgery also may be needed for placement of ventricular shunts to treat hydrocephalus secondary to arachnoiditis.[112,120]

NEUROSYPHILIS

Cases of syphilis have been documented since the late 1400s and, with the HIV epidemic in recent years, have had global resurgence. By the 1920s, more than 20% of patients in American mental hospitals had tertiary neurosyphilis (NS).[122] With the advent of antibiotics, such as penicillin, the incidence and prevalence of syphilis and resultant NS dropped significantly; however, in parallel with the HIV epidemic, rates of infection (largely by sexual intercourse) began to rise again. There has been an 81% increase in cases of syphilis infection among men since 2000, with an annual incidence of 0.2 to 2.1 cases per 100,000 immunocompetent individuals.[122–124] This has been an important health problem because syphilis facilitates coinfection with HIV.[124] HIV causes impaired cell-mediated immunity, which accelerates the progression of syphilis, so that patients with HIV have a greater frequency of neurosyphilis.[125]

Known as the original "great imitator," syphilis has a number of presentations in virtually all organ systems, including the CNS. Consequently, NS has been linked with a diverse array of cognitive and psychiatric syndromes. Untreated, symptomatic NS develops in 4% to 9% of patients infected with syphilis.[126]

NS is caused by *Treponema pallidum*, the spirochete responsible for syphilis. Infection may be either symptomatic or asymptomatic. Although NS classically presented with tabes dorsalis or general paresis, these are less common today. Instead, patients with NS are asymptomatic or may present with seizures, ocular symptoms, or with psychiatric and behavioral changes.[122] Early NS may occur within 5 years of infection, whereas late NS (involving the brain parenchyma) typically occurs within 5 to 25 years of infection. HIV infection, however, may accelerate the clinical progression to symptomatic NS.[126] The general paresis form of NS is the type most commonly associated with psychiatric symptoms.[122] The psychiatric presentation of NS typically begins insidiously, with mood changes including symptoms of mania or depression. Up to 27% of patients with the general paresis form of NS develop depression characterized by melancholia, suicidal ideation, and psychomotor retardation. Patients also may present with psychosis of acute or insidious onset that may mimic schizophrenia.[127] Personality changes in patients with NS can include emotional lability, antisocial behaviors, anhedonia, social withdrawal, explosive temper, giddiness, hypersexuality, or less attention to personal details. As NS progresses, however, intellectual functioning worsens. Ultimately, symptoms of dementia predominate, leading to disability and, finally, death.[122,127] NS often leads to cortical atrophy and brain lesions. Lesions imaged by MRI in the temporoparietal region have been associated with cognitive impairments as measured by the Mini Mental-State Examination, whereas lesions in the frontal lobes are associated with overall psychiatric morbidity.[128] Importantly, although prompt treatment of NS is necessary to halt the progression of the illness, it is not expected that patients' mental status will improve completely, because of neuronal loss.[122]

Diagnosis of NS is difficult, because unlike other infectious organisms, *T pallidum* cannot be grown in culture (see **Table 3**). Because so many cases of NS are asymptomatic, many infected patients are missed. If the index of suspicion is sufficiently high, however, NS is diagnosed serologically by the rapid plasma regain and Venereal Disease Research Laboratory tests; CSF may be used in the Venereal Disease Research Laboratory assay. If positive, results are confirmed with a microhemagglutination assay for *T pallidum* or with the fluorescent treponemal antibody-absorption assay.[122]

NS is treated with a 10-day to 14-day course of aqueous penicillin G (18–24 million units per day with 3–4 million units given intravenously every 4 hours). An alternative is to treat the patient with procaine penicillin (2.4 million units daily intramuscularly) combined with probenecid, 500 mg orally, 4 times daily, particularly if compliant with treatment; ceftriaxone may be used if the patient is allergic to penicillin.[122,124] Sexual partners of the patient also may need evaluation and treatment.[112] There has been little documentation specifically addressing treatment of psychiatric symptoms associated with NS. There is no consensus that antibiotic treatment of neurosyphilis produces a persistent improvement in cognition in persons with general paresis.[129] A recent study by Sanchez and Zisselman[124] recommended use of a typical antipsychotic, haloperidol, or the atypical agents, quetiapine or risperidone, to treat psychosis in patients with NS. An anticonvulsant, such as divalproex sodium, also was recommended to address agitation and for mood stabilization.[124] Smaller case reports supported atypical antipsychotics, such as olanzapine and quetiapine, in treatment of NS-associated psychosis.[130,131]

CREUTZFELDT-JAKOB DISEASE

Prion disorders have received much attention in the media given recent epidemics of bovine spongiform encephalopathy (also known as "mad cow disease") and the resulting health risks associated with possible transmission to humans. There are several diseases caused by the prion protein, a novel infectious agent composed of a protein ordinarily found in all humans. These diseases are known as "transmissible spongiform encephalopathies" and are found in many mammals, including cattle, in the form of bovine spongiform encephalopathy, in sheep (known as "scrapie"), and in humans. Prion diseases are believed to occur when the naturally occurring form of the prion protein acquires an abnormal conformational state that facilitates conversion of surrounding prion protein into the pathogenic form, ultimately leading to cell death.[132] In the CNS, this process leads to marked neurodegeneration causing spongiform changes, and, consequently, a reactive astrocytosis.[133]

Prion disease in humans was first noted in 1920 and 1921 by H G. Creutzfeldt and A.M. Jacob, respectively.[134] Human prion diseases occur in most of the developed world at a rate of 1.0 to 1.5 cases per million per year. In the United States, with a population of approximately 330 million, approximately 400 cases of prion disease are diagnosed per year, an incidence of 1.2 in 1.0 million. Of human prion diseases, 80% to 95% are sporadic Creutzfeldt-Jakob disease (CJD), 10% to 15% are genetic (often familial), and fewer than 1% are acquired.[135] Four forms of CJD exist: (1) sporadic CJD, (2) familial CJD, (3) variant CJD, and (4) iatrogenic CJD. Most CJD cases are sporadic in nature, constituting up to 80% to 95% of all reported CJD.[135] Sporadic CJD reportedly has a mean survival of approximately 6 months (median approximately 5 months), with 85% to 90% of patients dying within 1 year. The peak age of onset is 55 to 75 years of age, with median age of onset of approximately 67 years and mean of 64 years.[136,137] In sporadic CJD, the misfolding of the prion protein occurs likely because of a spontaneous mutation in the gene encoding the prion protein. Although the precise significance relating to pathogenesis is unknown, up to 85% of patients with sporadic CJD are homozygote for 2 copies of the methionine amino acid at codon 129 of the prion protein (Met/Met).[134]

Up to 10% to 15% of CJD cases are familial in origin. Genetic prion diseases historically have been divided into 3 forms based on clinicopathologic features: familial CJD, Gerstmann-Sträussler-Scheinker syndrome, and fatal familial insomnia. Familial CJD is inherited in an autosomal-dominant fashion. Most mutations causing genetic prion disease are caused by missense mutations, but several octapeptide repeat insertion mutations and at least 5 stop codon mutations exist.[138] Among the groups with the highest prevalence of familial CJD are Libyan Jews and clusters of families in Chile, Slovakia, Japan, and the United States.

Variant CJD (also known as "new-variant CJD") was first described in 1996 after several CJD cases in the United Kingdom were identified as having features that varied from the classic presentation of sporadic CJD. It is the only form of human prion disease known to be transmitted directly from animals to humans, in most cases through exposure to bovine spongiform encephalopathy.[139] It occurred because of the practice of feeding sheep products, some of which were unfortunately contaminated with the prion disease scrapie, to cattle, mostly in the United Kingdom but in other countries as well.[139,140] Food products derived from these infected cattle were consumed by humans, a portion of whom developed variant CJD. The clinical presentation of variant CJD usually begins with a psychiatric prodrome, often at least 6 months before the onset of traditional neurologic symptoms; cognitive dysfunction, dysesthesia, cerebellar dysfunction, and involuntary movements (eg, dystonia, myoclonus, or chorea) usually appear several months after psychiatric onset. Compared with sporadic CJD, the median age of onset of patients with variant CJD is much younger than most sporadic cases, approximately 27 years (range 12–74 years), with a longer median disease duration of 14.5 months.[140] Variant CJD also may be transmissible by blood, including transfusions.[133,134]

Last, iatrogenic CJD has been documented after exposure to tissues from patients infected with CJD or from surgical instruments that have come into contact with those infected. Cases have been reported of patients developing CJD after corneal transplantation or dura mater grafts from infected donors and by cadaveric pituitary growth hormone.[134] Clinically, sporadic CJD presents as a rapidly progressive dementia with average disease duration of only 1 year until death. Moreover, the neurologic and neuropsychiatric symptoms associated with CJD often mimic those found in other dementias, such as Alzheimer disease or Lewy body dementia. Common neurologic symptoms may include extrapyramidal signs, cerebellar ataxia, sensory complaints, myoclonus, and dysphagia. In advanced stages of illness, patients can exhibit akinetic mutism and may ultimately die from aspiration pneumonia.[132] Although sporadic CJD was classically believed to present with primarily neurologic manifestations with some psychiatric symptoms appearing late in the course of illness, more recently it has been demonstrated that psychiatric symptoms commonly occur at diagnosis and throughout progression of the disease. A retrospective review of 126 patients with sporadic CJD at the Mayo Clinic revealed that 80% of the cases demonstrated psychiatric symptoms within the first 100 days of illness, with 26% occurring at presentation.[141] In contrast to sporadic CJD, psychiatric and neuropsychiatric symptoms are often the most prominent aspects in the clinical presentation of variant CJD.[141]

Psychiatric sequelae of CJD include depressed mood and apathy.[142] A prodromal phase has been described characterized by fatigue, weight loss, impaired sleep, poor judgment, and unusual behavior. Patients also may display unusually intense emotional responses; anxiety; agitation; and psychotic symptoms, such as delusions and hallucinations.[141,143] At times, presentations of primarily depression or psychosis in CJD have made it difficult to distinguish from primary psychiatric disorders and led to misdiagnosis or delays in diagnosis of CJD.[144] Neuropsychologic testing revealed focal cortical deficits in sporadic CJD in contrast to more generalized deficits in variant CJD.[145]

Based on criteria suggested by the World Health Organization, definite diagnosis of sporadic CJD involves either neuropathologic examination or detection of the pathogenic scrapie form of the prion protein in brain samples by Western blot (see **Table 3**).[146] To receive a probable diagnosis of sporadic CJD, patients must have 2 of the following clinical signs: (1) cerebellar or visual signs; (2) myoclonus, pyramidal, or extrapyramidal signs; or (3) akinetic mutism. Additionally, patients must have detection of the 14-3-3 protein in the CSF or an EEG consistent with CJD coupled with disease duration leading to death in less than 2 years, or investigation not suggestive of an alternative diagnosis.[132]

Besides use of clinical symptoms, diagnosis is also based on EEG, imaging, and laboratory findings. Typical EEG findings in sporadic CJD include periodic sharp wave complexes that have either biphasic or triphasic waves or complexes with mixed spikes. In contrast, EEGs of patients with variant CJD do not show periodic sharp wave complexes, but rather have nonspecific slow-wave activity.[146] MRI has been used extensively in diagnosis of CJD. There are abnormalities in the basal ganglia and cortex and a unique pattern of "cortical ribboning." Patients with variant CJD prominently display a pattern of hyperintensity in the pulvinar thalami.[132] In applying laboratory testing for diagnosis, the detection of the 14-3-3 protein in the CSF of patients with CJD is both quite sensitive and specific for the sporadic form of the disease, although less so in the variant form.[147] A clear diagnosis of variant CJD also may be made by tonsil biopsy through detection of the scrapie form of the prion protein.[148]

Presently, there is no effective treatment for CJD. A focus of potential treatment strategies has been to block accumulation of the pathogenic scrapie form of the prion protein. The antimalarial agent quinacrine and the phenothiazines have been tried with little success in animal and human trials. Another recent approach has been development of vaccines to develop antibodies against the prion protein, although the results of these efforts have been unclear thus far.[133]

LYME DISEASE ENCEPHALOPATHY (NEUROBORRELIOSIS)

Lyme disease, caused by infection with the tic-borne spirochete *Borrelia burgdorferi*, has been associated with a variety of manifestations, including neuropsychiatric symptoms, or neuroborreliosis. Over the past 20 years, there has been significant controversy regarding the neuropsychiatric manifestations of neuroborreliosis, which is related to the fact that symptoms are often nonspecific (fatigue, sleep disturbance, generalized cognitive complaints, low mood, all symptoms of depression); serologic testing may show evidence of prior systemic exposure but cannot determine whether or not there is acute disease; and symptoms may persist after acute antibiotic treatment.[149,150] Further, the mechanisms of the neuropsychiatric manifestations are not precisely known, being possibly related to direct CNS infection with the organism, to acute or long-term inflammatory processes associated with systemic or CNS infection, or some combination of these. Over the past 10 years, there is accumulating evidence that *B burgdorferi* may adhere to endothelial cells at the blood-brain barrier, causing vasculitis and increased blood-brain barrier permeability, leading to CNS invasion and adherence to astrocytes, resulting in a deleterious inflammatory cascade.[151] The resulting changes in the CNS, including abnormalities in subcortical frontotemporal white matter and basal ganglia functioning,[152] may explain the more chronic neuropsychiatric symptoms and why antibiotic treatment of these chronic symptoms is generally not associated with improvement in symptoms or CNS pathology.[149–151]

In the early stages of acute Lyme disease, patients may present with meningitis, cranial neuritis, and radiculoneuritis.[150] In many such cases, there are positive CSF findings for *B burgdorferi* antibody (immunoglobulin G) and elevated protein. Cognitive deficits associated with acute and chronic Lyme disease include poor attention and concentration, impaired verbal memory, word-finding difficulties, psychomotor slowing, and executive dysfunction, all consistent with subcortical-frontal pathology. Interestingly, study of patients with Lyme disease with chronic cognitive complaints indicates that those with abnormal CSF are more likely than those with normal CSF to have actual neuropsychologic deficits. In those with normal CSF, cognitive complaints are more likely to be associated with concurrent depression.[150] Psychiatrically, patients with both acute and chronic symptoms of neuroborreliosis may present with depression, mood lability, irritability, anxiety, panic attacks, and more rarely, mania, psychosis, and obsessive-compulsive symptoms.[152] There are no large-scale well-controlled studies, however, to suggest that patients with Lyme disease have a greater burden of such symptoms than the general population.

In terms of diagnosis, neurologic examination is usually nonfocal. Bedside cognitive evaluation may be normal to mildly abnormal and more extensive neuropsychologic testing may be necessary to detect the characteristic deficits mentioned previously. Lumbar puncture and CSF evaluation may reveal *B burgdorferi* DNA detected by polymerase chain reaction and antibody to *B burgdorferi*, nonspecific protein elevation, and CSF pleocytosis. The CSF may be normal, however, in a substantial number of cases. Standard structural neuroimaging, including brain CT or MRI with contrast, is often normal in both the acute and chronic stages of the disease. Quantitative single-photon emission CT of the brain has proved more useful in detecting abnormality, including hypoperfusion in frontal subcortical and cortical regions.[153] This method has been used to follow response to antibiotic treatment.

In terms of treatment, intravenous infusion of ceftriaxone, 2 g daily for 30 days, followed by oral doxycycline, 200 mg daily for 60 days, has been tested.[149] Other regimens in the literature include intravenous penicillin or a derivative, amoxicillin.

Although such regimens have been helpful for neuroborreliosis with clear evidence of abnormal CSF in acute and chronic disease, results have been less favorable in patients with chronic symptoms and minimal objective evidence of CNS infection.

In terms of psychotropic medication treatment for psychiatric comorbidities, the literature is quite sparse. Treatment is generally symptomatic, addressing symptoms of depression (ie, with selective serotonin reuptake inhibitors), fatigue and cognitive complaints (ie, with psychostimulants or modafinil), and mood lability and psychosis (ie, with atypical neuroleptics). Given the subcortical involvement of the spirochete, however, it is important to assess for extrapyramidal side effects with the use of atypical neuroleptic medications.

SUMMARY

This article reviews the clinical characteristics and treatment of a number of infectious diseases that have prominent neuropsychiatric manifestations. Although each entity has unique characteristics, there are several common themes that are important for clinicians to remember. First, maintain an index of suspicion, especially when patients present with new-onset psychiatric symptoms without a history of prior psychiatric illness. It is commonplace to overlook medical or neurologic illness in assuming a primary psychiatric diagnosis, including sexual risk behavior, blood-borne exposures, and travel history. Third, although a thorough diagnostic workup is necessary to identify and treat the infection, equally important is a full characterization of the psychiatric and cognitive symptoms associated with the infection so as to track the effects of treatment. This becomes particularly important when patients have residual deficits that affect everyday function and ability to work. Finally, it is important to remember that concurrent treatment with antibiotics and psychotropic medications is often necessary. For most of these infectious diseases, formal study of psychotropic medications is relatively infrequent, so clinicians should be vigilant regarding potential drug-drug and drug-disease interactions. Fortunately, when these principles are followed, neuropsychiatric manifestations of infectious diseases can be successfully identified and treated.

REFERENCES

1. Fleishman JA, Hellinger FJ. Trends in HIV-related inpatient admissions from 1993–1997: a seven-state study. J Acquir Immune Defic Syndr 2001;28:73–80.
2. Fleishman JA, Hellinger FH. Recent trends in HIV-related inpatient admissions 1996–2000: a seven-state study. J Acquir Immune Defic Syndr 2003;34:102–10.
3. Paul S, Gilbert HM, Lande L, et al. Impact of antiretroviral therapy on decreasing hospitalization rates of HIV-infected patients in 2001. AIDS Res Hum Retroviruses 2002;18:501–6.
4. Cebo KA, Diener-West M, Moore RD. Hospitalization rates in an urban cohort after the introduction of highly active antiretroviral therapy. J Acquir Immune Defic Syndr 2003;27:143–52.
5. Adih W, Selik R, Hall H, et al. Associations and trends in cause-specific rates of death among persons reported with HIV infection, 23 U.S. jurisdictions, through 2011. Open AIDS J 2016;10(1):144–57.
6. Ferrando S, Tiamson M. HIV disease. In: Blumenfield M, Strain JJ, editors. Psychosomatic medicine. Philadelphia: Lippincott Williams and Wilkins; 2006. p. 277–96.
7. Perry S, Tross S. Psychiatric problems of aids inpatients at the New York Hospital: preliminary report. Public Health Rep 1984;99:200–5.

8. Dilley JW, Ochitill HN, Perl M, et al. Findings in psychiatric consultations with patients with acquired immune deficiency syndrome. Am J Psychiatry 1985;142: 82–6.

9. O'Dowd MA, McKegney FP. AIDS patients compared with others seen in psychiatric consultation. Gen Hosp Psychiatry 1990;12:50–5.

10. Bialer P, Wallack J, Prenzlauer S, et al. Psychiatric comorbidity among hospitalized AIDS patients vs. non-AIDS patients referred for psychiatric consultation. Psychosomatics 1996;37:469–75.

11. Ferrando SJ, Rabkin J, Rothenberg J. Psychiatric disorders and adjustment of HIV and AIDS patients during and after medical hospitalization. Psychosomatics 1998;39:214–5.

12. American Academy of Neurology AIDS Task Force. Nomenclature and research case definitions for neurologic manifestations of human immunodeficiency virus-type-1 (HIV-1) infection. Neurology 1991;41:778–85.

13. Antinori A, Arendt G, Becker JT, et al. Updated research nosology for HIV-associated neurocognitive disorders. Neurology 2007;69:1789–99.

14. Sacktor NC, Bacellar H, Hoover DR, et al. Psychomotor slowing in HIV infection: a predictor of dementia, AIDS and death. J Neurovirol 1996;2:404–10.

15. Wilkie FL, Goodkin K, Eisdorfer C, et al. Mild cognitive impairment and risk of mortality in HIV-1 infection. J Neuropsychiatry Clin Neurosci 1998;10:125–32.

16. Tozzi V, Balestra P, Serriano D, et al. Neurocognitive impairment and survival in a cohort of HIV-infected patients treated with HAART. AIDS Res Hum Retroviruses 2005;21:706–13.

17. Ragin A, Wu Y, Gao Y, et al. Brain alterations within the first 100 days of HIV infection. Ann Clin Transl Neurol 2014;2(1):12–21.

18. Anthony IC, Bell JE. The neuropathology of AIDS. Int Rev Psychiatry 2008;20: 15–24.

19. Smit TK, Brew BJ, Tourtellotte W, et al. Independent evolution of human immunodeficiency virus (HIV) drug resistance mutations in diverse areas of the brain in HIV-infected patients, with and without dementia, on antiretroviral treatment. J Virol 2004;78:10133–48.

20. Letendre S, Marquie-Beck J, Capparelli E, et al. Validation of the CNS penetration-effectiveness rank for quantifying antiretroviral penetration into the central nervous system. Arch Neurol 2008;65:65–70.

21. Nightingale S, Winston A, Letendre S, et al. Controversies in HIV-associated neurocognitive disorders. Lancet Neurol 2014;13(11):1139–51.

22. Sacktor N, Skolasky R, Seaberg E, et al. Prevalence of HIV-associated neurocognitive disorders in the multicenter AIDS cohort study. Neurology 2015; 86(4):334–40.

23. Sacktor N, Lyles RH, Skolasky R, et al. HIV-associated neurologic disease incidence changes: multicenter AIDS Cohort Study, 1990-1998. Neurology 2001;56: 257–60.

24. Beguelin C, Vazquez M, Bertschi M, et al. Viral escape in the CNS with multidrug-resistant HIV-1. J Int AIDS Soc 2014;17(4 Suppl 3):19745.

25. Filippi C, Sze G, Farber SJ, et al. Regression of HIV encephalopathy and basal ganglia signal intensity abnormality at MR imaging in patients with AIDS after the initiation of protease inhibitor therapy. Radiology 1998;206:491–8.

26. Sacktor N, Skolasky RL, Ernst T, et al. A multicenter study of two magnetic resonance spectroscopy techniques in individuals with HIV dementia. J Magn Reson Imaging 2005;21:325–33.

27. Tozzi V, Balestra P, Galgani S, et al. Positive and sustained effects of highly active antiretroviral therapy on HIV-1-associated neurocognitive impairment. AIDS 1999;13:1889–97.

28. Ferrando SJ, Rabkin JG, van Gorp WG, et al. Longitudinal improvement in psychomotor processing speed is associated with potent combination antiretroviral therapy in HIV-1 infection. J Neuropsychiatry Clin Neurosci 2003;15:208–14.

29. Mora-Peris B, Stevens E, Ferretti F, et al. Evolution of changes in cognitive function after the initiation of antiretroviral therapy. AIDS Res Ther 2016;13(1):20.

30. Ferrando S, van Gorp W, McElhiney M, et al. Highly active antiretroviral treatment (HAART) in HIV infection: benefits for neuropsychological function. AIDS 1998;12:F65–70.

31. Robertson KR, Smurzynski M, Parsons T, et al. The prevalence and incidence of neurocognitive impairment in the HAART era. AIDS 2007;21:1915–21.

32. Hinkin CH, Hardy DJ, Mason KL, et al. Medication adherence in HIV-infected adults: effect of patient age, cognitive status and substance abuse. AIDS 2004;18(Suppl 1):S19–25.

33. van Gorp WG, Rabkin JG, Ferrando SJ, et al. Neuropsychiatric predictors of return to work in HIV/AIDS. J Int Neuropsychol Soc 2007;13:80–9.

34. Perry S, Jacobsberg LB, Fishman B, et al. Psychiatric diagnosis before serological testing for the human immunodeficiency virus. Am J Psychiatry 1990;147: 89–93.

35. Williams JBW, Rabkin JG, Remien RH, et al. Multidisciplinary baseline assessment of homosexual men with and without human immunodeficiency virus infection II. Standardized clinical assessment of current and lifetime psychopathology. Arch Gen Psychiatry 1991;48:124–30.

36. Rifai M, Gleason O, Sabouni D. Psychiatric care of the patient with hepatitis C: a review of the literature. Prim Care Companion J Clin Psychiatry 2010;12(6): PCC.09r00877.

37. Abers M, Shandera W, Kass J. Neurological and psychiatric adverse effects of antiretroviral drugs. CNS Drugs 2013;28(2):131–45.

38. Staszewski S, Morales-Ramirez J, Tashima KT, et al. Efavirenz plus zidovudine and lamivudine, efavirenz plus indinavir, and indinavir plus zidovudine and lamivudine in treatment of HIV-1 infection in adults. Study 006 team. N Engl J Med 1999;341:1865–73.

39. Ji S, Jin C, Höxtermann S, et al. Prevalence and influencing factors of thyroid dysfunction in HIV-infected patients. Biomed Res Int 2016;2016:1–11.

40. Mylonakis E, Koutkia P, Grinspoon S. Diagnosis and treatment of androgen deficiency in human immunodeficiency virus-infected men and women. Clin Infect Dis 2001;33:857–64.

41. Mayo J, Callazos J, Martinez E, et al. Adrenal function in the human immunodeficiency virus-infected patient. Arch Intern Med 2002;162:1095–8.

42. Cassol E, Misra V, Morgello S, et al. Altered monoamine and acylcarnitine metabolites in HIV-positive and HIV-negative subjects with depression. J Acquir Immune Defic Syndr 2015;69(1):18–28.

43. Gonzalez JS, Batchelder AW, Psaros C, et al. Depression and HIV/AIDS treatment nonadherence: a review and meta-analysis. J Acquir Immune Defic Syndr 2011;58(2):181–7.

44. Bhatia M, Munjal S. Prevalence of depression in people living with HIV/AIDS undergoing ART and factors associated with it. J Clin Diagn Res 2014;8(10): WC01–4.

45. Mierlak D, Leon A, Perry S. Does physical improvement reduce depressive symptoms in HIV-infected medical inpatients? Gen Hosp Psychiatry 1995;17: 380–4.
46. Currier M, Nemeroff C. Inflammation and mood disorders: proinflammatory cytokines and the pathogenesis of depression. AntiInflamm Antiallergy Agents Med Chem 2010;9:212–20.
47. Rabkin JG, Williams JB, Remien RH, et al. Depression, distress, lymphocyte subsets and human immunodeficiency virus symptoms on two occasions in HIV-positive homosexual men. Arch Gen Psychiatry 1992;48:111–9.
48. Ferrando SJ, Goldman JG, Charness W. SSRI treatment of depression in symptomatic HIV infection and AIDS: improvements in affective and somatic symptoms. Gen Hosp Psychiatry 1997;19:89–97.
49. Steer RA, Cavalieri TA, Leonard DM, et al. Use of the Beck depression inventory for primary care to screen for major depression disorders. Gen Hosp Psychiatry 1999;21(2):106–11.
50. Watkins C, Treisman G. Cognitive impairment in patients with AIDS—prevalence and severity. HIV AIDS (Auckl) 2015;7:35–47.
51. Wagner GJ, Rabkin R. Effects of dextroamphetamine on depression and fatigue in men with HIV: a double-blind, placebo-controlled trial. J Clin Psychiatry 2000; 61:436–40.
52. Breitbart W, Rosenfeld B, Kaim M, et al. A randomized, double-blind, placebo-controlled trial of psychostimulants for the treatment of fatigue in ambulatory patients with human immunodeficiency virus disease. Arch Intern Med 2001;161: 411–20.
53. Rabkin J, McElhiney M, Rabkin R, et al. Modafinil treatment for fatigue in HIV/ AIDS. J Clin Psychiatry 2010;71(06):707–15.
54. Sonneville R, Ferrand H, Tubach F, et al. Neurological complications of HIV infection in critically ill patients: clinical features and outcomes. J Infect 2011; 62(4):301–8.
55. Breitbart W, Marotta R, Platt MM, et al. A double-blind trial of haloperidol, chlorpromazine, and lorazepam in the treatment of delirium in hospitalized AIDS patients. Am J Psychiatry 1996;153:231–7.
56. Brogan K, Lux J. Management of common psychiatric conditions in the HIV-positive population. Curr HIV/AIDS Rep 2009;6(2):108–15.
57. Valcour V, Watters M, Williams A, et al. Aging exacerbates extrapyramidal motor signs in the era of highly active antiretroviral therapy. J Neurovirol 2008;14(5): 362–7.
58. Dolder C, Patterson T, Jeste D. HIV, psychosis and aging. AIDS 2004;18(Suppl 1):35–42.
59. Itoh K, Mehrain P, Weis S. Neuronal damage of the substantia nigra in HIV-1 infected brains. Acta Neuropathol 2000;99(4):376–84.
60. Nakimuli-Mpungu E, Musisi S, Mpungu S, et al. Early-onset versus late-onset HIV-related secondary mania in Uganda. Psychosomatics 2008;49(6):530–4.
61. Mijch AM, Judd FK, Lyketsos CG, et al. Secondary mania in patients with HIV infection: are antiretrovirals protective? J Neuropsychiatry Clin Neurosci 1999; 11:475–80.
62. Acharjee S, Branton W, Vivithanaporn P, et al. HIV-1 Nef expression in microglia disrupts dopaminergic and immune functions with associated mania-like behaviors. Brain Behav Immun 2014;40:74–84.
63. Singer E, Thames A. Neurobehavioral manifestations of human immunodeficiency virus/AIDS. Neurol Clin 2016;34(1):33–53.

64. Siddiqi O, Birbeck G. Safe treatment of seizures in the setting of HIV/AIDS. Curr Treat Options Neurol 2013;15(4):529–43.

65. Birbeck G, French J, Perucca E, et al. Antiepileptic drug selection for people with HIV/AIDS: evidence-based guidelines from the ILAE and AAN. Epilepsia 2012;53(1):207–14.

66. Okulicz J, Grandits G, French J, et al. The impact of enzyme-inducing antiepileptic drugs on antiretroviral drug levels: a case-control study. Epilepsy Res 2013;103(2–3):245–53.

67. Spiegel D, Weller A, Pennell K, et al. The successful treatment of mania due to acquired immunodeficiency syndrome using ziprasidone: a case series. J Neuropsychiatry 2010;22(1):111–4.

68. McDaniel JS, for the Working Group on HIV/AIDS. Practice guideline for the treatment of patients with HIV/AIDS. Am J Psychiatry 2000;157:1–62.

69. Sewell DD, Jeste DV, Atkinson JH, et al. HIV-associated psychosis: a study of 20 cases. San Diego HIV neurobehavioral research center group. Am J Psychiatry 1994;151:237–42.

70. Alciati A, Fusi A, D'Arminio Monforte A, et al. New-onset delusions and hallucinations in patients infected with HIV. J Psychiatry Neurosci 2001;26(3):229–34.

71. Harris MJ, Jeste DV, Gleghorn A, et al. New-onset psychosis in HIV-infected patients. J Clin Psychiatry 1991;52(9):369–76.

72. Vergara-Rodriguez P, Vibhakar S, Watts J. Metabolic syndrome and associated cardiovascular risk factors in the treatment of persons with human immunodeficiency virus and severe mental illness. Pharmacol Ther 2009;124(3):269–78.

73. Sewell DD, Jeste DV, McAdams LA, et al. Neuroleptic treatment of HIV-associated psychosis. HNRC group. Neuropsychopharmacology 1994;10:223–9.

74. Lera G, Zirulnik J. Pilot study with clozapine in patients with HIV-associated psychosis and drug-induced parkinsonism. Mov Disord 1999;14:128–31.

75. Singh AN, Golledge H, Catalan J. Treatment of HIV-related psychotic disorders with risperidone: a series of 21 cases. J Psychosom Res 1997;42:489–93.

76. Meyer JM, Marsh J, Simpson G. Differential sensitivities to risperidone and olanzapine in a human immunodeficiency virus patient. Biol Psychiatry 1998;44:791–4.

77. Celesia BM, Nigro L, Pinzone MR, et al. High prevalence of undiagnosed anxiety symptoms among HIV-positive individuals on cART: a cross-sectional study. Eur Rev Med Pharmacol Sci 2013;17(15):2040–6.

78. Bing EG, Burnam MA, Longshore D, et al. Psychiatric disorders and drug use among human immunodeficiency virus-infected adults in the United States. Arch Gen Psychiatry 2001;58(8):721–8.

79. Kelly B, Raphael B, Judd F, et al. Posttraumatic stress disorder in response to HIV infection. Gen Hosp Psychiatry 1998;20(6):345–52.

80. Smith MY, Egert J, Winkel G, et al. The impact of PTSD on pain experience in persons with HIV/AIDS. Pain 2002;98(1–2):9–17.

81. Hsu AJ, Carson KA, Yung R, et al. Severe prolonged sedation associated with coadministration of protease inhibitors and intravenous midazolam during bronchoscopy. Pharmacotherapy 2012;32(6):538–45.

82. Clay PG, Adams MM. Pseudo-Parkinson disease secondary to ritonavir-buspirone interaction. Ann Pharmacother 2003;37(2):202–5.

83. Ammassari A, Trotta MP, Murri R, et al. Correlates and predictors of adherence to highly active antiretroviral therapy: overview of published literature. J Acquir Immune Defic Syndr 2002;31(Suppl 3):S123–7.

84. Freudenreich O, Goforth H, Cozza K, et al. Psychiatric treatment of persons with HIV/AIDS: an HIV-psychiatry consensus survey of current practices. Psychosomatics 2010;51(6):480–8.

85. Arciniegas DB, Anderson CA. Viral encephalitis: neuropsychiatric and neurobehavioral aspects. Curr Psychiatry Rep 2004;6:372–9.

86. Chaudhuri A, Kennedy PGE. Diagnosis and treatment of viral encephalitis. Postgrad Med J 2002;78:575–83.

87. Stahl JP, Mailles A, De Broucker T. Herpes simplex encephalitis and management of acyclovir in encephalitis patients in France. Epidemiol Infect 2012; 140:372–81.

88. Whitley RJ, Gnann JW. Viral encephalitis: familiar infections and emerging pathogens. Lancet 2002;359:507–14.

89. Steiner I, Benninger F. Update on herpes virus infections of the nervous system. Curr Neurol Neurosci Rep 2013;13(12):414.

90. Dagsdottir HM, Sigurethardottir B, Gottfreethsson M, et al. Herpes simplex encephalitis in Iceland 1987–2011. Springerplus 2014;3:524.

91. Widener RW, Whitley RJ. Herpes simplex virus. Handb Clin Neurol 2014;123: 251–63.

92. Gnann JW Jr, Skoldenberg B, Hart J, et al. Herpes simplex encephalitis: lack of clinical benefit of long-term valacyclovir therapy. Clin Infect Dis 2015;61(5): 683–91.

93. Vasconcelos-Moreno MP, Dargel AA, Goi PD, et al. Improvement of behavioural and manic-like symptoms secondary to herpes simplex virus encephalitis with mood stabilizers: a case report. Int J Neuropsychopharmacol 2011;14(5): 718–20.

94. Pavone P, Parano E, Rizzo R, et al. Autoimmune neuropsychiatric disorders associated with streptococcal infection: Sydenham's chorea, PANDAS, and PANDAS variants. J Child Neurol 2006;21:727–36.

95. Schneider RK, Robinson MJ, Levenson JL. Psychiatric presentations of non-HIV infectious diseases: neurocysticercosis, Lyme disease, and pediatric autoimmune neuropsychiatric disorder associated with streptococcal infection. Psychiatr Clin North Am 2002;25:1–16.

96. Swedo SE. Pediatric autoimmune neuropsychiatric disorders associated with streptococcal infections (PANDAS). Mol Psychiatry 2002;7:S24–5.

97. Perlmutter SJ, Garvey MA, Castellanos X, et al. A case of pediatric autoimmune neuropsychiatric disorders associated with streptococcal infections. Am J Psychiatry 1998;155:1592–8.

98. Swedo S, Leckman J, Rose N. From research subgroup to clinical syndrome: modifying the PANDAS criteria to describe PANS (pediatric acute-onset neuropsychiatric syndrome). Pediatr Ther 2012;2:1–8.

99. Singer HS, Gilbert DL, Wolf DS, et al. Moving from PANDAS to CANS. J Pediatr 2012;160(5):725–31.

100. Johnson DR, Kurlan R, Leckman J, et al. The human immune response to streptococcal extracellular antigens: clinical, diagnostic, and potential pathogenetic implications. Clin Infect Dis 2010;50:481–90.

101. Pavone P, Bianchini R, Parano E, et al. Anti-brain antibodies in PANDAS versus uncomplicated streptococcal infection. Pediatr Neurol 2004;30:107–10.

102. Giedd JN, Rapoport JL, Garvey MA, et al. MRI assessment of children with obsessive-compulsive disorder or tics associated with streptococcal infection. Am J Psychiatry 2000;157:281–3.

103. Chang K, Frankovich J, Cooperstock M, et al. Clinical evaluation of youth with pediatric acute-onset neuropsychiatric syndrome (PANS): recommendations from the 2013 PANS consensus conference. J Child Adolesc Psychopharmacol 2015;25(1):3–13.

104. Perlmutter SJ, Leitman SF, Garvey MA, et al. Therapeutic plasma exchange and intravenous immunoglobulin for obsessive-compulsive disorder and tic disorders in childhood. Lancet 1999;354:1153–8.

105. Kalra SK, Swedo SE. Children with obsessive-compulsive disorder: are they just "little adults"? J Clin Invest 2009;119(4):737–46.

106. Cortese I, Chaudhry V, So YT, et al. Evidence-based guideline update: plasmapheresis in neurologic disorders: report of the therapeutics and technology assessment subcommittee of the American Academy of Neurology. Neurology 2011;76(3):294–300.

107. Garvey MA, Perlmutter SJ, Allen AJ, et al. A pilot study of penicillin prophylaxis for neuropsychiatric exacerbations triggered by streptococcal infections. Biol Psychiatry 1999;45:1564–71.

108. Snider LA, Lougee L, Slattery M, et al. Antibiotic prophylaxis with azithromycin or penicillin for childhood-onset neuropsychiatric disorders. Biol Psychiatry 2005; 57:788–92.

109. de Oliveira SK, Pelajo CF. Pediatric autoimmune neuropsychiatric disorders associated with streptococcal infection (PANDAS): a controversial diagnosis. Curr Infect Dis Rep 2010;12(2):103–9.

110. Swedo SE, Leonard HL, Rapoport JL. The pediatric autoimmune neuropsychiatric disorders associated with streptococcal infection (PANDAS) subgroup: separating fact from fiction. Pediatrics 2004;113(4):907.

111. Kurlan R, Kaplan EL. The pediatric autoimmune neuropsychiatric disorders associated with streptococcal infection (PANDAS) etiology for tics and obsessive-compulsive symptoms: hypothesis or entity? Practical considerations for the clinician. Pediatrics 2004;113(4):883.

112. Del Brutto OH. Neurocysticercosis. Semin Neurol 2005;25:243–51.

113. Ndimubanzi PC, Carabin H, Budke CM, et al. A systematic review of the frequency of neurocysticercosis with a focus on people with epilepsy. PLoS Negl Trop Dis 2010;4(11):e870.

114. Carabin H, Ndimubanzi PC, Budke CM. Clinical manifestations associated with neurocysticercosis: a systematic review. PLoS Negl Trop Dis 2011;5(5):e1152.

115. Tavares AR. Psychiatric disorders in neurocysticercosis. Br J Psychiatry 1993; 163:839.

116. Meza NW, Rossi NE, Galeazzi TN, et al. Cysticercosis in chronic psychiatric inpatients from a Venezuelan community. Am J Trop Med Hyg 2005;73:504–9.

117. Signore RJ, Lahmeyer HW. Acute psychosis in a patient with cerebral cysticercosis. Psychosomatics 1988;29:106–8.

118. Almeida SM, Gurjão SA. Frequency of depression among patients with neurocysticercosis. Arq Neuropsiquiatr 2010;68(1):76–80.

119. Singh G, Rajshekhar V, Murthy JM, et al. A diagnostic and therapeutic scheme for a solitary cysticercus granuloma. Neurology 2010;75(24):2236–45.

120. Nash TE, Singh G, White AC, et al. Treatment of neurocysticercosis: current status and future research needs. Neurology 2006;67:1120–7.

121. Baird RA, Wiebe S, Zunt JR, et al. Neurology 2013;80(15):1424–9.

122. Hutto B. Syphilis in clinical psychiatry: a review. Psychosomatics 2001;46: 453–60.

123. Conde-Sendín MA, Amela-Peris R, Aladro-Benito Y, et al. Current clinical spectrum of neurosyphilis in immunocompetent patients. Eur Neurol 2004;52:29–35.

124. Sanchez FM, Zisselman MH. Treatment of psychiatric symptoms associated with neurosyphilis. Psychosomatics 2007;48:440–5.

125. Berger JR, Dean D. Neurosyphilis. Handb Clin Neurol 2014;121:1461–72.

126. Carmo RA, Moura AS, Christo PP, et al. Syphilitic meningitis in HIV-patients with meningeal syndrome: report of two cases and review. Braz J Infect Dis 2001;5: 280–7.

127. Sobhan T, Rowe HM, Ryan WG, et al. Unusual case report: three cases of psychiatric manifestations of neurosyphilis. Psychiatr Serv 2004;55:830–2.

128. Russouw HG, Roberts MC, Emsley RA, et al. Psychiatric manifestations and magnetic resonance imaging in HIV-negative neurosyphilis. Biol Psychiatry 1997;41:467–73.

129. Moulton CD, Koychev I. The effect of penicillin therapy on cognitive outcomes in neurosyphilis: a systematic review of the literature. Gen Hosp Psychiatry 2015 Jan-Feb;37(1):49–52.

130. Taycan O, Ugur M, Ozmen M. Quetiapine vs. risperidone in treating psychosis in neurosyphilis: a case report. Gen Hosp Psychiatry 2006;8:359–61.

131. Turan S, Emul M, Duran A, et al. Effectiveness of olanzapine in neurosyphilis related organic psychosis: a case report. J Psychopharmacol 2007;21:556–8.

132. Martindale JL, Geschwind MD, Miller BL. Psychiatric and neuroimaging findings in Creutzfeldt-Jakob disease. Curr Psychiatry Rep 2003;5:43–6.

133. Caramelli M, Ru G, Acutis P, et al. Prion diseases: current understanding of epidemiology and pathogenesis and therapeutic advances. CNS Drugs 2006; 20:15–28.

134. Pederson NS, Smith E. Prion diseases: epidemiology in man. APMIS 2002;110: 14–22.

135. Maddox RA, Person M, Minino A, et al. P.85: improving Creutzfeldt-Jakob disease incidence estimates by incorporating results of neuropathological analyses, United States, 2003–2011. Presented at Prion 2015 International Research Congress; Prion. Fort Collins, May 26–29, 2015. p. S55–6.

136. Puoti G, Bizzi A, Forloni G, et al. Sporadic human prion diseases: molecular insights and diagnosis. Lancet Neurol 2012;11(7):618–28.

137. Collins SJ, Sanchez-Juan P, Masters CL, et al. Determinants of diagnostic investigation sensitivities across the clinical spectrum of sporadic Creutzfeldt-Jakob disease. Brain 2006;129(pt 9):2278–87.

138. Geschwind M. Prion diseases. Continuum (Minneap Minn) 2015;21:1612–38.

139. Brown K, Mastrianni JA. The prion diseases. J Geriatr Psychiatry Neurol 2010; 23(4):277–98.

140. Heath CA, Cooper SA, Murray K, et al. Diagnosing variant Creutzfeldt-Jakob disease: a retrospective analysis of the first 150 cases in the UK. J Neurol Neurosurg Psychiatry 2011;82(6):646–51.

141. Wall CA, Rummans TA, Aksamit AJ, et al. Psychiatric manifestations of Creutzfeldt-Jakob disease: a 25-year analysis. J Neuropsychiatry Clin Neurosci 2005;17(4):489–95.

142. Jiang TT, Moses H, Gordon H, et al. Sporadic Creutzfeldt-Jakob disease presenting as major depression. South Med J 1999;92:807–8.

143. Moellentine CK, Rummans TA. The varied neuropsychiatric presentations of Creutzfeldt- Jakob disease. Psychosomatics 1999;40:260–3.

144. Jadri R, DiPaola C, Lajugie C, et al. Depressive disorder with psychotic symptoms as psychiatric presentation of sporadic Creutzfeldt-Jakob disease: a case report. Gen Hosp Psychiatry 2006;28:452–4.
145. Kapur N, Abbot P, Lowman A, et al. The neuropsychological profile associated with variant Creutzfeldt-Jakob disease. Brain 2003;126:2693–702.
146. Wieser HG, Schindler K, Zumsteg D. EEG in Creutzfeldt-Jakob disease. Clin Neurophysiol 2006;117:935–51.
147. Green AJE. Use of 14-3-3 in the diagnosis of Creutzfeldt-Jacob disease. Biochem Soc Trans 2002;30:382–6.
148. Collinge J. Molecular neurology of prion disease. J Neurol Neurosurg Psychiatry 2005;76:906–19.
149. Kaplan RF, Trevino RP, Johnson GM, et al. Cognitive function in post-treatment Lyme disease: do additional antibiotics help? Neurology 2003;60(12):1888–9.
150. Kaplan RF, Jones-Woodward L. Lyme encephalopathy: a neuropsychological perspective. Semin Neurol 1997;17:31–7.
151. Oksi J, Kalimo H, Marttila RJ, et al. Inflammatory brain changes in Lyme borreliosis: a report on three patients and review of literature. Brain 1996;119:2143–54.
152. Garakani A, Mitton A. New-onset panic, depression with suicidal thoughts, and somatic symptoms in a patient with a history of Lyme disease. Case Rep Psychiatry 2015;2015:1–4.
153. Logigian EL, Johnson KA, Kijewski MF, et al. Reversible cerebral hypoperfusion in Lyme encephalopathy. Neurology 1997;49(6):1661–70.

Medical Complications of Psychiatric Treatment
An Update

Sheila C. Lahijani, MD[a],*, Kirk A. Harris, MD[b]

KEYWORDS

- Complications of psychiatric medications • Psychiatry and critical illness
- Psychiatric medications in hospitalized patients

KEY POINTS

- The use of psychiatric medications is common and frequently indicated in the management of critically ill patients.
- Medical complications from these medications may occur and can range from being minor to life-threatening.
- Careful consideration of their toxicity, interactions with other treatments, and intoxication or withdrawal syndromes should be made in the care of the critically ill patient.
- This article discusses the most significant medical complications of psychiatric treatment and is organized by each organ system.

Psychiatric medications are used commonly in critically ill patients and may be indispensable to manage many conditions, including preexisting disorders, emotional and behavioral symptoms due to medical illness, disruption of sleep, and to facilitate successful weaning from sedation. Such treatment should be closely monitored, however, as medical complications may arise. These complications may occur due to direct toxicity, drug-drug interactions, or intoxication or withdrawal from psychotropic medications. They range from life-threatening reactions, such as neuroleptic malignant syndrome and Stevens-Johnson Syndrome (SJS),

This article is an update of an article previously published in *Critical Care Clinics*, Volume 24, Issue 4, October 2008.
Disclosure Statement: The authors have nothing to disclose.
[a] Department of Psychiatry and Behavioral Sciences, Stanford University School of Medicine, 401 Quarry Road, Palo Alto, CA 94305, USA; [b] Department of Psychiatry, Rush University, 1725 West Harrison Street, Suite 955, Chicago, IL 60612, USA
* Corresponding author. Department of Psychiatry and Behavioral Sciences, Stanford University School of Medicine, 401 Quarry Road, Palo Alto, CA 94305.
E-mail address: lahijani@stanford.edu

Crit Care Clin 33 (2017) 713–734
http://dx.doi.org/10.1016/j.ccc.2017.03.008
0749-0704/17/© 2017 Elsevier Inc. All rights reserved.

criticalcare.theclinics.com

to minor syndromes (electrolyte disturbances or elevations in liver function testing), to mild adverse effects, such as sedation. This article discusses the most significant medical complications of psychiatric treatment and is organized by each organ system.

CENTRAL NERVOUS SYSTEM
Neuroleptic Malignant Syndrome

Neuroleptic malignant syndrome (NMS) is an idiosyncratic, potentially life-threatening reaction caused by the administration of antipsychotics and other medications that block dopamine in the central nervous system. The syndrome is characterized by the onset of fever, autonomic instability, extrapyramidal signs, and altered mental status (**Box 1**).[1] Incidence rates range from 0.01% to 0.02%. Historically, typical antipsychotics with strong dopamine blockade have caused NMS, but atypical antipsychotics with lower dopamine receptor affinity and phenothiazine antiemetics have also been implicated.[2] Onset is usually within 24 hours to 1 month after drug initiation, with altered mental status and neurologic signs, such as rigidity, generally preceding other features. Duration is limited once the drug is discontinued; however, mortality rates have been reported as high as 10% to 20% when NMS has not been recognized.[3] In the intensive care unit (ICU), several risk factors exist for NMS, including the use of antipsychotics for management of agitation or delirium, use of higher doses of antipsychotics in the parenteral formulation, rapid dose escalation, switching from one agent to another, use of these agents in treatment-naïve individuals, and compromised metabolism.[2–4]

Box 1
Neuroleptic malignant syndrome

Major Features

Exposure to dopamine antagonist within 72 hours before symptom development

"Lead pipe" muscle rigidity

Hyperthermia (>100°F or 38°C, measured orally × 2)

Associated Features

Altered mental status

Autonomic instability (tachycardia, hypertension, tachypnea)

Associated with profuse diaphoresis

Creatinine kinase >4 times upper limit

Evaluation

Leukocytosis

Metabolic acidosis

Hypoxia

Respiratory distress from hypermetabolism, chest wall restriction, metabolic acidosis, aspiration pneumonia, pulmonary emboli

Decreased serum iron concentrations

Elevations in serum muscle enzymes and catecholamines

Electroencephalographic generalized slowing

Treatment of NMS generally includes discontinuation of all dopamine blockers and supportive care. Additionally, there is some evidence for the use benzodiazepines, dopaminergic agents, dantrolene, and, in severe cases, electroconvulsive therapy.[5] A form of NMS (known as NM-like syndrome or parkinsonism hyperpyrexia syndrome) is also seen in individuals treated with dopamine agonists (amantadine, levodopa), following rapid discontinuation of the agents. Supportive care may be administered as in NMS; however, reinitiation of dopamine agonist treatments for parkinsonism should be highly considered (**Box 2**).[6]

Box 2
Examples of medications associated with neuroleptic malignant syndrome

Typical antipsychotics

Haloperidol, droperidol, fluphenazine, perphenazine, chlorpromazine, trifluoperazine, thiothixene, thioridazine, pimozide, loxapine, molindone

Atypical antipsychotics

Clozapine, olanzapine, risperidone, paliperidone, ziprasidone, quetiapine, aripiprazole

Dopamine blockers

Metoclopramide, promethazine, prochlorperazine

Serotonin Syndrome

Serotonin syndrome (SS) is a potentially life-threatening reaction caused by excessive activity of postsynaptic serotonin receptors. It is characterized by altered mental status, autonomic excitation, and neuromuscular abnormalities, and may develop in patients who are receiving serotonergic agents for a range of indications, including emesis, pain, or depression. The syndrome is diagnosed based on these clinical findings as well as the Hunter Serotonin Toxicity Criteria.[7,8] Patients with SS may present with altered mental status or some kind of toxidrome. Severe SS should be managed in the ICU, although little literature exists on the complications experienced in the ICU by patients with SS. In a retrospective study, Pedavally and colleagues[9] reviewed patients admitted to the ICU for presentations of SS as well as those admitted for another reason who developed SS in the ICU. Most patients were exposed to multiple serotonergic agents; antidepressants (selective serotonin reuptake inhibitors [SSRIs], venlafaxine, trazodone), opioids, and antiemetics were the most common. A range of presentations were reported. Altered mental status was noted in all cases; however, fever was not. Clonus, rigidity, and hyperreflexia were the most common neurologic signs. SS should therefore be judiciously considered, and serotonergic agents promptly discontinued, in any patient who develops altered mental status with signs of neuromuscular disinhibition (**Box 3**).

As with NMS, treatment includes discontinuation of all suspected causative agents, and supportive care. Use of benzodiazepines and serotonin antagonists (eg, cyproheptadine) may be considered. Differentiating SS from NMS can be challenging, particularly in patients receiving both a serotonin agonist and a dopamine antagonist. According to a review of the literature, low serum iron, proteinuria, creatine kinase, lactate dehydrogenase, aspartate transaminase, and leukocytosis can infer NMS in at least 75% of cases. Thus, it is worthwhile to review laboratory data in differentiating between SS and NMS.[10]

Box 3
Drugs and drug-drug interactions associated with moderate-severe toxicity

Monoamine oxidase inhibitors

Irreversible inhibitors: phenelzine, isocarboxazid

Reversible inhibitors: moclobemide

Nonpsychotropic agents: linezolid, methylene blue

Serotonergic agents

Selective serotonin reuptake inhibitors: fluoxetine, fluvoxamine, paroxetine, sertraline, citalopram, escitalopram

Serotonin-norepinephrine reuptake inhibitors: venlafaxine, desvenlafaxine, duloxetine

Tricyclic antidepressants: clomipramine, imipramine

Opioid analgesics: tramadol, fentanyl, dextromethorphan

Synthetic stimulants: ecstasy, bath salts

St John's wort

Amphetamine, methylphenidate, phentermine

Fenfluramine, sibutramine

Dopamine blockers

Metoclopramide, promethazine, prochlorperazine

Miscellaneous

Lithium

Buspirone

Tryptophan

From Buckley NA, Dawson AH, Isbister GK. Serotonin syndrome. BMJ 2014;348:g1626; with permission.

Delirium

The *Diagnostic and Statistical Manual, 5th edition* definition describes delirium as a change in attention or awareness that develops over a short time span, fluctuates, and is accompanied by other disturbances in cognition. A diagnosis requires evidence that the change is caused by a medical condition, substance intoxication, withdrawal state, or medication side effect. Profound disturbances in psychomotor activity and emotion often accompany the syndrome, and delirium is also associated with disruption in the sleep-wake cycle.[3] The prevalence of delirium in medical and surgical ICU cohort studies has ranged between 20% and 80%, depending on both the severity and the diagnostic methods. Delirium is often unrecognized and identified inappropriately as another disorder, such as depression or dementia. This is partly attributable to the different subtypes of delirium, which include hypoactive, mixed, and hyperactive. Delirium in the ICU is associated with complications and adverse outcomes.[1] Delirium pathways are discussed in detail elsewhere in this issue. Risk factors for delirium with the strongest evidence include the following: age, dementia, hypertension, coma, Acute Physiology and Chronic Health Evaluation II score, previous delirium, emergency surgery, mechanical ventilation, organ failure, trauma, and metabolic acidosis.[11] Careful consideration of the use of psychotropic medications as treatment for delirium should be made as well as potentially causing delirium in some causes of toxicity or withdrawal.

Delirium in patients taking valproic acid should raise concern for hyperammonemic encephalopathy, which has been reported during both initiation of the drug and stable chronic treatment. Elevations of ammonia occur at therapeutic serum levels of valproic acid and are unrelated to liver function. Depletion of carnitine stores may play a role in pathophysiology, and L-carnitine is often administered as treatment. Most patients will recover following discontinuation of the agent; however, progression to fatal coma has been reported.[12]

The relationship between sleep disturbance and delirium has not been well established. Sleep in the ICU is characterized by fragmentation, more light sleep, and decrease in both slow-wave sleep and rapid eye movement sleep. Sleep disorders in the ICU include parasomnias and dyssomnias. Parasomnias are physiologic or behavioral events that are not associated with the sleep-wake cycle and take place during sleep phases or sleep-wake transition phases. Dyssomnias include the inability to initiate or maintain sleep; this includes circadian rhythm sleep disorder. Disrupted sleep in the ICU is caused by many factors, including noise, patient care, and mechanical ventilation. The literature suggests similar mechanisms for both, including imbalances in neurotransmitters and alterations in melatonin. Both the administration and withdrawal of benzodiazepines and opioids may affect sleep and delirium.[13]

Seizures

There are numerous neurochemical pathways identified in the provocation of seizures. Agents that block adenosine, histamine, and GABA receptors may result in seizures. Agents that stimulate cholinergic and glutamatergic receptors may trigger seizures. Noradrenergic and serotonergic effects of antidepressants used at therapeutic doses are known to be anticonvulsant. With larger doses of antidepressants, such as in overdose, other neurochemical pathways are activated, which may result in seizures (**Box 4**).[14]

Antipsychotics traditionally have been associated with a high risk of seizures by blocking the dopamine 2 (D2) receptor. Dopamine 1 (D1) antagonists are known to be protective against seizures. Because each neuroleptic has a different affinity for each of the dopamine receptors, there are variable effects as well on seizure threshold. Chlorpromazine and clozapine carry the highest risk of seizures among the first generation antipsychotics. Among the second generation antipsychotics, olanzapine and quetiapine can portend a higher risk.[15,16]

Box 4
Seizure risks with psychotropic medications

Low (less than 5%)

Isocarboxazid, moclobemide, phenelzine, selegiline, tranylcypromine, selective serotonin reuptake inhibitors except citalopram, mirtazapine, trazodone

Intermediate risk (5 – 10%)

Amitriptyline, clomipramine, doxepin, trimipramine, protriptyline, citalopram, venlafaxine

High risk (greater than 10%)

Imipramine, desipramine, nortriptyline, amoxapine, maprotiline, bupropion

Unknown risk

Duloxetine

Data from the World Health Organization adverse drug reactions database reveals that some of the most frequently associated neuroactive medications with seizures included the following antipsychotics and cholinomimetics: escitalopram, bupropion, clozapine, amoxapine, donepezil, rivastigmine, and quetiapine.[15]

Cerebrovascular Events

Increasingly more antipsychotic medications are being used to treat behavioral dysregulation and agitation in individuals with dementia. Over time, regulatory agencies have warned about the use of antipsychotics in patients with dementia as causes for cerebrovascular events and death. Potential mechanisms include orthostatic hypotension, tachycardia, atherosclerosis accelerated by hyperprolactinemia, and venous thromboembolism. Higher doses, older age, a diagnosis of dementia (especially vascular dementia), and atrial fibrillation have been noted as risk factors for cerebrovascular events. In a systematic review of the literature, the risk of cerebrovascular events in those treated with antipsychotics was noted to be approximately 1.3 to 2.0 times. No one antipsychotic was noted to be safer. Risk of death with typical and atypical antipsychotics was approximately 1.2 to 1.6 times higher in those treated with antipsychotics. Risk of death was found to be similar between antipsychotic categories. Older men with severe dementia and functional impairment were at highest risk of death.[17] In a more recent review of observational studies, the highest risk of mortality was reported for haloperidol and chlorpromazine, whereas the lowest risk was reported from olanzapine, quetiapine, and ziprasidone. The evidence was noted to be less clear for risk of cerebrovascular events.[18] Management of agitation and behavioral disturbances in patients with dementia should include weighing the risks and the benefits of treatment.

Reversible Cerebral Vasoconstriction Syndrome

Stroke also may occur as a consequence of diffuse, segmental cerebral vasoconstriction, which has been associated with serotonergic antidepressants. This reversible cerebral vasoconstriction syndrome (RCVS) usually presents with sudden headache, and also has been associated with pseudoephedrine, bromocriptine, hormone therapies, and immunosuppressive agents, including cyclophosphamide and tacrolimus. It occurs more commonly in women, and more than half of reported cases occurred in the first week postpartum. Significant hypertension was present in most cases.[19,20] Intracerebral hemorrhage has been rarely reported, and only a minority of cases will present with focal neurologic deficits. Because maximum vasoconstriction is reached at an average of 16 days after symptom onset, stroke may more commonly occur as a late complication, with subarachnoid hemorrhage occurring a week after symptom onset, and ischemic stroke after more than 2 weeks.[21] Clinicians must take care to distinguish RCVS from cerebral vasculitis because use of glucocorticoids has been suggested as a poor prognostic factor in RCVS.[22,23]

Extrapyramidal Syndromes

Extrapyramidal syndromes (EPSs) are caused by administration of antipsychotic medications and include acute manifestations (dystonia and akathisia) and subacute or chronic forms (parkinsonism and tardive dyskinesia). Acute dystonia involves contraction of involuntary muscles and is manifested in the neck as well as the eyes (oculogyric crisis). Akathisia is a subjective sensation of inner restlessness. Both of these may be treated by discontinuation of the offending agent and administration of an anticholinergic agent or a beta blocker. Parkinsonism and tardive dyskinesia are also caused by antipsychotics and other dopamine blockers. Parkinsonism includes bradykinesia, rigidity, and tremor. Quetiapine and clozapine are least associated with parkinsonism.

Tardive dyskinesia is the most chronic form of EPS and generally presents with involuntary movements of the muscles of the tongue, lips, mouth, and face.[24] In a review of the literature, EPS was associated with different classes of antidepressants. The reports included duloxetine, sertraline, escitalopram, and bupropion.[25] Given the association with increased morbidity and mortality, as well as decreased quality of life, monitoring for EPS is always indicated when using psychotropic medications for any duration of time.

Discontinuation Syndromes

Discontinuation of treatment with antipsychotics and antidepressants can cause the rapid onset of a range of symptoms that are often self-limiting and distinct from the psychiatric disorder for which they are being used. Antidepressant discontinuation syndrome develops with discontinuation of all major classes of antidepressants, including SSRIs, serotonin-norepinephrine reuptake inhibitors (SNRIs), tricyclic antidepressants (TCAs), monoamine oxidase inhibitors (MAOIs), and mirtazapine. The risk is highest for paroxetine and lowest for fluoxetine due to its long half-life and active metabolite. Symptoms are vast and primarily physical and may include the characteristic electric shock–like sensations in the scalp, back, and arms, as well as noises in the ears with vertigo and unsteadiness. These generally resolve spontaneously. However, benzodiazepines, as well as fluoxetine, can suppress the discontinuation syndrome.[26]

Antipsychotic discontinuation symptoms include delirium, anxiety, restlessness, insomnia, nausea, vomiting, and diaphoresis. They have been associated with chlorpromazine and clozapine. Cases of withdrawal dystonias, dyskinesias, and tics have been described with other antipsychotics.[26]

Sedation

Sedation is a noted side effect of many psychotropic medications, such as benzodiazepines, mood stabilizers, some antipsychotics and some antidepressants. In critical care settings, where patients are often on other sedating agents, there is a higher risk of oversedation and thus medical complications, such as pneumonia, aspiration, and malnutrition. Although many psychotropic medications are useful in the management of critically ill patients, caution should be used in terms of dosing and titration schedules.

Myoclonus

Myoclonus is the second most common involuntary nonepileptic involuntary movement in the critical care setting. It is a sudden, brief, abrupt twitching of the face, extremities, and/or trunk. A vast group of medications may trigger or aggravate myoclonus in the ICU. Exposures to opioids, mood stabilizers, antidepressants, dopaminergic agents, and illicit drugs affect the cerebral cortex causing myoclonus. Cortical myoclonus is elicited by tendon taps, touching, posturing, passive or voluntary movements, and emotional excitation. The recognition and treatment of cortical myoclonus is important to prevent the progression to generalized seizures or status epilepticus. Discontinuation of medications and treatment of any metabolic derangements may resolve myoclonus.[27]

Thermoregulation

Psychotropic medications may interfere with temperature regulation. Drug-induced hyperthermic syndromes are organized into 7 main categories: (1) adrenergic fever from cocaine, ecstasy, thyroxine, or abrupt withdrawal of sedative hypnotics; (2) anticholinergic fever; (3) antidopaminergic fever (NMS); (4) SS; (5) malignant hyperthermia; (6)

uncoupling of oxidative-phosphorylation, which occurs with salicylate overdose; and (7) baclofen withdrawal from abrupt discontinuation of baclofen.[28] Given the variability of these syndromes, it is imperative that a thorough history is taken, especially in the ICU where patients may be even more susceptible to these conditions given their comorbidities.

CARDIOVASCULAR SYSTEM

Cardiovascular effects of psychotropic treatment most commonly include changes in blood pressure, heart rate, and changes in cardiac conduction that increase risks of arrhythmia. In a minority of patients, anticholinergic properties of clozapine cause benign tachycardia, which is not elevated above the intrinsic rate of the sinus node (approximately 110 beats per minute). Elevated serum lithium levels are associated with bradycardia. Rarely, myocarditis and cardiomyopathy result from treatment with specific agents.

Arrhythmia

Tricyclic antidepressants
TCAs are known to increase heart rate, and cause fatal arrhythmia in overdose. They act as Vaughan Williams class Ia antiarrhythmics, which delay depolarization and widen the QRS complex. The resulting prolongation of PR and QT intervals can contribute to heart block and ventricular dysrhythmias in patients with preexisting conduction delay. Class I antiarrhythmic drugs also increase the risk of ventricular dysrhythmia when given to patients with atrial fibrillation and of sudden death after myocardial infarction. Caution is warranted in patients at high cardiac risk.[29,30]

QT prolongation
Prolongation of the QT interval is recognized as a marker of risk for torsades de pointes (TdP) and other ventricular arrhythmias. Although the incidence of TdP in the general population is extremely low, monitoring of QT interval has become increasingly common practice during treatment with psychotropic medications. A wide variety of nonpsychotropic and psychotropic medications prolong the QT interval, some of which are in **Box 5**. Among psychotropic agents, antipsychotics have the highest propensity to prolong the QT, especially ziprasidone, iloperidone, pimozide, and amisulpride.[24,31] Other second-generation antipsychotics and haloperidol are generally thought to be safer, and several agents with minimal or no risk of QT prolongation are available (**Box 6**).[31]

Risk factors for TdP include female gender, age, hypokalemia, hypomagnesemia, human immunodeficiency virus infection, and underlying heart conditions, including known conduction defects or cardiomyopathy.[32,33] Psychotropic medications are known to contribute to risk of TdP from an extensive literature of case reports and epidemiologic study; however, in nearly all cases, multiple QT-prolonging medications were administered, usually in patients at high medical risk. Other population studies suggest treatment with methadone and antiarrhythmic agents substantially increase risk of TdP, whereas antipsychotic medications and other agents causing moderate QT prolongation do not.[33] Periodically monitoring the electrocardiogram and maintaining potassium and magnesium in high normal ranges is recommended in at-risk patients.

Orthostatic hypotension

Orthostatic hypotension is a common side effect of a variety of psychotropic medications that act as antagonists at a1-adrenergic receptors. These notably include

---

Box 5
Medications associated with QT prolongation

Antiarrhythmics
  Class I
    Disopyramide, quinidine, procainamide
  Class III
    Amiodarone, dofetilide, sotalol

Antibiotics
  Macrolides
    Azithromycin, clarithromycin, erythromycin
  Quinolones
    Ciprofloxacin, levofloxacin, moxifloxacin

Furosemide

Methadone

Antidepressants
  Tricyclic antidepressants
    Amitriptyline, nortriptyline, imipramine, desipramine
  Citalopram

Antipsychotics
  See **Box 6**

---

low-potency first-generation antipsychotics (eg, chlorpromazine and thioridazine),[34] and a number of second-generation antipsychotics, including clozapine, olanzapine, quetiapine, and risperidone.[35] Likewise, orthostatic hypotension may result more frequently with tertiary amine TCAs (eg, amitriptyline, imipramine), paroxetine, and the atypical antidepressants trazodone and mirtazapine.[36] Hypotensive effects should diminish rapidly as tachyphylaxis develops but may still pose considerable risk of falls or hemodynamic compromise, especially in elderly or medically ill patients.[37]

Box 6
Clinically significant QT prolongation of selected antipsychotics

Greatest

Amisulpride

Ziprasidone

Iloperidone

Modest

Risperidone

Olanzapine

Quetiapine

Haloperidol

None

Paliperidone

Aripiprazole

Lurasidone

Hypertension

Hypertension occurs as a side effect of a number of medications that promote the effects of dopamine or norepinephrine, including bupropion, stimulants, and SNRI antidepressants. Where detectable, these increases are small, and clinically significant only at the highest doses. For instance patients taking SNRIs are more likely to convert from prehypertension to hypertension.[38] Statistically and clinically significant elevations in blood pressure persist during treatment with high doses of venlafaxine[39]; however, treatment with venlafaxine does not complicate control of blood pressure in patients with preexisting hypertension.[39] Sustained hypertension has not been observed in studies of levomilnacipran or duloxetine,[38,40,41] even with escalation of dose.[42]

Severe hypertensive complications from psychotropic treatment are rarely seen. Life-threatening hypertensive crisis may be caused by MAOIs if patients are exposed to tyramine-containing foods, or a variety of medications including vasopressor monoamines, phenylpiperidine opioids, stimulants, and over-the-counter cold remedies. Autonomic instability and marked hypertension also may occur during NMS and SS, which are described in detail earlier in this article.

Cardiotoxicity

Cardiotoxicity from psychotropic treatment may occur as acute myocarditis or a more chronic cardiomyopathy. Although small numbers of reports have associated cardiotoxicity with several agents, it has been best characterized in the form of acute myocarditis following the initiation of clozapine. Incidence is estimated at between 0.7% and 1.2% of treated patients, generally occurs within a few weeks after the start of treatment, and is not dependent on dose.[43] Based on timing and typical findings of peripheral eosinophilia, an immunoglobulin E hypersensitivity reaction is considered the most likely mechanism.[44] Common symptoms, including tachycardia and flulike symptoms, are nonspecific and often missed. Fever after starting treatment may raise concern, and may precede development of myocarditis by several days.[35,45] Nonspecific symptoms also may accompany the development of cardiomyopathy with chronic use of clozapine, the incidence of which remains uncertain. Incidence is estimated as negligible in some sources, and as high as 3% in recent Australian investigations.[45–47] A recent review of published cases documented a mean onset of cardiomyopathy 14.4 months after the start of treatment, which is considerably longer than the average for reports to national sentinel-event databases.[48]

GASTROINTESTINAL
Gastrointestinal Symptoms

Gastrointestinal symptoms, including abdominal discomfort, nausea, vomiting, constipation, loose stools, and diarrhea, are among the most widely reported effects of psychotropic treatment. These occur most commonly with use of SSRI antidepressants. Nausea and loose stools/diarrhea each occur in 20% to 25% of individuals. For most patients, these symptoms are merely unpleasant and resolve early in the course of treatment. Incidence of vomiting is less than 5%. Severe or persistent symptoms may occur as part of SS and therefore should prompt investigation for other signs of serotonin toxicity. Lithium is also known to cause significant gastrointestinal distress, and loose stools are both a common symptom after initiation of treatment, as well as a symptom of lithium toxicity. Constipation caused by psychotropic medication most commonly results from anticholinergic activity and is generally mild and easily managed. Clozapine, however, has potent anticholinergic activity, and may cause more significant constipation. Fatal cases of paralytic ileus and toxic megacolon have also been reported.

Pancreatitis

Pancreatitis is a rare serious consequence of psychiatric treatment. In general, occurrence of pancreatitis may be early or late in treatment, and clear causal mechanisms or dose-dependent relationships have not been established. Valproic acid has been most commonly implicated. Atypical antipsychotics have also been associated with pancreatitis. In data reported by the Food and Drug Administration (FDA), clozapine, olanzapine, and risperidone accounted for 90% of all reports related to antipsychotics.[49] In a review of published cases, clozapine, olanzapine, and quetiapine accounted for more than 80%.[50] Among antidepressants, a very small number of case reports have implicated sertraline and mirtazapine.[51,52] Broad surveillance of adverse event databases suggests no association between SSRI antidepressants and pancreatitis,[51] and a case-control design found no association with pancreatitis after controlling for confounding factors.[53]

Hepatic Dysfunction

A number of psychotropic medications have hepatic effects, ranging from abnormalities in laboratory tests to severe hepatocellular injury. Among these, valproic acid is most notoriously linked with hepatic toxicity, most often reported in the first 6 months of treatment. Although later onset is less common, monitoring of liver function tests (LFTs) is recommended throughout treatment. Hepatic injury and failure also have occurred with other anticonvulsants commonly used as mood stabilizers.

Antipsychotic drugs commonly produce mild and transient elevations in LFTs. Clinically significant elevations occur in fewer than 5% of patients. Severe hepatitis and fatal injury are reported very rarely for both first-generation and second-generation antipsychotics.[54,55] Reports of toxicity are most commonly reported during treatment with chlorpromazine, which may cause jaundice in 0.1% of patients, and for which cases of severe or fatal hepatitis exceed other antipsychotics by an order of magnitude. Among second-generation antipsychotics, rates of LFT elevation are higher for those medications with structural similarity to chlorpromazine (i.e., clozapine, olanzapine, and quetiapine).[56]

All antidepressant drugs have been reported to cause elevations in LFTs, with more severe reactions reported in cases of MAOIs, TCAs, duloxetine, venlafaxine, sertraline, bupropion, trazodone, and agomelatine.[57]

IMMUNOLOGIC

Psychotropic medications are not extensively linked to immunologic complications. Drug-induced systemic lupus erythematosus has been associated with medications of all types. Among psychotropics, several case reports and case-control analyses implicate carbamazepine.[58] Isolated cases associate clozapine, lithium, valproic acid, sertraline, citalopram, and bupropion with drug-induced systemic lupus erythematosus.[59–63] Phenothiazine antipsychotics have been associated with positive tests for antinuclear antibodies, without consistent progression to systemic lupus erythematosus.[64]

RENAL

Complications of psychiatric mediation involving the kidney commonly occur in the form of electrolyte disturbances and changes in genitourinary function. In addition to causing problems with electrolyte balance, lithium is well known to cause direct renal toxicity.

Lithium

Lithium is associated with both acute and chronic renal toxicity. Tubular atrophy and interstitial fibrosis are well-described consequences of renal treatment.[65] An increase in number of sclerotic glomeruli also has been described; however, it remains controversial whether lithium treatment is a direct cause of decreased glomerular function. As many as 20% of patients treated with lithium will have a decline in renal function, usually after decades of treatment.[24,65] Duration of lithium therapy has been identified as an independent risk factor.[66] Other risk factors include age, female sex, smoking, hypertension, medical comorbidity, psychotic disorder, and lithium serum level.[67] Large cohort studies provide mixed evidence about whether this risk is due to routine lithium treatment, episodes of toxicity, or confounding factors. Lithium treatment has been associated with an increased risk of renal failure diagnosis (identified by use of International Classification of Diseases, 10th Revision codes).[68,69] Alternatively, direct measurements of renal function in a large cohort over 12 years observed no relationship between lithium treatment and decline in glomerular filtration rate when episodes of lithium toxicity were accounted for.[70] Lithium is also the most widely recognized cause of nephrogenic diabetes insipidus, occurring in up to 20% of patients treated chronically. Onset of diabetes insipidus has been reported after 1 year and as late as 3 decades after start of treatment. Median onset is 6 years from start of treatment.[71]

Hyponatremia

Hyponatremia has been frequently associated with the mood-stabilizing anticonvulsants carbamazepine and oxcarbazepine. Incidence has been estimated at 13.5% for carbamazepine and 29.9% for oxcarbazepine. Monitoring of sodium is recommended during oxcarbazepine treatment. The mechanism of the disorder is unknown. Antidepressants may be associated with hyponatremia by causing a syndrome of inappropriate antidiuretic hormone secretion (SIADH). Estimates of the frequency of SIADH vary with definition, with incidence estimated at 9% to 40% for sodium less than 135 mEq/dL and 0.06% to 2.6% for sodium less than 130 mEq/dL.[72] Although SIADH is likely to be broadly associated with all classes of antidepressant, it is particularly noted for SSRIs, and the incidence may be lower for TCAs and mirtazapine.[72] The risk of hyponatremia is significantly higher among patients using diuretic medications and with increasing age. Other risk factors include female gender, low body weight, and low baseline sodium level.

Urinary Symptoms

Many psychiatric medications have been associated with urinary symptoms, including retention, frequency, and incontinence. Implicated medications generally include those with significant anticholinergic activity, which is a significant cause of urinary retention (Box 7). A number of psychotropic medications also cause urinary retention by significant antagonism at alpha-1 adrenergic receptors, including antipsychotics (haloperidol, risperidone, quetiapine, and olanzapine), TCAs, and mirtazapine. The alpha-1 antagonist prazosin has grown in popularity in the treatment of posttraumatic stress disorder. Urinary symptoms also have been attributed to SSRI and SNRI antidepressants, with serotonergic mechanisms speculated; however, incidence of these side effects remains very low.[36]

Box 7
Common psychotropics with anticholinergic properties

Benztropine

Trihexyphenidyl

Antipsychotics
  Clozapine
  Chlorpromazine
  Olanzapine

Selective serotonin reuptake inhibitors
  Paroxetine

Tricyclic antidepressants (tertiary amine)
  Amitriptyline
  Clomipramine
  Doxepin
  Imipramine

ENDOCRINOLOGIC
Weight Gain and Diabetic Ketoacidosis

Current evidence suggests that several neurotransmitter receptors are implicated in weight gain and glucose dysregulation in individuals treated with antipsychotics, including the serotonin 5-HT2c, histamine H1, and muscarinic M3 receptors. It also has been proposed that antipsychotics may increase appetite and food intake by actions on dopamine D2-mediated reward pathway.[73] Weight gain and metabolic sequelae are two of the most notable side effects of the atypical antipsychotics; clozapine and olanzapine have carried the greatest risk, whereas aripiprazole, lurasidone, and ziprasidone carry the lowest risk. Of the typical antipsychotics, chlorpromazine carries highest risk of weight gain and metabolic effects of the first generation antipsychotics, whereas fluphenazine, haloperidol, and pimozide show the lowest risk. Although this is noted to be a class effect, reports of diabetic ketoacidosis (DKA) have argued against weight gain being the sole mechanism by which atypical antipsychotics cause glucose dysregulation. DKA may occur at any point in time of treatment with an antipsychotic and is independent of weight gain. All atypical antipsychotics are at risk of causing DKA. Furthermore, DKA has also been reported with typical antipsychotics and lithium.[74] More than half of the reports of second generation antipsychotics-associated DKA have involved individuals on polypharmacy. The incidence of DKA has been noted to be 10 times higher in patients with schizophrenia than the general population. Although the underlying mechanism is not entirely clear, there is evidence for both increased appetite and altered metabolism, which may increase the susceptibility in patients with schizophrenia by treating with these agents.[75]

Thyroid Disorders

The etiology of lithium-associated hypothyroidism is related to the inhibition of synthesis and release of thyroid hormones. The risk of developing lithium-induced hypothyroidism has been demonstrated to be significantly higher in women older than 50, and those with family history of thyroid disorders. Lithium is also reported to induce hyperthyroidism, although less frequently, due to direct toxic effects on the thyroid gland and possible autoimmunity. Thyroid function tests and assessment of the thyroid gland on examination and by ultrasound should be performed when starting lithium and later every year. More frequent assessment should be done in patients at higher risk.[76] Monitoring of clinical symptoms is warranted in this patient population. Treatment of hypothyroidism associated with lithium may be managed conservatively by reducing the dose of lithium, stopping it, or administering thyroid supplementation (**Box 8**).[77]

HEMATOLOGIC
Blood Dyscrasias

Medication-induced hematologic effects include neutropenia, agranulocytosis, eosinophilia, thrombocytopenia, purpura, and anemia. Leukocytosis, thrombocytosis, and altered platelet function are other side effects. If hematologic problems occur while a patient is on a psychotropic agent, other contributory factors, such as medical illnesses, use of other medications, and poor nutrition, should be considered. More often, hematologic side effects occur at the inception of treatment. Other than aplastic anemia, most of these effects cease on discontinuation of the drug.[78]

Neutropenia was recognized first as a side effect of chlorpromazine in the early 1950s. Since then, antidepressants, benzodiazepines, antipsychotics, anticonvulsants, and mood stabilizers all have been associated with blood dyscrasias. Neutropenia and agranulocytosis are the most common drug-related blood dyscrasias.[79] The risk of developing neutropenia and agranulocytosis related to clozapine is 3.0% and 0.8%, respectively. The mechanisms by which each of these takes place may be different. Proposed mechanisms include immune-mediated response against neutrophils, apoptosis of neutrophils, and direct toxicity against the bone

---

Box 8
Endocrine effects of psychotropic medications

Hyperprolactinemia

Antipsychotics, risperidone, paliperidone

Hyponatremia, syndrome of inappropriate antidiuretic hormone secretion

Carbamazepine, oxcarbazepine, selective serotonin reuptake inhibitors, N-methyl-D-aspartate receptor antagonists

Nephrogenic diabetes insipidus

Lithium, clozapine

Hypothyroidism, hyperthyroidism

Lithium

Sexual dysfunction

Selective serotonin reuptake inhibitors

Polycystic ovarian syndrome

Valproic acid

Metabolic syndrome

Antipsychotics, mood stabilizers, antidepressants, sedatives

Weight loss

Psychostimulants, topiramate

Adapted from Bhuvaneswar CG, Baldessarini RJ, Harsh VL, et al. Adverse endocrine and metabolic effects of psychotropic drugs. CNS Drugs 2009;23(12):1003–21; with permission.

marrow. Clozapine also may cause anemia, eosinophilia, leukocytosis, lymphope-nia, thrombocytopenia, and thrombocytosis. Use of clozapine in the United States requires registration in the national registry, and weekly blood draws when cloza-pine is initiated. Other significant psychotropic-related blood dyscrasias include carbamazepine (neutropenia and agranulocytosis), phenytoin (neutropenia and agranulocytosis), mirtazapine (agranulocytosis), and valproic acid (thrombocytopenia).[80]

Bleeding

SSRIs and non-SSRIs, such as venlafaxine and duloxetine, have been associated with the risk of abnormal gastrointestinal bleeding. The following etiologic mechanisms have been implicated: (1) inhibition of serotonin uptake into platelets, which prevents serotonin-mediated vasoconstriction and platelet aggregation; (2) increase in gastric acid secretion by SSRIs; and (3) CYP450 inhibition by SSRIs, which would alter the levels of other drugs that would cause bleeding. Bleeding related to SSRIs may be life-threatening, and therefore patients at risk for abnormal bleeding (those with peptic ulcer or liver disease, those undergoing surgical or dental procedures, those on other antiplatelet medications or on nonsteroidal anti-inflammatory drugs [NSAIDs]) should be closely monitored.[81] In a recent meta-analysis and systematic review, it was concluded that the risk of upper gastrointestinal bleeding with SSRIs in patients who are at high risk and taking NSAIDs is substantial and to reduce the risk of bleeding, proton pump inhibitor therapy should be prescribed. Therefore, the risk of a gastrointestinal bleed should be highly considered in this patient population before the prescription or continuation of SSRIs.[82]

RESPIRATORY
Respiratory Depression

Benzodiazepines decrease respiratory frequency due to their alteration of central ner-vous system (CNS) response to hypoxia. This effect is greater with long-acting agents, and shorter-acting benzodiazepines, such as lorazepam, may be preferred. The addi-tive effects of benzodiazepines and other CNS depressants, such as antipsychotics and sedating TCAs, should be carefully considered. Patients at higher risk of respira-tory depression, including those with sleep apnea, respiratory dysfunction, or pneu-monia, should be monitored closely while on sedating psychotropics.[24]

Respiratory Dyskinesia

Respiratory dyskinesia is a side effect of chronic antipsychotic use as a manifestation of tardive dyskinesia. It presents as irregular respiration, dyspnea, grunting or gasping, and abnormal chest or esophageal movements.[83] There have been cases of respira-tory dyskinesia on discontinuation of or withdrawal from metoclopramide and risper-idone.[84,85] Thus, for patients who have multiple risk factors for tardive dyskinesia, particular attention should be made to the use of these agents.

Pulmonary Embolism

Antipsychotic medications have been associated with venous thromboembolism since the introduction of chlorpromazine. The proposed mechanisms include weight gain, sedation, platelet aggregation, increased levels of antiphospholipid antibodies, hyperprolactinemia, and hyperhomocysteinemia. The increased risk appears to be related to clozapine and low-potency first-generation antipsychotics. Olanzapine, ris-peridone, and typical antipsychotics may carry a smaller risk.[86]

DERMATOLOGIC

Cutaneous drug reactions may be attributed to non–immune-mediated mechanisms as well as the direct release of mediators, accumulation of toxic metabolites, and phototoxicity. Type A drug reactions are the most common and attributable to the toxic effects of the drug. Type B drug reactions are idiosyncratic. Risk factors associated with cutaneous drug reactions include the following: female gender, advanced age, African American race, HLA subtype, winter months, and a high loading dose of the drug.[87]

Psychotropic-induced dermatologic reactions range from benign to potentially life-threatening. The incidence has been reported to be 0.1%. The most clinically relevant reactions are due to mood stabilizers (39%), antidepressants (29%), and neuroleptics (19%).[87] Data from a multicenter surveillance program reported that substances with the highest and statistically significant cutaneous adverse reactions risk were the antiepileptic drugs ($P<.0001$), particularly lamotrigine and carbamazepine.[88] The most important types of cutaneous drug reactions are exanthematous eruptions, urticarial, fixed drug eruptions, drug-induced hypersensitivity syndrome, and epidermal necrolysis, which includes SJS and toxic epidermal necrolysis (TEN).[87] The severe and life-threatening reactions that can occur with psychotropics are erythema multiforme, SJS, and TEN. Drug rash with eosinophilia and systemic symptoms presents as a triad of fever, rash, and internal organ involvement. It has been associated with antiepileptic medications, desipramine, amitriptyline, imipramine, fluoxetine, olanzapine, perphenazine, carbamazepine, lamotrigine, oxcarbazepine, and valproic acid.[89]

The character of cutaneous skin reactions may be associated with the amount of the drug and the rate at which it is administered. Additionally, cross reactions of medications within the same drug class may occur. Treatment usually involves the discontinuation of the agent, and symptomatic management with antihistamines and steroids. Lowering the dose of certain agents, such as lithium or carbamazepine, may result in resolution of the skin reaction.[87] It is important to note that lithium is associated with a wide range of cutaneous reactions, including inflammation, disorders of the hair and nails, keratinization, infection, and autoimmune disorders. Careful attention should be paid to these reactions with appropriate management of lithium to minimize any significant psychiatric decompensation.[90]

REPRODUCTIVE
Sexual Dysfunction

A number of neurotransmitters and hormones are involved in sexual activity. The three stages of the sexual response cycle are desire, arousal, and orgasm. Sexual dysfunction at any of these stages has been associated with both psychiatric illness and psychotropic medications. Antidepressant-related sexual dysfunction is due mostly to a sexual inhibitory action. Although the mechanism remains unclear, the evidence supports activation of a serotonin receptor subtype. The reported prevalence of antidepressant-related sexual dysfunction ranges from 10% to 80%. Many of the studies are limited by flaws in methodology. The most remarkable associations have been found with use of SSRIs and SNRIs.[91] In a systematic review of patients being treated with second-generation antidepressants for major depressive disorder, a similar risk of sexual dysfunction was shown among them. However, the following three main patterns were observed: a statistically significant lower risk of sexual dysfunction with bupropion and a statistically significant higher risk of sexual function for both escitalopram and paroxetine.[92]

With respect to antipsychotics, there is more evidence that sexual dysfunction is common and that all antipsychotics can cause sexual dysfunction. Different mechanisms of action have been proposed, including dopamine antagonist action, increased prolactin, antiadrenergic action, anticholinergic action, serotonin antagonist action, and antihistaminic. The antipsychotics that are most frequently cited in the literature include some of the conventional antipsychotics, including haloperidol, chlorpromazine, pimozide, thioridazine, and thiothixene. Of the antipsychotics, risperidone and paliperidone are associated with the highest rates, and aripiprazole is associated with the lowest rate.[93] With regard to the effects of mood stabilizers and anxiolytic agents on sexual function, the studies have not been robust and thus the evidence is inconclusive.[94,95]

Priapism

Priapism is a painful sustained penile erection, and is considered another potentially serious side effect of psychotropic medications. Traditionally, trazodone has been associated with this; however, more evidence suggests that antipsychotics also induce priapism. Priapism may develop soon after starting typical or atypical antipsychotic medications, after a period of stable usage, with changes in doses, or with the addition of another agent. The mechanism is not clear, but is thought to be related to alpha-adrenergic blockage by the alpha receptors in the corpora cavernosa of the penis.[96] Particular attention should be given to patients who are at higher risk of developing priapism due to low flow states, such as those with sickle cell anemia, leukemia, hypercoagulable states, and autonomic dysfunction. Priapism should be treated as a neurologic emergency due to its potential morbidity.[24]

Pregnancy

There is extensive literature on the outcomes for infants exposed to psychotropic medications in utero. Approximately 15% of pregnant women have a psychiatric diagnosis and approximately 10% to 13% of fetuses are exposed to psychotropic medications. All psychotropic medications can pass through the placenta. Although there may be risks associated with exposure to some psychotropic agents, there is evidence that untreated psychiatric illness of pregnant women is associated with poorer outcomes for the exposed fetus. Among the complications associated with psychotropics are teratogenesis, cardiovascular malformations, persistent pulmonary hypertension, spontaneous abortion, preterm birth, and low birth weight, and autism.[97] The FDA is in the process of changing its drug labeling about medication use in pregnancy and lactation, which will be referred to as the "Pregnancy and Lactation Labeling Rule." Drugs approved on or after June 30, 2001, will now include a risk summary. Previously used drugs will include revised labeling.[90]

SUMMARY

Psychiatric medications are used with frequency in hospitalized patients and are of particular benefit in the critically ill patient. Due to their systemic effects, close monitoring and assessment of these agents is indicated to minimize any toxicity, drug-drug interactions, and complications. The risks and benefits always should be of consideration when making clinical decisions surrounding the use of these agents to provide comprehensive care for patients.

REFERENCES

1. Girard TD, Pandharipande PP, Ely EW. Delirium in the intensive care unit. Crit Care 2008;12(Suppl 3):S3.

2. Sevransky JE, Bienvenu OJ, Neufeld KJ, et al. Treatment of four psychiatric emergencies in the intensive care unit. Crit Care Med 2012;40(9):2662–70.
3. Association AP. Diagnostic and statistical manual of mental disorders. Arlington (VA): American Psychiatric Publishing; 2013.
4. Seitz DP, Gill SS. Neuroleptic malignant syndrome complicating antipsychotic treatment of delirium or agitation in medical and surgical patients: case reports and a review of the literature. Psychosomatics 2009;50(1):8–15.
5. Trollor JN, Sachdev PS. Electroconvulsive treatment of neuroleptic malignant syndrome: a review and report of cases. Aust N Z J Psychiatry 1999;33(5):650–9.
6. Newman EJ, Grosset DG, Kennedy PGE. The parkinsonism-hyperpyrexia syndrome. Neurocrit Care 2008;10(1):136–40.
7. Buckley NA, Dawson AH, Isbister GK. Serotonin syndrome. BMJ 2014;348:g1626.
8. Boyer EW, Shannon M. The serotonin syndrome. N Engl J Med 2005;352(11):1112–20.
9. Pedavally S, Fugate JE, Rabinstein AA. Serotonin syndrome in the intensive care unit: clinical presentations and precipitating medications. Neurocrit Care 2013;21(1):108–13.
10. Perry PJ, Wilborn CA. Serotonin syndrome vs neuroleptic malignant syndrome: a contrast of causes, diagnoses, and management. Ann Clin Psychiatry 2012;24(2):155–62.
11. Zaal IJ, Devlin JW, Peelen LM, et al. A systematic review of risk factors for delirium in the ICU. Crit Care Med 2015;43(1):40–7.
12. Chopra A, Kolla BP, Mansukhani MP, et al. Valproate-induced hyperammonemic encephalopathy: an update on risk factors, clinical correlates and management. Gen Hosp Psychiatry 2012;34(3):290–8.
13. Figueroa-Ramos MI, Arroyo-Novoa CM, Lee KA, et al. Sleep and delirium in ICU patients: a review of mechanisms and manifestations. Intensive Care Med 2009;35(5):781–95.
14. Judge BS, Rentmeester LL. Antidepressant overdose–induced seizures. Neurol Clin 2011;29(3):565–80.
15. Kumlien E, Lundberg PO. Seizure risk associated with neuroactive drugs: data from the WHO adverse drug reactions database. Seizure 2010;19(2):69–73.
16. Lertxundi U, Hernandez R, Medrano J, et al. Antipsychotics and seizures: higher risk with atypicals? Seizure 2013;22(2):141–3.
17. Mittal V, Kurup L, Williamson D, et al. Risk of cerebrovascular adverse events and death in elderly patients with dementia when treated with antipsychotic medications: a literature review of evidence [review]. Am J Alzheimers Dis Other Demen 2011;26(1):10–28.
18. Trifiró G, Sultana J, Spina E. Are the safety profiles of antipsychotic drugs used in dementia the same? An updated review of observational studies. Drug Saf 2014;37(7):501–20.
19. Ducros A. Reversible cerebral vasoconstriction syndrome. Lancet Neurol 2012;11(10):906–17.
20. Velez A, McKinney JS. Reversible cerebral vasoconstriction syndrome: a review of recent research. Curr Neurol Neurosci Rep 2012;13(1):319.
21. Ducros A, Boukobza M, Porcher R, et al. The clinical and radiological spectrum of reversible cerebral vasoconstriction syndrome. A prospective series of 67 patients. Brain 2007;130(12):3091–101.
22. Singhal AB, Caviness VS, Begleiter AF, et al. Cerebral vasoconstriction and stroke after use of serotonergic drugs. Neurology 2002;58(1):130–3.

23. Singhal AB. Reversible cerebral vasoconstriction syndromes. Arch Neurol 2011; 68(8):1005.

24. Smith FA, Wittmann CW, Stern TA. Medical complications of psychiatric treatment. Crit Care Clin 2008;24(4):635–56.

25. Madhusoodanan S. Extrapyramidal symptoms associated with antidepressants—a review of the literature and an analysis of spontaneous reports. Ann Clin Psychiatry 2010;22(3):148–56.

26. Haddad PM, Dursun SM. Neurological complications of psychiatric drugs: clinical features and management. Hum Psychopharmacol Clin Exp 2007;23(S1): S15–26.

27. Sutter R, Ristic A, Rüegg S, et al. Myoclonus in the critically ill: diagnosis, management, and clinical impact. Clin Neurophysiol 2016;127(1):67–80.

28. McAllen KJ, Schwartz DR. Adverse drug reactions resulting in hyperthermia in the intensive care unit. Crit Care Med 2010;38:S244–52.

29. Nelson JC. Tricyclic and tetracyclic drugs. In: Schatzberg AF, Nemeroff CB, editors. The American psychiatric publishing textbook of psychopharmacology. Washington, DC: American Psychiatric Publishing, Inc; 2009. p. 263.

30. Robinson M. Psychopharmacology. In: Levenson JA, editor. The American Psychiatric Publishing textbook of psychosomatic medicine. Washington, DC: American Psychiatric Publishing; 2005. p. 871–922.

31. Leucht S, Cipriani A, Spineli L, et al. Comparative efficacy and tolerability of 15 antipsychotic drugs in schizophrenia: a multiple-treatments meta-analysis. The Lancet 2013;382(9896):951–62.

32. Beach SR, Celano CM, Noseworthy PA, et al. QTc prolongation, torsades de pointes, and psychotropic medications. Psychosomatics 2013;54(1):1–13.

33. Romero J, Baldinger SH, Goodman-Meza D, et al. Drug-induced torsades de pointes in an underserved urban population. Methadone: is there therapeutic equipoise? J Interv Card Electrophysiol 2015;45(1):37–45.

34. Gugger JJ. Antipsychotic pharmacotherapy and orthostatic hypotension. CNS Drugs 2011;25(8):659–71.

35. Mackin P. Cardiac side effects of psychiatric drugs. Hum Psychopharmacol Clin Exp 2007;23(S1):S3–14.

36. Carvalho AF, Sharma MS, Brunoni AR, et al. The safety, tolerability and risks associated with the use of newer generation antidepressant drugs: a critical review of the literature. Psychother Psychosom 2016;85(5):270–88.

37. Buckley NA, Sanders P. Cardiovascular adverse effects of antipsychotic drugs. Drug Saf 2000;23(3):215–28.

38. Citrome L. Levomilnacipran for major depressive disorder: a systematic review of the efficacy and safety profile for this newly approved antidepressant–what is the number needed to treat, number needed to harm and likelihood to be helped or harmed? Int J Clin Pract 2013;67(11):1089–104.

39. Thase ME. Effects of venlafaxine on blood pressure: a meta-analysis of original data from 3744 depressed patients. J Clin Psychiatry 1998;59(10):502–8.

40. Raskin J, Wiltse CG, Dinkel JJ, et al. Safety and tolerability of duloxetine at 60 mg once daily in elderly patients with major depressive disorder. J Clin Psychopharmacol 2008;28(1):32–8.

41. Dell'Osso B. Duloxetine in affective disorders: a naturalistic study on psychiatric and medical comorbidity, use in association and tolerability across different age groups. Clin Pract Epidemiol Ment Health 2012;8(1):120–5.

42. Wohlreich MM, Mallinckrodt CH, Prakash A, et al. Duloxetine for the treatment of major depressive disorder: safety and tolerability associated with dose escalation. Depress Anxiety 2006;24(1):41–52.
43. Haas SJ, Hill R, Krum H, et al. Clozapine-associated myocarditis. Drug Saf 2007; 30(1):47–57.
44. Kilian JG, Kerr K, Lawrence C, et al. Myocarditis and cardiomyopathy associated with clozapine. The Lancet 1999;354(9193):1841–5.
45. Ronaldson KJ, Fitzgerald PB, McNeil JJ. Clozapine-induced myocarditis, a widely overlooked adverse reaction. Acta Psychiatr Scand 2015;132(4):231–40.
46. Khan A, Baker D, Savage L, et al. Clozapine and incidence of myocarditis and sudden death–a regional Australian experience. Heart Lung Circ 2016;25: S103–4.
47. Youssef DL, Narayanan P, Gill N. Incidence and risk factors for clozapine-induced myocarditis and cardiomyopathy at a regional mental health service in Australia. Australas Psychiatry Bull R Aust N Z Coll Psychiatr 2016;24(2):176–80.
48. Alawami M, Wasywich C, Cicovic A, et al. A systematic review of clozapine induced cardiomyopathy. Int J Cardiol 2014;176(2):315–20.
49. Koller EA, Cross JT, Doraiswamy PM, et al. Pancreatitis associated with atypical antipsychotics: from the Food and Drug Administration's MedWatch surveillance system and published reports. Pharmacotherapy 2003;23(9):1123–30.
50. Silva MA, Key S, Han E, et al. Acute pancreatitis associated with antipsychotic medication. J Clin Psychopharmacol 2016;36(2):169–72.
51. Spigset O, Hägg S, Bate A. Hepatic injury and pancreatitis during treatment with serotonin reuptake inhibitors. Int Clin Psychopharmacol 2003;18(3):157–61.
52. Hussain A, Burke J. Mirtazapine associated with recurrent pancreatitis–a case report. J Psychopharmacol (Oxf) 2008;22(3):336–7.
53. Ljung R, Rück C, Mattsson F, et al. Selective serotonin reuptake inhibitors and the risk of acute pancreatitis. J Clin Psychopharmacol 2012;32(3):336–40.
54. Marwick KFM, Taylor M, Walker SW. Antipsychotics and abnormal liver function tests. Clin Neuropharmacol 2012;35(5):244–53.
55. Derby L, Gutthann S, Jick H, et al. Liver disorders in patients receiving chlorpromazine or isoniazid. Pharmacotherapy 1993;13(4):353–8.
56. Slim M, Medina-Caliz I, Gonzalez-Jimenez A, et al. Hepatic safety of atypical antipsychotics: current evidence and future directions. Drug Saf 2016;39(10): 925–43.
57. Voican CS, Corruble E, Naveau S, et al. Antidepressant-induced liver injury: a review for clinicians. Am J Psychiatry 2014;171(4):404–15.
58. Schoonen WM, Thomas SL, Somers EC, et al. Do selected drugs increase the risk of lupus? A matched case-control study. Br J Clin Pharmacol 2010;70(4):588–96.
59. Rami AF. Clozapine-induced systemic lupus erythematosus. Ann Pharmacother 2006;40(5):983–5.
60. Boussaadani Soubai R, Lahlou M, Tahiri L, et al. Valproate-induced systemic lupus erythematous: a case report. Rev Neurol (Paris) 2013;169(3):278–9.
61. Hussain HM, Zakaria M. Drug-induced lupus secondary to sertraline. Aust N Z J Psychiatry 2008;42(12):1074–5.
62. Röhrs S, Geiser F, Conrad R. Citalopram-induced subacute cutaneous lupus erythematosus—first case and review concerning photosensitivity in selective serotonin reuptake inhibitors. Gen Hosp Psychiatry 2012;34(5):541–5.
63. Cassis TB, Callen JP. Bupropion-induced subacute cutaneous lupus erythematosus. Australas J Dermatol 2005;46(4):266–9.

64. Delluc A, Rousseau A, Le Galudec M, et al. Prevalence of antiphospholipid anti-bodies in psychiatric patients users and non-users of antipsychotics. Br J Hae-matol 2013;164(2):272–9.
65. Hansen HE. Renal toxicity of lithium. Drugs 1981;22(6):461–76.
66. Bocchetta A, Ardau R, Fanni T, et al. Renal function during long-term lithium treat-ment: a cross-sectional and longitudinal study. BMC Med 2015;13(1):12.
67. Castro VM, Roberson AM, McCoy TH, et al. Stratifying risk for renal insufficiency among lithium-treated patients: an electronic health record study. Neuropsycho-pharmacology 2015;41(4):1138–43.
68. Kessing LV, Gerds TA, Feldt-Rasmussen B, et al. Use of lithium and anticonvul-sants and the rate of chronic kidney disease. JAMA Psychiatry 2015;72(12):1182.
69. Close H, Reilly J, Mason JM, et al. Renal failure in lithium-treated bipolar disorder: a retrospective cohort study. van Os J. PLoS One 2014;9(3):e90169.
70. Clos S, Rauchhaus P, Severn A, et al. Long-term effect of lithium maintenance therapy on estimated glomerular filtration rate in patients with affective disorders: a population-based cohort study. Lancet Psychiatry 2015;2(12):1075–83.
71. Garofeanu CG, Weir M, Rosas-Arellano MP, et al. Causes of reversible nephro-genic diabetes insipidus: a systematic review. Am J Kidney Dis 2005;45(4): 626–37.
72. De Picker L, Van Den Eede F, Dumont G, et al. Antidepressants and the risk of hyponatremia: a class-by-class review of literature. Psychosomatics 2014;55(6): 536–47.
73. Deng C. Effects of antipsychotic medications on appetite, weight, and insulin resistance. Endocrinol Metab Clin North Am 2013;42(3):545–63.
74. Guenette MD, Hahn M, Cohn TA, et al. Atypical antipsychotics and diabetic ke-toacidosis: a review. Psychopharmacology (Berl) 2013;226(1):1–12.
75. Correll CU, Detraux J, De Lepeleire J, et al. Effects of antipsychotics, antidepres-sants and mood stabilizers on risk for physical diseases in people with schizo-phrenia, depression and bipolar disorder. World Psychiatry 2015;14(2):119–36.
76. Kibirige D, Luzinda K, Ssekitoleko R. Spectrum of lithium induced thyroid abnor-malities: a current perspective. Thyroid Res 2013;6(1):3.
77. Bhuvaneswar CG, Baldessarini RJ, Harsh VL, et al. Adverse endocrine and meta-bolic effects of psychotropic drugs. CNS Drugs 2009;23(12):1003–21.
78. Oyesanmi O, Kunkel EJS, Monti DA, et al. Hematologic side effects of psychotro-pics. Psychosomatics 1999;40(5):414–21.
79. Flanagan RJ, Dunk L. Haematological toxicity of drugs used in psychiatry. Hum Psychopharmacol Clin Exp 2007;23(S1):S27–41.
80. Nooijen PMM, Carvalho F, Flanagan RJ. Haematological toxicity of clozapine and some other drugs used in psychiatry. Hum Psychopharmacol Clin Exp 2011; 26(2):112–9.
81. Andrade C, Sandarsh S, Chethan KB, et al. Serotonin reuptake inhibitor antide-pressants and abnormal bleeding: a review for clinicians and a reconsideration of mechanisms. J Clin Psychiatry 2010;71(12):1565–75.
82. Anglin R, Yuan Y, Moayyedi P, et al. Risk of upper gastrointestinal bleeding with selective serotonin reuptake inhibitors with or without concurrent nonsteroidal anti-inflammatory use: a systematic review and meta-analysis. Am J Gastroen-terol 2014;109(6):811–9.
83. Kruk J, Sachdev P, Singh S. Neuroleptic-induced respiratory dyskinesia. J Neuropsychiatry Clin Neurosci 1995;7(2):223–9.
84. Muzyk AJ, Cvelich RG, Rivelli SK. Metoclopramide-induced tardive respiratory dyskinesia. J Neuropsychiatry Clin Neurosci 2012;24(3):E37–8.

85. Komatsu S, Kirino E, Inoue Y, et al. Risperidone withdrawal-related respiratory dyskinesia. Clin Neuropharmacol 2005;28(2):90–3.
86. Jönsson AK, Spigset O, Hägg S. Venous thromboembolism in recipients of antipsychotics. CNS Drugs 2012;26(8):649–62.
87. Mitkov MV, Trowbridge RM, Lockshin BN, et al. Dermatologic side effects of psychotropic medications. Psychosomatics 2014;55(1):1–20.
88. Lange-Asschenfeldt C, Grohmann R, Lange-Asschenfeldt B, et al. Cutaneous adverse reactions to psychotropic drugs. J Clin Psychiatry 2009;70(9):1258–65.
89. Bliss SA, Warnock JK. Psychiatric medications: adverse cutaneous drug reactions. Clin Dermatol 2013;31(1):101–9.
90. Jafferany M. Lithium and skin: dermatologic manifestations of lithium therapy. Int J Dermatol 2008;47(11):1101–11.
91. La Torre A, Giupponi G, Duffy D, et al. Sexual dysfunction related to psychotropic drugs: a critical review—part I: antidepressants. Pharmacopsychiatry 2013; 46(05):191–9.
92. Reichenpfader U, Gartlehner G, Morgan LC, et al. Sexual dysfunction associated with second-generation antidepressants in patients with major depressive disorder: results from a systematic review with network meta-analysis. Drug Saf 2013; 37(1):19–31.
93. La Torre A, Conca A, Duffy D, et al. Sexual dysfunction related to psychotropic drugs: a critical review part II: antipsychotics. Pharmacopsychiatry 2013; 46(06):201–8.
94. Clayton AH, Balon R. Continuing medical education: the impact of mental illness and psychotropic medications on sexual functioning: the evidence and management (CME). J Sex Med 2009;6(5):1200–11.
95. La Torre A, Giupponi G, Duffy D, et al. Sexual dysfunction related to psychotropic drugs: a critical review. Part III: mood stabilizers and anxiolytic drugs. Pharmacopsychiatry 2013;47(01):1–6.
96. Sood S, James W, Bailon M-J. Priapism associated with atypical antipsychotic medications: a review. Int Clin Psychopharmacol 2008;23(1):9–17.
97. Chisolm MS, Payne JL. Management of psychotropic drugs during pregnancy. BMJ 2016;532:h5918.

Psychiatric and Palliative Care in the Intensive Care Unit

Stephanie M. Harman, MD

KEYWORDS

- Palliative care • Palliative psychiatry • End-of-life care • Comfort care
- Intensive care • ICU communication • Family meeting

KEY POINTS

- Palliative care is a core component of critical care and addresses the multiple domains of suffering that patients and families experience.
- Current models of palliative care in the intensive care unit (ICU) combine consultative and integrative approaches to ensure standard palliative care quality measures and continuity of care if the patient moves out of the ICU.
- Communication behaviors that are family centered can improve both patient and family outcomes.
- Patients with preexisting severe mental illness present as a unique and vulnerable population in the ICU and require a palliative psychiatric approach to ensure ethical decision making.

INTRODUCTION

Why consider palliative care in the setting of critical care? Palliative care is an essential component of the clinical practice of critical care. Although trends in place of death have shifted over time, with more patients dying outside of the hospital, 1 in 5 deaths still occur in the intensive care unit (ICU) or just after an ICU stay.[1] The World Health Organization defines palliative care as "an approach that improves the quality of life of patients and their families facing the problem associated with life-threatening illness, through the prevention and relief of suffering by means of early identification and impeccable assessment and treatment of pain and other problems, physical, psychosocial and spiritual."[2] The Center to Advance Palliative Care commissioned a national polling firm to conduct a public opinion survey regarding palliative care in 2011. Based

Disclosure: The author has nothing to disclose.
Department of Medicine, Stanford University School of Medicine, 1265 Welch Road, MC 5475, Stanford, CA 94305, USA
E-mail address: smharman@stanford.edu

Crit Care Clin 33 (2017) 735–743
http://dx.doi.org/10.1016/j.ccc.2017.03.010   criticalcare.theclinics.com

on preferences for communication and language, they described palliative care as "specialized medical care for people living with serious illness" with a focus on "providing relief from the symptoms and stress" and a goal "to improve quality of life for both the patient and the family."[3] Palliative care is often confused with hospice, but the two are distinct. Palliative care can be delivered at any point in the course of a serious illness, whereas hospice requires a prognosis of 6 months or less.[3] In the setting of the ICU, palliative care can be applied to any patient with serious illness, particularly with the high stakes and significant emotional distress that often accompany decision making regarding treatment goals in the ICU.

This article describes the psychiatric aspects of providing palliative care for patients and their families. In the ICU, palliative care has historically centered on care for the dying and support for their families. With the increase of chronic critical illness, palliative care for ICU patients is beginning to extend beyond the experience in the ICU with persisting physical and psychiatric symptoms after hospital discharge.

PALLIATIVE CARE EVALUATION OF INTENSIVE CARE UNIT PATIENTS AND FAMILIES

Although palliative care in the ICU is not exclusive to end-of-life care, the development of the domains of high-quality palliative care have stemmed from work focused on what constitutes high-quality end-of-life care. The Robert Wood Johnson Foundation Critical Care End-of-Life Peer Workgroup, a group originally convened in 1998 for the foundation's Promoting Excellence in End-of-Life Care project, synthesized the literature and expert opinion to develop domains for high-quality end-of-life care. They identified the following 7 domains: (1) patient-centered and family-centered decision making; (2) communication within the team and with patients and families; (3) continuity of care; (4) emotional and practical support for patients and families; (5) symptom management and comfort care; (6) spiritual support for patients and families; (7) emotional and organizational support for ICU clinicians.[4]

Although management of common psychiatric complications and syndromes in the ICU are addressed elsewhere in this issue, it is important to acknowledge the tension that sometimes arises in treating symptoms of critically ill patients who are at the end of life while the goals of care remain uncertain. Families can struggle with the conceptual model of comfort care with the misunderstanding that comfort is not attended when the patient is in a curative mode of care. In other instances, while a patient is sedated to maintain comfort while on a ventilator, families may request that sedation be discontinued so that they can speak with the patient about their wishes; or, they may attribute a patient's neurologic impairment to medications rather than an underlying fatal or deteriorating condition (**Box 1**).

Box 1
Common psychiatric symptoms in the intensive care unit for patients at the end of life

Delirium

Agitation

Anxiety

Pain (both neuropathic and nonneuropathic)

Data from Akgun KM, Capo JM, Siegel MD. Critical care at the end of life. Semin Respir Crit Care Med 2015;36:921–33.

Evaluation and Management of Patients with Preexisting Chronic Mental Illness

Patients with preexisting psychiatric illness can present a unique challenge for symptom management, particularly if they have chronic severe mental illness. This population of patients may involve more complicated decision making if there is the presence of a conservator or guardian for those patients who do not have the capacity to make decisions regarding their medical care globally, or who may be under a Lanterman-Petris-Short conservatorship. Depending on the rules and regulations of individual states, conservators may have limited authority for medical decision making and some medical decisions require court orders, including the placement of a do-not-resuscitate order or discontinuation of life-sustaining treatment. Chronic mental illness has a high prevalence among patients who are homeless, as high as 47% to 57%; this is another population of patients who are particularly vulnerable in an ICU setting, because homeless persons are more likely than the general population to be socially isolated and not have a family member or close friend that they can name as a surrogate decision maker.[5–7]

Spiritual Care Needs

Spirituality, faith, and religion play a significant role in the experience of patients and families in an ICU, particularly in the context of end-of-life care. Compared with physicians and other health professionals, patients cite prayer and being at peace with God as major factors that are important at the end of life.[8] Spiritual support is a quality indicator of palliative care in the ICU; assessment for spiritual care needs is a routine part of a palliative care assessment.[4] Encouraging and facilitating spiritual practices can serve to comfort patients and families.[4]

MODELS OF PALLIATIVE CARE IN THE INTENSIVE CARE UNIT

There are several models of palliative care in the ICU: consultative, integrative, and a combined approach. All of them have some evidence to support their use to improve palliative care in the ICU; the choice of model depends on resources and local factors for individual institutions.

The Consultative Model

For the first time, more than 90% of large hospitals (>300 beds) have a palliative care program and every state has at least 20% or more of its hospitals reporting a palliative care program.[9] The consultative model uses the specialty palliative care team and generally focuses their efforts on a subset of ICU patients who are at the highest risk of death.[10] The members of the palliative care consult team varies by institution and resources; in some institutions, there is a single consultant, often an advanced practice nurse, who provides consultation. In others, the palliative care consult team is multidisciplinary and includes a physician, an advanced practice nurse, a social worker, a chaplain, and (to a lesser extent) a psychologist.[10] Depending on their resources, the consult team may be available 24 hours a day, 7 days a week; the scope of the consult may include all of the domains listed earlier.

Within the consultative model, some services use formal triggers to prompt consults. These triggers can range from patient factors such as age or stage of disease (ie, metastatic cancer), the acute diagnoses requiring ICU-level care and health care use (eg, length of stay, request for tracheostomy and gastrostomy tube placement). Triggers can be used as initial screening tools rather than an automatic consult. Some services have a palliative care consultant present in the ICU at a regular interval (eg, rounds) and that person serves to screen and identify patients who would benefit from a palliative care consult. In other ICUs, the trigger is more ad hoc and relies on the judgment of the critical care physician to consult palliative care.

The Integrative Model

The integrative model relies on the primary ICU team to provide palliative care and emphasizes the needs of virtually all patients and families in the ICU for basic palliative care. Integrated models either incorporate or assume palliative care training for ICU clinicians. They can include the use of systems-based tools to assess for palliative care needs (a screening protocol or checklist) as well as treatment-directed interventions such as a comfort care order set or triggered family meetings (based on length of stay, severity of illness, and so forth). Similar to a sepsis bundle, a palliative care bundle approach has been used with a checklist of palliative care processes and interventions, including the identification of the surrogate decision maker, review of any existing advance care planning documents, social work and/or chaplaincy services, and a family meeting to discuss the patient's current condition and goals of care.

The Combined Consultative-Integrative Model

Although each of these models have clear advantages, there are disadvantages to each one in isolation. The consultative model requires adequate palliative care staffing and resources and introduces a new set of clinicians to each patient and family's care. There is currently a shortage of palliative care specialists, with an approximate gap of at least 6000 physicians.[11] With the routine involvement of a palliative care consultant, there may be less incentive for primary ICU team members to improve their palliative care knowledge and skills. Alternatively, the integrative model places additional requirements on the ICU staff and needs a cultural commitment in the ICU. Most institutions arrive at some combination of the two, which becomes heavily influenced by local culture and resources (**Box 2**).

COMMUNICATION AND PALLIATIVE CARE IN THE INTENSIVE CARE UNIT

Communication between ICU clinicians and patients and families is crucial, in light of the high stakes of mortality in the ICU and the need to incorporate patient values into decision making. Families have reported communication from the clinicians as inadequate and of poor quality.[12] However, communication approaches to improve communication between patients, families, and clinicians has been shown to improve the quality of care for patients and their families.[11,13] A 2011 systematic review of interventions to improve communication in the ICU described improvements in family emotional outcomes as well as ICU length of stay and treatment intensity. In that review, Scheunemann and colleagues included trials in which the communication intervention was delivered by the primary ICU team, ethics consultants, or palliative care consultants[14–20]; written information and structured communication through family conferences improved emotional distress, family comprehension, and timely decision making.[14]

Several recent studies evaluated the impact of communication interventions on the surrogate decision maker/family experience. A 2016 study from Mt Sinai and Duke noted that having palliative care–led family meetings versus standard ICU-led family meetings for patients with chronic critical illness (defined by >7 days on a ventilator) did not show any difference in depression or anxiety of the surrogate decision makers 3 months after the family meetings; there was a higher incidence of posttraumatic stress disorder (PTSD) symptoms in the intervention group.[21] However, these

Box 2
Models of palliative care in the intensive care unit

Feature	Consultative	Integrative	Combined
Delivered by	Palliative care specialists	ICU frontline clinicians	Collaboration between palliative care and the ICU
Training requirements	No additional training	Training sessions needed to address palliative care knowledge and skills	Moderate training needed for frontline clinician skills in palliative care
Continuity post-ICU (if patient survives ICU discharge)	Yes; palliative care consultant can follow as patient transitions to the floor	No	Yes
Relationship centered?	Challenging, because palliative care team has to build rapport quickly	Yes	Yes
Access to palliative care	Limited to only those for whom palliative care is consulted	All ICU patients have access as palliative care practices are integrated into routine ICU care	Allows for broad access, with the option for specialty-level palliative care if needed
Cost and resources	Requires multidisciplinary palliative care team and adequate staffing	No additional staffing but does require training for existing staff and creation of standard work	Requires a palliative care consult service; needs to be tailored to the needs/ resources of the institution

Data from Nelson JE, Bassett R, Boss RD, et al. Improve palliative care in the intensive care unit project. Models for structuring a clinical initiative to enhance palliative care in the intensive care unit: a report from the IPAL-ICU Project (improving palliative care in the ICU). Crit Care Med 2010;38:1765–72.

palliative care family meetings were not true palliative care consults, because they involved solely a single palliative care clinician who attended 2 family meetings as the meeting facilitator. Another randomized controlled trial of the use of communication facilitators from the University of Washington in 2016 showed a decrease in family members' reported depression symptoms at 6 months, but no difference in anxiety or PTSD.[22] There was a notable decrease in ICU cost and length of stay with the use of a communication facilitator who interviewed families regarding their needs, concerns, and communication preferences and then communicated with the ICU team about how best to communicate with the family. These facilitators consisted of a nurse and a social worker who were trained for these conversations[22] (**Boxes 3 and 4**).

PALLIATIVE PSYCHIATRY IN THE INTENSIVE CARE UNIT

There are no formal guidelines or quality metrics regarding the provision of palliative care for patients with severe persistent mental illness in the ICU setting. Medical illness and its treatment can compromise optimal therapy for mental illness; for example, in the ICU, home antipsychotic medications may be held when a patient is sedated on a ventilator. This option prompts consideration of how to approach quality end-of-life

> **Box 3**
> **Approach to family meetings in the intensive care unit: common elements**
>
> Premeet (clinicians)
>
> Introductions
>
> Assess family understanding/expectations
>
> Elicit patient values/preferences
>
> Acknowledge emotion, empathize
>
> Align treatment plan with patient values, make recommendation
>
> Plan next steps
>
> *Adapted from* Refs.[23–26]

care for this population of patients in the ICU. A palliative psychiatric approach seeks to address the psychosocial dimensions in the context of serious medical illness; in the absence of standard guidelines for patients with severe mental illness, this palliative psychiatric approach ensures attention to the psychological suffering of ICU patients at the end of life with preexisting severe mental illness.[27–29] Palliative psychiatry acknowledges that the severe persistent mental illness can be incurable and offers support to both the patient and the family to cope with distressing psychiatric symptoms.[29] Family members and surrogate decision makers as well as clinicians caring for patients with severe persistent mental illness may not have the benefit of having discussed or understood their wishes in the context of a terminal condition compared with other patients.[29] A palliative care team can offer support for both family members and clinicians dealing with decision making for this patient population.

PSYCHIATRIC AND PALLIATIVE CARE IN THE POST–INTENSIVE CARE UNIT SETTING
The Patient Experience

Patients who survive their critical illness continue to have significant symptoms and suffering in the months and years after their discharge. A systematic review of

> **Box 4**
> **Best practices for communication in the intensive care unit**
>
> Assess patient and family's information and decision-making preferences
>
> Identify the patient's health care proxy or surrogate decision maker
>
> Meet as an interdisciplinary team of ICU and consultants regarding patient's condition and goals of treatment before meeting with family, to address potential conflicts
>
> Conduct routine interdisciplinary conferences with the family
>
> Use structured communication approaches for family meetings
>
> Communicate with patients and families with clear language, avoiding medical jargon
>
> *Adapted from* Davidson JE, Aslakson RA, Long AC, et al. Guidelines for family-centered care in the neonatal, pediatric, and adult ICU. Crit Care Med 2017;45:103–28; and Levin TT, Moreno B, Silvester W, et al. End-of-life communication in the intensive care unit. Gen Hosp Psychiatry 2010;32:433–42.

Box 5
Common psychiatric symptoms and disorders of intensive care unit survivors

Depression

Anxiety

Posttraumatic stress disorder

Pain

Data from Refs.[30–33]

---

quality of life in ICU survivors found that although there was overall improvement in quality of life over time, that was not universally true across different domains of quality of life. Functional status overall improved over time from the point of hospital discharge, but mental health symptoms (anxiety and depression, pain) did not change.[30] Clinically significant depression is reported at rates as high 33%, which is higher than that of the general population and other hospitalized populations, such as patients post–myocardial infarction, who report a prevalence of 14% of substantial depressive symptoms.[31] Anxiety and posttraumatic stress disorders following critical illness are addressed extensively elsewhere. However, this is an emerging population of patients who can benefit from community-based palliative care services and psychiatry; community-based palliative care is increasing in access but remains less common than hospital-based palliative care programs (**Box 5**).

The Family Experience

The experience of the ICU for family members and caregivers takes its toll both during and after the ICU stay, for both bereaved and nonbereaved family members. A 2008 study of family members of ICU patients noted that, 6 months after the ICU stay, 35% had posttraumatic stress regardless of whether their loved one had died in the ICU.[34] Of those who were bereaved, 38% had complicated grief.[34] Another study of solely bereaved family members found that 34% met criteria for at least 1 psychiatric disorder, with major depressive disorder being the most common and with some family members having multiple psychiatric disorders.[35] Although grief and bereavement counseling are included for families of patients who die on a hospice program, this is not universally available to bereaved families of ICU patients and is an area for further exploration in delivering quality palliative care.

SUMMARY/DISCUSSION

- Palliative care is a core component of critical care and addresses the multiple domains of suffering that patients and families experience.
- Current models of palliative care in the ICU combine consultative and integrative approaches to ensure standard palliative care quality measures and continuity of care if the patient moves out of the ICU.
- Communication behaviors that are family centered can improve both patient and family outcomes.
- Patients with preexisting severe mental illness present as a unique and vulnerable population in the ICU and require a palliative psychiatric approach to ensure ethical decision making.

REFERENCES

1. Angus DC, Barnato AE, Linde-Zwirble WT, et al, Robert Wood Johnson Foundation ICU End-Of-Life Peer Group. Use of intensive care at the end of life in the United States: an epidemiologic study. Crit Care Med 2004;32:638–43.
2. World Health Organization definition of palliative care. Available at: http://www.who.int/cancer/palliative/definition/en/. Accessed January 2, 2017.
3. Center to Advance Palliative Care. A new definition of palliative care. In: 2011 public opinion research on palliative care: a report based on research by public opinion strategies. Available at: https://media.capc.org/filer_public/18/ab/18ab708c-f835-4380-921d-fbf729702e36/2011-public-opinion-research-on-palliative-care.pdf. Accessed January 2, 2017.
4. Clarke EB, Curtis JR, Luce JM, et al, Robert Wood Johnson Foundation Critical Care End-of-Life Peer Workgroup Members. Quality indicators for end-of-life care in the intensive care unit. Crit Care Med 2003;31:2255–62.
5. Baggett TP. The unmet health care needs of homeless adults: a national study. Am J Public Health 2010;100(7):1326–33.
6. Burt M, Aron L, Lee E. Helping America's homeless: emergency shelter or affordable housing? Washington, DC: Urban Institute Press; 2001.
7. Kushel MB, Miaskowski C. End-of-life care for homeless patients: "She says she is there to help me in any situation". JAMA 2006;296(24):2959–66.
8. Steinhauser KE, Christakis NA, Clipp EC, et al. Factors considered important at the end of life by patients, family, physicians, and other care providers. JAMA 2000;284:2476–82.
9. Morrison RS, Meier DE, Dumanovsky T, et al. America's care of serious illness: 2015 state-by-state report card on access to palliative care in our nation's hospitals. Available at: https://reportcard.capc.org/wp-content/uploads/2015/08/CAPC-Report-Card-2015.pdf. Accessed January 2, 2017.
10. Nelson JE, Bassett R, Boss RD, et al, Improve Palliative Care in the Intensive Care Unit Project. Models for structuring a clinical initiative to enhance palliative care in the intensive care unit: a report from the IPAL-ICU project (improving palliative care in the ICU). Crit Care Med 2010;38:1765–72.
11. Lupu D. American Academy of Hospice and Palliative Medicine Workforce Task Force. Estimate of current hospice and palliative medicine physician workforce shortage. J Pain Symptom Manage 2010;40:899–911.
12. Azoulay E, Chevret S, Leleu G, et al. Half the families of intensive care unit patients experience inadequate communication with physicians. Crit Care Med 2000;28(8):3044–9.
13. Hua M, Li G, Blinderman C, et al. Estimates of the need for palliative care consultation across United States intensive care units using a trigger-based model. Am J Respir Crit Care Med 2014;189:428–36.
14. Scheunemann LP, McDevitt M, Carson SS, et al. Randomized, controlled trials of interventions to improve communication in intensive care: a systematic review. Chest 2011;139:543–54.
15. Curtis JR, Vincent JL. Ethics and end-of-life care for adults in the intensive care unit. Lancet 2010;376:1347–53.
16. Schneiderman LJ, Gilmer T, Teetzel HD, et al. Effect of ethics consultations on nonbeneficial life-sustaining treatments in the intensive care setting: a randomized controlled trial. JAMA 2003;290:1166–72.

17. Lautrette A, Darmon M, Megarbane B, et al. A communication strategy and brochure for relatives of patients dying in the ICU. N Engl J Med 2007;356: 469–78.
18. Dowdy MD, Robertson C, Bander JA. A study of proactive ethics consultation for critically and terminally ill patients with extended lengths of stay. Crit Care Med 1998;26:252–9.
19. Schneiderman LJ, Gilmer T, Teetzel HD. Impact of ethics consultations in the intensive care setting: a randomized, controlled trial. Crit Care Med 2000;28: 3920–4.
20. Campbell ML, Guzman JA. A proactive approach to improve end-of-life care in a medical intensive care unit for patients with terminal dementia. Crit Care Med 2004;32:1839–43.
21. Carson SS, Cox CE, Wallenstein S, et al. Effect of palliative care–led meetings for families of patients with chronic critical illness: a randomized clinical trial. JAMA 2016;316(1):51–62.
22. Curtis JR, Treece PD, Nielsen EL, et al. Randomized trial of communication facilitators to reduce family distress and intensity of end-of-life care. Am J Respir Crit Care Med 2016;193(2):154–62.
23. Wysham NG, Mularski RA, Schmidt DM, et al. Long-term persistence of quality improvements for an intensive care unit communication initiative using the VALUE strategy. J Crit Care 2014;29(3):450–4.
24. Billings JA. The end-of-life family meeting in intensive care part II: family-centered decision making. J Palliat Med 2011;14(9):1051–7.
25. Talking map for the family conference. Available at: http://vitaltalk.org/sites/ default/files/quick-guides/FamilyConfForVitaltalkV1.0_0.pdf. Accessed January 17, 2017.
26. Levin TT, Moreno B, Silvester W, et al. End-of-life communication in the intensive care unit. Gen Hosp Psychiatry 2010;32:433–42.
27. Irwin SA, Ferris FD. The opportunity for psychiatry in palliative care. Can J Psychiatry 2008;53:713–24.
28. Fairman N, Irwin SA. Palliative care psychiatry: update on an emerging dimension of psychiatric practice. Curr Psychiatry Rep 2013;15(7):374.
29. Trachsel M, Irwin SA, Biller-Andorno N, et al. Palliative psychiatry for severe persistent mental illness as a new approach to psychiatry? Definition, scope, benefits, and risks. BMC Psychiatry 2016;16:260.
30. Dowdy DW, Eid MP, Sedrakyan A, et al. Quality of life in adult survivors of critical illness: a systematic review of the literature. Intensive Care Med 2005;31:611–20.
31. Davydow DS, Gifford JM, Desai SV, et al. Depression in general intensive care unit survivors: a systematic review. Intensive Care Med 2009;35:796–809.
32. Davydow DS, Gifford JM, Desai SV, et al. Posttraumatic stress disorder in general intensive care unit survivors: a systematic review. Gen Hosp Psychiatry 2008;30: 421–34.
33. Myhren H, Ekeberg O, Toien K, et al. Posttraumatic stress, anxiety and depression symptoms in patients during the first year post intensive care unit discharge. Crit Care 2010;14:R14.
34. Anderson WG, Arnold RM, Angus DC, et al. Posttraumatic stress and complicated grief in family members of patients in the intensive care unit. J Gen Intern Med 2008;23:1871–6.
35. Siegel MD, Hayes E, Vanderwerker LC, et al. Psychiatric illness in the next of kin of patients who die in the intensive care unit. Crit Care Med 2008;36:1722–8.

Index

Note: Page numbers of article titles are in **boldface** type.

A

Acetylcholinesterase inhibitors
    in delirium management, 500–501
    in delirium prevention, 486, 494
Acute alcohol hepatitis
    in transplant patients, 666
Acute brain failure, **461–519**. *See also* Delirium
AEDs. *See* Antiepileptic drugs (AEDs)
Affective dysregulation
    PCI in ICU and, 452
Aggression
    post-TBI, 430–431
Agitation
    PCI in ICU and, 449
    substance use–related
        in ICU, 544–545
Alcohol
    neurobiological effects of, 560
Alcohol use disorders (AUDs)
    background of, 559–560
    described, 559–560
Alcohol withdrawal
    in heart disease patients in ICU, 627–628
Alcohol withdrawal syndromes (AWSs), **559–599**
    background of, 559–560
    overview of, 560–563
    treatment of, 563–587
        AEDs in, 565–571
        alpha-2 adrenergic receptor agonist in, 571–581
        γ-aminobutyric acid-ergic agents in, 565
        benzodiazepine-sparing alternative in, 563–581
        clinical dilemma related to, 563
        development of novel algorithm for, 581–587
Alpha-2 adrenergic receptor agonist
    in AWS management, 571–581
Alpha-2 agonists
    in delirium management, 491, 500
    in delirium prevention, 483
Alpha-2 antagonists

Crit Care Clin 33 (2017) 745–761
http://dx.doi.org/10.1016/S0749-0704(17)30037-4
0749-0704/17

Moving?

Make sure your subscription moves with you!

To notify us of your new address, find your **Clinics Account Number** (located on your mailing label above your name), and contact customer service at:

Email: journalscustomerservice-usa@elsevier.com

800-654-2452 (subscribers in the U.S. & Canada)
314-447-8871 (subscribers outside of the U.S. & Canada)

Fax number: 314-447-8029

Elsevier Health Sciences Division
Subscription Customer Service
3251 Riverport Lane
Maryland Heights, MO 63043

*To ensure uninterrupted delivery of your subscription, please notify us at least 4 weeks in advance of move.

Printed and bound by CPI Group (UK) Ltd, Croydon, CR0 4YY

07/10/2024

01040504-0011